MW01118604

Handbook of
Dermatologic Drug Therapy

Handbook of
Dermatologic Drug Therapy

Steven R. Feldman MD PhD
Wake Forest University School of Medicine,
Winston-Salem, North Carolina, USA

Kathy C. Phelps PharmD BCPS
Wake Forest University Baptist Medical Center,
Winston-Salem, North Carolina, USA

&

Kelly C. Verzino PharmD BCPS
DCH Regional Medical Center,
Tuscaloosa, Alabama, USA

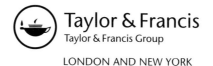

Taylor & Francis
Taylor & Francis Group

LONDON AND NEW YORK

Our knowledge in clinical sciences is constantly changing. As new information becomes available, changes in treatment and in the use of drugs become necessary. The authors and the publisher of this volume have taken care to make certain that the doses of drugs and schedules of treatment are correct and compatible with the standards generally accepted at the time of publication. The reader is advised to consult carefully the instruction and information material included in the package insert of each drug or therapeutic agent before administration. This advice is especially important when using new or infrequently used drugs.

© 2005 Taylor & Francis, an imprint of the Taylor & Francis Group
First published in the United Kingdom in 2005
by Taylor & Francis,
an imprint of the Taylor & Francis Group,
2 Park Square, Milton Park
Abingdon, Oxon OX14 4RN, UK

Tel: +44 (0)20 7017 6000
Fax: +44 (0)20 7017 6699
Email: info.medicine@tandf.co.uk
Website: http://www.tandf.co.uk/medicine

British Library Cataloguing in Publication Data

Data available on application

Library of Congress Cataloging-in-Publication Data

Data available on application

ISBN10: 1-84214-260-7
ISBN13: 9-78-1-84214-260-8

Distributed in North and South America by

Taylor & Francis
2000 NW Corporate Blvd
Boca Raton, FL 33431, USA

Within Continental USA
Tel: 800 272 7737; Fax: 800 374 3401
Outside Continental USA
Tel: 561 994 0555; Fax: 561 361 6018
E-mail: orders@crcpress.com

Distributed in the rest of the world by
Thomson Publishing Services
Cheriton House
North Way
Andover, Hampshire SP10 5BE, UK
Tel: +44 (0) 1264 332424
E-mail: salesorder.tandf@thomsonpublishingservices.co.uk

Composition by Parthenon Publishing
Printed and bound by Antony Rowe Ltd., Chippenham, Wiltshire, UK

Contents

Preface   xi

Acknowledgments   xiii

Drug Administration Abbreviations   xiv

Acne and Rosacea Medications   1
  Adapalene   2
  Azelaic acid   3
  Benzoyl peroxide   4
  Isotretinoin   6
  Norgestimate–ethinyl estradiol   8

  Topical   10
    Clindamycin   10
    Erythromycin   12
    Metronidazole   14
    Sodium sulfacetamide   15
    Sulfacetamide/sulfur   16
    Tretinoin   17

Antibiotics   19
  Penicillins and cephalosporins   19
    Ampicillin   20
    Cefuroxime axetil   22
    Cephalexin   24
    Penicillin   26

  Macrolides   29
    Azithromycin   29
    Clarithromycin   31
    Erythromycin   33

  Fluoroquinolones   36
    Ciprofloxacin   36
    Ofloxacin   38

  Tetracyclines   40
    Doxycycline   40
    Minocycline   42
    Tetracycline   44

  Sulfa   46
    Dapsone   46
    Trimethoprim–sulfamethoxazole   48

Contents

Clindamycin phosphate   50
Clofazimine   52
Topical antibiotics   53
    Mupirocin   53
    Polymyxin B/bacitracin/neomycin   54
    Polymyxin B/bacitracin   55

Anticancer and Immunosuppressant Drugs   **57**
    Adalimumab   58
    Alefacept   59
    Alitretinoin   61
    Aminolevulinic acid   62
    Azathioprine   63
    Bexarotene   65
    Bexarotene, topical   67
    Colchicine   68
    Cyclophosphamide   70
    Cyclosporine   71
    Denileukin diftitox   73
    Efalizumab   75
    Etanercept   76
    Fluorouracil   78
    Hydroxychloroquine   80
    Hydroxyurea   82
    Infliximab   84
    Interferon α-2a   86
    Interferon α-2b   88
    Leflunomide   91
    Leucovorin   92
    Mechlorethamine   93
    Methotrexate   95
    Methyl aminolevulinate   97
    Mycophenolate mofetil/mycophenolic acid   100
    Pimecrolimus   101
    Quinacrine   102
    Sulfapyridine   103
    Sulfasalazine   105
    Tacrolimus, systemic   107
    Tacrolimus, topical   109
    Thalidomide   110
    Thioguanine   112

Contents

Antifungals   **113**
- Oral   114
  - Fluconazole   114
  - Griseofulvin   116
  - Itraconazole   118
  - Ketoconazole   120
  - Terbinafine   122
- Topical   123
  - Ciclopirox   123
  - Clotrimazole   124
  - Table of topical antifungal agents   126
  - Table of vaginal preparations for vaginal candidiasis   130

Antihistamines   **133**
- Cetirizine   134
- Chlorpheniramine   135
- Cromolyn   136
- Desloratadine   137
- Diphenhydramine   138
- Fexofenadine   139
- Hydroxyzine   140
- Loratadine   142
- Table of histamine-2 receptor antagonists   143

Anti-inflammatory Agents   **145**
- Ibuprofen   146
- Naproxen   148
- Prednisone   150
- Table of nonsteroidal anti-inflammatory drugs   152
- Topical corticosteroids   155
- Triamcinolone (for injection)   160

Antiparasitics   **161**
- Ivermectin   162
- Lindane   163
- Malathion   165
- Permethrin   166

Antipruritics and Topical Anesthetics   **167**
- Capsaicin   168
- Diphenhydramine, topical   169
- Doxepin topical   170
- Lidocaine patch   171

Contents

Lidocaine/prilocaine 172
Table of topical anesthetics 175

Antiviral and Wart Treatments 179
Acyclovir, systemic 180
Acyclovir, topical 183
Bleomycin 184
Docosanol 186
Famciclovir 187
Imiquimod 189
Penciclovir 191
Podofilox 192
Podophyllin 194
Topical salicylic acid preparations 195
Trichloroacetic acid 197
Valacyclovir 198

Hair Growth and Reduction Medications 201
Eflornithine 202
Finasteride 203
Minoxidil, topical 204
Spironolactone 205

Ophthalmic and Otic Preparations 207
Ophthalmic 208
Ciprofloxacin 208
Erythromycin 209
Neomycin/polymyxin B/bacitracin/hydrocortisone 210
Neomycin/polymyxin B/hydrocortisone 211
Sulfacetamide 212
Trifluridine 213
Table of ophthalmic antibiotics, corticosteroids, and combinations 214
Table of ophthalmic decongestants 218

Otic 221
Ciprofloxacin/dexamethasone 221
Ciprofloxacin/hydrocortisone 222
Hydrocortisone/neomycin/colistin 223
Hydrocortisone/neomycin/polymyxin B 224
Ofloxacin 225
Table of miscellaneous otic preparations 226

Pigmenting and Depigmenting Agents 227
β-Carotene 228
Dihydroxyacetone 229

Contents

Fluocinolone acetonide/hydroquinone/tretinoin   231
Hydroquinone   232
Hydroquinone/retinol   234
Mequinol and tretinoin   235
Monobenzone   236

Psoriasis Agents   **237**
Acitretin   238
Anthralin   240
Calcipotriene   241
Methoxsalen   243
Tazarotene   246

Psychotropic Medications and Sedatives   **247**
Antidepressants   248
Amitriptyline   248
Doxepin   250
Table of selective serotonin reuptake inhibitors   252
Table of atypical antidepressants   255

Anxiolytics   257
Alprazolam   257
Buspirone   259
Lorazepam   261
Midazolam   263
Temazepam   265

Antipsychotics   266
Haloperidol   266
Pimozide   268

Miscellaneous Agents   **271**
Alendronate   272
Cevimeline   274
Gabapentin   275
Glycopyrrolate   276
Pentoxifylline   277
Risedronate   278
Table of topical antiseptics   279
Table of topical burn preparations   283

Appendix
Amount of topical medication to prescribe based on body surface   284
area affected
Index   285

Preface

It is our hope that this handbook will be a useful resource for the practicing dermatologist. An expanding pharmaceutical market and evolving indications warranted a single reference with collated use, safety, and availability of information. Drugs included in this manual are those we anticipated most dermatologists may use or be exposed to use in clinical practice, including those for dermatologic uses as well as commonly encountered co-morbid conditions. Feedback is welcome, in order that we can optimize future editions.

SRF
KCP
KCV

Acknowledgments

The authors are appreciative of the able assistance of Katie Rau, Sarah Melissa Godfrey, Erica Smithberger, Heather Greist, Kevin Stein, Brian Price, Johanna Su and Erin Eades.

Dr Phelps would additionally like to acknowledge the leadership of North Carolina Baptist Hospital, its dedication to excellence in patient care, and continued support of the provision of evidence-based and patient-centered drug information.

Drug Administration Abbreviations

ACHS	before meals and at bedtime
BID	twice daily
HS	at bedtime
IM	intramuscular
IV	intravenous
PO	by mouth
prn	as needed
q	every
qam	every morning
QD	every day
QHS	each bedtime
QID	four times daily
SC	subcutaneous
TID	three times daily

Acne and Rosacea Medications

Adapalene (Differin)

Dose and Administration

Apply to cleansed affected area once a day in the evening.

Uses

Treatment of acne vulgaris.

Pharmacology

Adapalene is a retinoid-like compound that binds to retinoic acid nuclear receptors. Although its exact mechanism of action is not known, it is thought to normalize follicular epithelial cell function leading to decreased microcomedone formation. It is a modulator of cellular differentiation, keratinization, and the inflammatory process, all of which are seen in acne vulgaris.

Adverse Effects/Precautions

Local irritation is the most frequent adverse reaction. Erythema, dryness, scaling, burning, or pruritus may be seen. These effects usually occur within the first 2 to 4 weeks of therapy and will usually lessen with continued use. Exposure to cold or windy environments and sunlight, including sunlamps, should be avoided if possible. Use of sunscreen products and protective clothing is recommended to avoid serious skin reactions.

Pregnancy: FDA category C.

Special Considerations

Acne exacerbation may occur when therapy is initiated. Acne improvement should occur within 8 to 12 weeks of therapy.

Preparation *Rx*

Cream	0.1%	Differin	45 g
Gel	0.1%	Differin	15 & 45 g
Pledgets	0.1%	Differin	#60 per box
Solution	0.1%	Differin	30 ml

Selected References

Cunliffe WJ, Poncet M, Loesche C, Verschoore M. A comparison of the efficacy and tolerability of adapalene 0.1% gel versus tretinoin 0.025% gel in patients with acne vulgaris: a meta-analysis of five randomized trials. Br J Dermatol 1998; 139(Suppl 52): 48–56.

Haider A, Shaw JC. Treatment of acne vulgaris. JAMA 2004; 292: 726–35.

Waugh J, Noble S, Scott LJ. Adapalene. A review of its use in the treatment of acne vulgaris. Drugs 2004; 64: 1465–78.

Azelaic Acid (Azelex, Finacea)

Dose and Administration

Apply a thin film and gently but thoroughly massage into the cleansed affected area twice daily.

Uses

FDA-approved: Treatment of mild to moderate inflammatory acne vulgaris and inflammatory papules and pustules of mild to moderate rosacea. It is also used for hyperpigmentary disorders, including melasma.

Pharmacology

The exact mechanism of azelaic acid is not known. Azelaic acid displays antibacterial activity against *Propionibacterium acnes* and *Staphylococcus aureus,* which may be due to inhibition of protein synthesis. Normalization of keratinization is also thought to be involved, which results in decreased comedone formation. Azelaic acid also has an anti-inflammatory action mediated via its oxygen radical scavenging properties.

Adverse Effects/Precautions

Adverse reactions are generally mild and transient. Pruritus, burning, stinging, scaling, dry skin, and tingling are the most frequent adverse effects. Hypo-pigmentation may occur; the effect of azelaic acid has not been evaluated in dark complexions.

Pregnancy: FDA category B.

Special Considerations

Reduction in inflammatory lesions generally occurs within 4 to 8 weeks. Broad-spectrum sunscreens should be used adjunctively for hyperpigmentary disorders. Response may not be evident until at least 6 months of therapy.

Preparation *Rx*

| Cream | 20% | Azelex | 30 & 50 g |
| Gel | 15% | Finacea | 30 g |

Selected References

Fitton A, Goa KL. Azelaic acid. A review of its pharmacological properties and therapeutic efficacy in acne and hyperpigmentary skin disorders. Drugs 1991; 41: 780–98.

Graupe K, Cunliffe WJ, Gollnick HP, Zaumseil RP. Efficacy and safety of topical azelaic acid (20 percent cream): an overview of results from European clinical trials and experimental reports. Cutis 1996; 57(Suppl 1): 20–35.

Haider A, Shaw JC. Treatment of acne vulgaris. JAMA 2004; 292: 726–35.

Benzoyl Peroxide (various)

Dose and Administration

Cleansers: Wash face with product once or twice daily.

Cream, lotion, gel: Apply to cleansed affected area once daily initially.

Increase frequency of application to twice daily if tolerated.

Uses

Treatment of acne vulgaris.

Pharmacology

Benzoyl peroxide is an oxidizing agent with antibacterial activity against *Propionibacterium acnes*. Concentrations of *P. acnes,* free fatty acids and sebum are reduced on the skin surface after use. These actions result in decreased comedone formation and inflammation.

Adverse Effects/Precautions

Local irritation is the most frequent adverse event. The frequency of application or drug concentration should be decreased if excessive erythema, drying, or peeling of skin occurs. Since benzoyl peroxide is an oxidizing agent, it may bleach hair.

Pregnancy: FDA category C.

Preparation *Rx*

Cream	5%	Benzashave	120 g
	10%	Benzashave	120 g
Gel	2.5%	Benzac AC	60 & 90 g
		Benzac W	60 g
		Desquam-E	45 g
		Generic	60 g
	3%	Triaz	42.5 g
		Triaz Cleanser	170.3 & 340.2 g
	4%	Brevoxyl 4	42.5 & 90 g
	5%	Benzamycin (with erythromycin 3%)	46.6 g
		Generic	23.3 & 46.6 g
		Benzamycin Pak (with erythromycin 3%)	#60
		BenzaClin (with clindamycin 1%)	25 & 50 g
		Duac (with clindamycin 1%)	45 g
		Benzagel-5	45 g
		Benzac AC 5	60 & 90 g
		Benzac W 5	60 g
		Desquam-E 5	45 g
		Desquam-X 5	45 & 90 g

Benzoyl Peroxide (various)

		Generic	60 & 90 g
	6%	Triaz	42.5 g
		Triaz Cleanser	170.3 & 340.2 g
	7%	Clinac BPO	45 g
	8%	Brevoxyl-8	42.5 & 90 g
	9%	Triaz	42.5 g
		Triaz Cleanser	170.3 & 340.2 g
	10%	Benzac AC 10	60 & 90 g
		Benzac W 10	60 g
		Benzagel Wash	60 g
		Benzagel-10	45 g
		Desquam-E 10	45 g
		Desquam-X 10	45 & 90 g
		Generic	60 & 90 g
Liquid	2.5%	Benzac AC Wash	240 ml
		Benzoyl Peroxide Wash	237 ml
	5%	Benzac AC Wash 5	240 ml
		Benzac W Wash 5	240 ml
		Desquam-X 5	150 ml
		Benzoyl Peroxide Wash	118, 148 & 237 ml
	10%	Benzac AC Wash 10	240 ml
		Benzac W Wash 10	240 ml
		Desquam-X 10	150 ml
		Benzoyl Peroxide Wash	150 & 240 ml
Lotion	4%	Brevoxyl-4 Creamy Wash	170 g
		Brevoxyl-4	297 g
	5%	Various generics	
		Sulfoxyl Regular (with sulfur 2%)	59 ml
	8%	Brevoxyl-8 Creamy Wash	170 g
		Brevoxyl-8	297 g
	10%	Various generics	
		Sulfoxyl Strong (with sulfur 5%)	59 ml
Pads	3, 6, & 9%	Triaz	#30
Soap	5%	Various OTC products	
	10%	Various OTC products	
		Desquam-X 10	

Selected References

Haider A, Shaw JC. Treatment of acne vulgaris. JAMA 2004; 292: 726–35.

Mills OH, Kligman AM, Pochi P, Comite H. Comparing 2.5%, 5%, and 10% benzoyl peroxide on inflammatory acne vulgaris. Int J Dermatol 1986; 25: 664–7.

White GM. Acne therapy. Adv Dermatol 1999; 14: 29–58, discussion 59.

Isotretinoin (Accutane)

Dose and Administration

Severe recalcitrant nodular acne: 0.5 to 2 mg/kg administered by mouth in two divided doses per day for 15 to 20 weeks. Isotretinoin should be administered with food to maximize absorption. Most patients should receive 0.5 to 1 mg/kg total doses; however, patients with very severe acne with scaring or acne manifested primarily on the trunk may require 2 mg/kg dosing. The drug may be discontinued before 20 weeks of therapy if total nodules have been reduced by 70%. If symptoms recur after 2 months of discontinuing therapy, a second course of therapy may be given.

Other indications: 0.5 to 2 mg/kg by mouth per day in two divided doses.

Uses

FDA-approved: Treatment of severe recalcitrant nodular acne (lesions with a diameter of 5 mm or greater) in patients who have not responded adequately to other therapies.

Other indications: acne conglobata, ichthyosis, Darier's disease, psoriasis, dissecting folliculitis, lichen planus, hidradenitis suppurativa, pityriasis rubra pilaris, refractory rosacea.

Monitoring

Blood lipid parameters and liver function tests should be performed prior to therapy initiation and at weekly or biweekly intervals until the response to isotretinoin has been established (usually 4 weeks).

Pharmacology

Its exact mechanism in acne is unknown yet its primary effect is on epithelial cell proliferation and differentiation. Isotretinoin is a synthetic retinoid that inhibits sebaceous gland differentiation and proliferation, reduces sebaceous gland size, decreases sebum production, and normalizes follicular epithelial desquamation. Additionally, *Propionibacterium acnes* concentrations on the skin are reduced, which may contribute to its efficacy in acne. Isotretinoin absorption is improved with food or milk. It is eliminated in both the urine and the feces.

Adverse Effects/Precautions

Frequent adverse reactions include cheilitis, dry skin, skin fragility, pruritus, epistaxis, and dry nose and mouth.

Depression, psychosis, suicidal ideation, suicide attempts, suicide, and aggressive and/or violent behavior have been reported.

Musculoskeletal complaints, including arthralgia, have occurred.

Skeletal hyperostosis manifested as premature closure of the epiphysis in children has been noted with higher isotretinoin doses. Additionally, osteoporosis, osteopenia, bone fractures, and delayed healing of bone fractures have been reported.

Pseudotumor cerebri characterized by papilledema, headache, nausea and vomiting, and visual disturbances has occurred. The risk is increased with concomitant use of tetracyclines.

Night vision may be decreased, and patients should be warned of this potential problem to prevent accidents.

Corneal opacities may occur and are more frequent with higher doses. If visual problems occur, therapy should be discontinued and an ophthalmologic examination should be performed.

Isotretinoin (Accutane)

Patients with a history of inflammatory bowel disease may develop a flare of their disease while receiving isotretinoin. Therapy should be discontinued if rectal bleeding or severe abdominal pain develops.

Plasma lipids may be altered with isotretinoin. Specific changes include elevated triglycerides, decreased high-density lipoproteins (HDL), and increased total cholesterol. Cardiovascular consequences of the lipid alterations are unknown.

Acute pancreatitis has been reported in patients with both normal and elevated triglycerides. Discontinue isotretinoin if the triglyceride elevation cannot be controlled.

Hepatitis has been reported in addition to mild to moderate elevations of liver enzymes.

Pregnancy: FDA category X. Isotretinoin is contraindicated in females of childbearing age unless the patient is willing to comply with mandatory contraceptive measures, which should include use of two reliable methods. A pregnancy test should be performed prior to isotretinoin use. A consent form, which is provided by the manufacturer, should be completed by female patients and their physician prior to initiating therapy. Two forms of birth control are required while taking isotretinoin starting 1 month prior to therapy and ending 1 month after therapy has been stopped.

Drug Interactions

Isotretinoin may increase the clearance of carbamazepine. If used concomitantly, carbamazepine serum monitoring should be performed.

Special Considerations

A single course of therapy for 15 to 20 weeks results in complete and prolonged remission in many patients. If a second course of treatment is needed, it should not be initiated until at least 8 weeks after completion of the first course, because many patients may continue to improve while off isotretinoin.

Patients should not donate blood while receiving isotretinoin or within 1 month after discontinuing therapy, since their blood could be administered to a pregnant female. The product contains parabens and is contraindicated in patients with paraben hypersensitivity.

Isotretinoin can be dispensed only as a 30-day supply. A written prescription containing a yellow Accutane Qualification Sticker must be presented within 7 days of the qualification date to obtain isotretinoin. Refills require a new written prescription and sticker. An Accutane Medication Guide must be given to the patient each time Accutane is dispensed.

Preparation Rx

Capsules	10, 20 & 40 mg	Accutane

Selected References

Goldsmith LA, Bolognia JL, Callen JP, et al. American Academy of Dermatology Consensus Conference on the safe and optimal use of isotretinoin: summary and recommendations. J Am Acad Dermatol 2004; 50: 900–6.

Haider A, Shaw JC. Treatment of acne vulgaris. JAMA 2004; 292: 726–35.

Ward A, Brogden RN, Heel RC, et al. Isotretinoin: a review of its pharmacological properties and therapeutic efficacy in acne and other skin disorders. Drugs 1984; 28: 6–37.

Norgestimate–Ethinyl Estradiol (Ortho Tri-Cyclen)

Dose and Administration

Take one active tablet by mouth once a day for 21 days followed by a placebo pill once per day for 7 days. Repeat cycle every 28 days. Generally therapy should be initiated on the first Sunday after menstruation begins.

Uses

FDA-approved: (1) Prevention of pregnancy, and (2) treatment of moderate acne vulgaris in female patients who have achieved menarche and are not responsive to topical antiacne therapies.

Pharmacology

This triphasic oral contraceptive consists of a combination of an estrogenic component, ethinyl estradiol, and a progestational component, norgestimate. Norgestimate has low androgenic activity as compared with other progestins contained in combination oral contraceptives. It is proposed that the combination of ethinyl estradiol and norgestimate increases sex hormone binding globulin with resultant increased protein binding of testosterone. Additionally, ethinyl estradiol may decrease ovarian production of testosterone by suppressing the secretion of pituitary gonadotropins. These combined effects result in lower concentrations of circulating testosterone and improvement in acne.

Adverse Effects/Precautions

Common adverse reactions include nausea, vomiting, bloating, abdominal cramping, edema, melasma, breast tenderness, and breakthrough bleeding.

Use of oral contraceptives increases the risk for thromboembolic events, hypertension, gallbladder disease, and hepatic adenomas or benign liver tumors. Patients at greatest risk include cigarette smokers, those with hyperlipidemia, hypertension, diabetes mellitus, obesity, and age greater than 35 years.

Contraindications for use include patients with thromboembolic disorders (current or past history), cerebrovascular or coronary artery disease, carcinoma of the breast, endometrium or liver, cholestatic jaundice, or pregnancy.

Drug Interactions

Reduced contraceptive efficacy and unplanned pregnancies have occurred with the combination of oral contraceptives and other medications. These include, but are not limited to, rifampin, barbiturates, phenytoin, carbamazepine, griseofulvin, ampicillin, and tetracyclines. Patients should be instructed to utilize an alternative (or additional) form of contraception while receiving these concomitant medications.

Special Considerations

Following initiation, patients should use a second form of birth control until 7 days of consecutive oral contraceptive therapy has been administered. Advise patients to avoid cigarette smoking while receiving this therapy because of increased cardiovascular risk (e.g. myocardial infarction, stroke) with the combination.

Norgestimate–Ethinyl Estradiol (Ortho Tri-Cyclen)

Preparation *Rx*

| Ethinyl estradiol | Ortho Tri-Cyclen | 21-day Dialpak |
| & norgestimate | | 28-day Dialpak |

	Phase 1 (Days 1–7)	Phase 2 (Days 8–14)	Phase 3 (Days 15–21)	Phase 4 (Days 22–28)
21 day	180 µg NG & 35 µg EE	215 µg NG & 35 µg EE	250 µg NG & 35 µg EE	None
28 day	180 µg NG & 35 µg EE	215 µg NG & 35 µg EE	250 µg NG & 35 µg EE	Inert ingredients

NG, norgestimate; EE, ethinyl estradiol

Selected References

Haider A, Shaw JC. Treatment of acne vulgaris. JAMA 2004; 292: 726–35.

Redmond GP, Olson WH, Lippman JS, et al. Norgestimate and ethinyl estradiol in the treatment of acne vulgaris: a randomized, placebo-controlled trial. Obstet Gynecol 1997; 89: 615–22.

Runnebaum B, Brunwald K, Rabe T. The efficacy and tolerability of norgestimate/ethinyl estradiol (250 mcg of norgestimate/35 mcg of ethinyl estradiol): results of an open, multicenter study of 59,701 women. Am J Obstet Gynecol 1992; 166: 1963–8.

Clindamycin Phosphate Topical (various)

Dose and Administration

Apply to cleansed affected area twice a day. The 1% foam should be applied once per day.

Uses

FDA-approved: Treatment of acne vulgaris.

Pharmacology

Clindamycin is a lincosamide antibiotic that inhibits bacterial protein synthesis in susceptible organisms by reversibly binding to the 50S ribosomal subunit. The exact mechanism of action for clindamycin in acne is unknown but may be due to its antibacterial activity. Skin surface growth of the anaerobe *Propionibacterium acnes* and free fatty acid concentrations in sebum are decreased with topical clindamycin application. These actions result in decreased inflammation and microcomedo formation. Inhibition of leukocyte chemotaxis may also be involved.

Adverse Effects/Precautions

Local irritation is the most frequent adverse event. Diarrhea, bloody diarrhea, and pseudomembranous colitis have been reported rarely in patients receiving topical clindamycin therapy. Overgrowth of nonsusceptible organisms on the skin surface may occur.

Pregnancy: FDA category B.

Special Considerations

Reduction in inflammatory lesions generally occurs within 2 to 6 weeks with a maximal benefit noted after 12 weeks of therapy.

Preparation Rx

Foam	1%	Evoclin	50 & 100 g
Gel	1%	Cleocin T	30 & 60 g
		ClindaMax	
		Generic	
		Clindagel	40 & 75 ml
		BenzaClin (with benzoyl peroxide 5%)	25 & 50 g
		Duac (with benzoyl peroxide 5%)	45 g
Lotion	1%	Cleocin T	60 ml
		ClindaMax	
		Generic	
Pledgets	1%	Cleocin T	60 pledgets
		Clindets	69 pledgets
		Generic	60 pledgets

Clindamycin Phosphate Topical (various)

Solution	1%	Cleocin T	30 & 60 ml
		Clinda-Derm	60 ml
		Generic	30 & 60 ml

Selected References

Haider A, Shaw JC. Treatment of acne vulgaris. JAMA 2004; 292: 726–35.

Schachner L. The treatment of acne: a contemporary review. Pediatr Clin North Am 1983; 30: 501–10.

Shahlita AR, Smith EB, Bauer E. Topical erythromycin vs. clindamycin therapy for acne. A multicenter, double-blind comparison. Arch Dermatol 1984; 120: 351–5.

Erythromycin Topical (various)

Dose and Administration

Apply a thin film to the cleansed affected area each morning and evening.

Uses

FDA-approved: Treatment of inflammatory acne vulgaris.

Pharmacology

Erythromycin is a macrolide antibiotic that inhibits bacterial protein synthesis in susceptible organisms by reversibly binding to the 50S ribosomal subunit. The exact mechanism of action for erythromycin in acne is unknown but is thought to be related to its antibacterial activity. Growth of the anaerobe *Propionibacterium acnes* on the skin surface and free fatty acid concentrations in sebum are decreased with topical erythromycin application. These actions result in decreased inflammation and microcomedo formation.

Adverse Effects/Precautions

Local irritation is the most frequent adverse event. Hypersensitivity has been reported infrequently.
Pregnancy: FDA category B and C.

Special Considerations

Reduction in inflammatory lesions generally occurs within 3 to 8 weeks with a maximal benefit noted after 12 weeks of therapy.

Preparation Rx

Gel	2%	A/T/S	30 g
		Emgel	27 & 50 g
		Erygel	30 & 60 g
		Generic	30 & 60 g
	3%	Benzamycin (with 5% benzoyl peroxide)	23.3 & 46.6 g
		Benzamycin Pak (with 5% benzoyl peroxide)	#60
		Generic	
Ointment	2%	Akne-Mycin	25 g
Pledgets	2%	Erycette	60 pledgets
		T-Stat Pads	60 pads
		Ery 2% Pads	60 pads
		Erythromycin Pledgets	60 pledgets
Solution	1.5%	Staticin	60 ml
		Generic	60 ml
	2%	A/T/S	60 ml
		EryDerm	60 ml
		Theramycin Z	60 ml
		T-Stat	60 ml
		Generic	60 ml

Erythromycin Topical (various)

Selected References

Haider A, Shaw JC. Treatment of acne vulgaris. JAMA 2004; 292: 726–35.

Schachner L. The treatment of acne: a contemporary review. Pediatr Clin North Am 1983; 30: 501–10.

Shahlita AR, Smith EB, Bauer E. Topical erythromycin vs. clindamycin therapy for acne. A multicenter, double-blind comparison. Arch Dermatol 1984; 120: 351–5.

Metronidazole Topical
(MetroCream, MetroGel, MetroLotion, Noritate)

Dose and Administration

Apply a thin film twice a day (gel & lotion) or once a day (cream) to the cleansed affected area.

Uses

FDA-approved: Treatment of inflammatory papules, pustules, and erythema of acne rosacea.

Pharmacology

Metronidazole is a nitroimidazole antibiotic and antiprotozoal agent. Its exact mechanism of action in rosacea is unknown but may be due to its anti-inflammatory and immunosuppressive activity and not its antimicrobial activity. Specifically, metronidazole affects neutrophil motility, lymphocyte transformation and cell-mediated immunity. Systemic absorption following topical application is limited.

Adverse Effects/Precautions

Local irritation is the most frequent adverse event. Metallic taste, tingling or numbness of extremities, and nausea may also occur. Ocular tearing and irritation may result if applied too close to the eyes.

Pregnancy: FDA category B.

Special Considerations

Clinical improvement generally occurs within 3 weeks and continues through 9 weeks of therapy. Relapse is common following metronidazole discontinuation. Cosmetics and moisturizers may be applied over metronidazole as early as 5 minutes after application.

Preparation *Rx*

Gel	0.75%	MetroGel	30 & 45 g
Cream	0.75%	MetroCream	45 g
	1%	Noritate	30 g
Lotion	0.75%	MetroLotion	59 ml

Selected References

Lowe NJ, Henderson T, Millikan LE, et al. Topical metronidazole for severe and recalcitrant rosacea: a prospective open trial. Cutis 1989; 43: 283–6.

Schmadel LK, McEvoy GK. Topical metronidazole: a new therapy for rosacea. Clin Pharm 1990; 9: 94–101.

Thiboutot DM. Acne and rosacea. New and emerging therapies. Dermatol Clin 2000; 18: 63–71.

Sodium Sulfacetamide Topical (Klaron)

Dose and Administration

Apply a thin film twice daily to cleansed affected areas.

Uses

FDA-approved: Treatment of acne vulgaris.

Pharmacology

Sodium sulfacetamide is a sulfonamide with antibacterial activity that is exerted via competitive antagonism of para-aminobenzoic acid (PABA). The exact mechanism of sodium sulfacetamide in the treatment of acne is unknown but is thought to be related to its antibacterial activity against *Propionibacterium acnes*.

Adverse Effects/Precautions

Local irritation is the most frequent adverse event. The product is contraindicated in patients with sulfonamide hypersensitivity.

Pregnancy: FDA category C.

Preparation *Rx*

Lotion	10%	Klaron	118 ml

Selected References

Haider A, Shaw JC. Treatment of acne vulgaris. JAMA 2004; 292: 726–35.

Thiboutot D. New treatments and therapeutic strategies for acne. Arch Fam Med 2000; 9: 179–87.

Sulfur and Sodium Sulfacetamide Topical (various)

Dose and Administration

Apply a thin film to cleansed affected areas one to three times daily.

Uses

FDA-approved: Treatment of acne vulgaris, acne rosacea, and seborrheic dermatitis.

Pharmacology

Sodium sulfacetamide is a sulfonamide with antibacterial activity; sulfur acts as a keratolytic agent. The exact mechanism of sulfur and sodium sulfacetamide in the treatment of acne is unknown. It is suspected that the combination promotes keratolysis and inhibits the growth of *Propionibacterium acnes* and the formation of free fatty acids. These combined actions result in decreased inflammation and comedone formation.

Adverse Effects/Precautions

Local irritation is the most frequent adverse event. The product is contraindicated in patients with sulfonamide or sulfur hypersensitivity.

Pregnancy: FDA category C.

Preparation *Rx*

5% sulfur and 10% sodium sulfacetamide

Cream	Avar-E	45 g
	Clenia	28 g
	Plexion SCT	120 g
	Rosanil	170 g
	Rosac Cream with Sunscreens	45 g
Gel	Avar Gel	45 g
	Rosula Aqueous Gel	45 g
Lotion	Avar Cleanser	226.8 g
	Nicosyn	45 g
	Plexion	170.3 & 340.2 g
	Sulfacet-R	25 g
	Zetacet	25 & 30 g
	Generic	25, 30, 45 & 60 g
Soap	Prascion	170.3 & 340.2 g
Suspension	Plexion TS	30 g
	Generic	30 g

Selected References

Breneman DL, Ariano MC. Successful treatment of acne vulgaris in women with a new topical sodium sulfacetamide/sulfur lotion. Int J Dermatol 1993; 32: 365–7.

Olansky S. Old drug in a new system revisited. Cutis 1977; 19: 852–4.

Tarimci N, Sener S, Kilinc T. Topical sodium sulfacetamide/sulfur lotion. J Clin Pharm Ther 1997; 22: 301.

Tretinoin Topical
(Avita, Retin-A, Retin-A Micro, Renova)

Dose and Administration

Lightly apply to affected cleansed area once daily at bedtime.

Uses

FDA-approved: Acne vulgaris (Avita, Retin-A, Retin-A Micro) and mitigation of fine wrinkles, mottled hyperpigmentation, and tactile roughness of facial skin unrelieved by comprehensive skin care and sun avoidance (Renova). Other uses include flat warts and melasma.

Pharmacology

Tretinoin, or all-*trans*-retinoic acid, is a vitamin A derivative. Its exact mechanism of action is unknown; however, tretinoin affects keratinization by stimulating follicular epithelium turnover. This action causes decreased follicular cell cohesiveness, which facilitates removal of existing comedones and subsequently decreases micro-comedone formation. Tretinoin also inhibits melanogenesis. Systemic absorption is minimal following topical application.

Adverse Effects/Precautions

Local irritation is the most frequent adverse reaction. Reversible hyper- or hypo-pigmentation may also occur. Exposure to cold or windy environments and sunlight, including sunlamps, should be avoided if possible. Use of sunscreen products and protective clothing is recommended to avoid serious skin reactions.

Pregnancy: FDA category C.

Drug Interactions

Other medications with the potential to cause photosensitivity (e.g. fluoroquinolones, tetracyclines, sulfonamides, thiazides, phenothiazines) should be co-administered with caution.

Special Considerations

Therapy should be initiated at the lowest concentration and titrated upward as needed. Initially symptom exacerbation may occur but therapy should not be discontinued. For acne, therapeutic results should become apparent within 2 to 3 weeks, but 6 weeks of therapy may be required before improvement is noted. At least 6 months of therapy may be required before the effects are seen on photodamaged skin.

For many patients with acne and photodamage, maintenance therapy will generally be required. Cosmetics may be used but the affected area should be cleansed prior to tretinoin application for maximal benefit. Avoid contact with the eyes, paranasal creases, mouth, and mucous membranes.

Preparation *Rx*

Cream	0.02%	Renova	40 g
	0.025%	Avita	20 & 45 g

Tretinoin Topical
(Avita, Retin-A, Retin-A Micro, Renova)

		Retin-A	20 & 45 g
		Generic	20 & 45 g
	0.05%	Retin-A	20 & 45 g
		Generic	20 & 45 g
		Renova	40 & 60 g
	0.1%	Retin-A	20 & 45 g
		Generic	20 & 45 g
Gel	0.01%	Retin-A	15 & 45 g
		Generic	15 & 45 g
	0.025%	Retin-A	15 & 45 g
		Avita	20 & 45 g
		Generic	15 & 45 g
Gel with	0.04%	Retin-A Micro	20 & 45 g
microspores			
	0.1%	Retin-A Micro	20 & 45 g
Solution	0.05%	Retin-A	28 ml

Selected References

Haider A, Shaw JC. Treatment of acne vulgaris. JAMA 2004; 292: 726–35.

Kang S. Photoaging and tretinoin. Dermatol Clin 1998; 16: 357–64.

Shapiro SS, Latriano L. Pharmacokinetic and pharmacodynamic considerations of retinoids: tretinoin. J Am Acad Dermatol 1998; 39: S13–16.

Webster GF. Topical tretinoin in acne therapy. J Am Acad Dermatol 1998; 39: S38–44.

Antibiotics

Ampicillin (Principen)

Dose and Administration

Usual oral dose: Give 250 to 500 mg orally every 6 hours depending on the site of infection. Children weighing more than 20 kg can receive the adult dose. For smaller children, give 50 to 100 mg/kg per day divided every 6 hours depending on the site and severity of the infection.

Usual parenteral dose: For adults, give 500 to 1500 mg IM every 4 to 6 hours or 500 to 3000 mg IV every 4 to 6 hours (maximum 12 g/day). For infants and children, 100 to 400 mg/kg per day IM/IV divided every 4 to 6 hours.

Endocarditis prophylaxis: Give 2 g (adults) or 50 mg/kg (children) IM/IV 30 minutes prior to the procedure. For high-risk patients, concomitant gentamicin administration is recommended.

Uses

Treatment of enterococcal infections (e.g. urinary tract infections, endocarditis); respiratory tract infections; skin and skin structure infections; urinary tract infections; infections due to susceptible strains of *Listeria monocytogenes* (e.g. meningitis), *Proteus mirabilis, Escherichia coli*, and *Eikenella corrodens*. It is also recommended for prophylaxis of bacterial endocarditis in patients with cardiac risk factors undergoing certain genitourinary and gastrointestinal (nonesophageal) procedures and those undergoing dental, oral, esophageal or respiratory tract procedures who cannot take oral medications (i.e. amoxicillin).

Pharmacology

The penicillins are β-lactam antibiotics that inhibit bacterial cell wall synthesis via binding to penicillin proteins. The affinity for these proteins as well as their activity against different bacteria varies among the penicillin class members. Ampicillin is classified as an aminopenicillin. It has greater activity than the natural penicillins against enterococci and *Haemophilus influenzae* but slightly lower activity against *Streptococcus pyogenes*, *Streptococcus pneumoniae*, *Neisseria* species, and *Clostridium* species. Ampicillin also demonstrates activity against some gram-negative organisms, including *Escherichia coli*, *Proteus mirabilis*, *Salmonella*, *Shigella*, and *Listeria* species; resistance to these organisms has occurred in multiple areas, however.

Ampicillin is stable in the presence of gastric acid and is well absorbed following oral administration. To maximize absorption, it should be taken on an empty stomach. It is primarily excreted in the urine. Dose adjustment is recommended in renal insufficiency.

Adverse Effects/Precautions

Hypersensitivity reactions may occur with ampicillin. These reactions most commonly present as eosinophilia or rash. Serum sickness-type reactions have also been reported. Anaphylaxis can occur but is rare.

Patients who have developed hypersensitivity to ampicillin may experience cross reactivity if exposed to other β-lactam antibiotics, including cephalosporins and carbapenems.

Generalized erythematous, maculopapular rashes are common with ampicillin. The rash generally develops 3 to 14 days after therapy is initiated and appears on the trunk and spreads to most parts of the body. The rash is frequently seen in patients with a concomitant viral illness (e.g. infectious mononucleosis). It is suspected that the rash is nonimmunologically mediated and should not preclude subsequent use of ampicillin.

Gastrointestinal adverse effects, including nausea, vomiting, abdominal pain, and diarrhea, are common with ampicillin administration. Black hairy tongue, glossitis, stomatitis, and sore tongue may also occur.

Rare hematologic adverse effects include hemolytic anemia, transient neutropenia, leukopenia, and thrombocytopenia.

Pregnancy: FDA category B.

Drug Interactions

Probenecid interferes with the tubular secretion of ampicillin. Ampicillin may decrease the efficacy of oral contraceptives. Concomitant therapy with allopurinol may increase the risk of developing an ampicillin rash.

Preparation *Rx*

Capsules	250 & 500 mg	Principen	
		Various generics	
Oral suspension	125 mg/5 ml	Principen	100 & 200 ml
		Various generics	
Oral suspension	250 mg/5 ml	Principen	100, 150 & 200 ml
		Various generics	
Injections	125, 250 & 500 mg	Various generics	
Injections	1 g & 2 g	Various generics	

Selected References

Anon. The choice of antimicrobial drugs. Med Lett Drugs Ther 1999; 41: 95–104.

Wright AJ. The penicillins. Mayo Clin Proc 1999; 74: 290–307.

Cefuroxime Axetil (Ceftin)

Dose and Administration

Adults: Usual dose is 250 to 500 mg orally every 12 hours depending on the site of infection. For uncomplicated urinary tract infection, 125 to 250 mg every 12 hours is recommended. A single dose of 1000 mg is given for gonorrhea.

Children: Usual dose is 20 to 30 mg/kg per day orally divided every 12 hours depending on the site of infection.

Uses

FDA-approved: Treatment of pharyngitis and tonsillitis caused by *Streptococcus pyogenes*; impetigo caused by *Staphylococcus aureus* or *S. pyogenes*; otitis media caused by *Streptococcus pneumoniae, Haemophilus influenzae, Moraxella catarrhalis*, or *S. pyogenes*; acute bacterial maxillary sinusitis caused by *S. pneumoniae* or *H. influenzae*; acute bacterial exacerbations of chronic bronchitis caused by *S. pneumoniae, H. influenzae*, or *Haemophilus parainfluenzae*; uncomplicated skin and skin-structure infections caused by *S. aureus* or *S. pyogenes*; uncomplicated urinary tract infections caused by *Escherichia coli* or *Klebsiella pneumoniae*; uncomplicated gonorrhea caused by *Neisseria gonorrhoeae*; and early Lyme disease (erythema migrans) caused by *Borrelia burgdorferi*.

Pharmacology

Cefuroxime is a β-lactam antimicrobial that is classified as a second-generation cephalosporin. The cephalosporins exert their antibacterial effects via interference with the synthesis of peptidoglycan, a major structural component of the bacterial cell wall. Defective bacterial cell walls are ultimately formed resulting in cell lysis and bacterial death.

Cefuroxime demonstrates activity against aerobic gram-positive cocci including methicillin-susceptible *S. aureus* and *Staphylococcus epidermidis* (including β-lactamase-producing strains), *S. pyogenes, Streptococcus agalactiae*, and *S. pneumoniae*. Cefuroxime has improved gram-negative activity as compared with the first-generation cephalosporins. Susceptible gram-negative organisms generally include *Proteus mirabilis, E. coli, M. catarrhalis* (including β-lactamase-producing strains), *N. gonorrhoeae, K. pneumoniae, H. influenzae* (including β-lactamase-producing strains), and *H. parainfluenzae*. Cefuroxime also exhibits activity against the spirochete *B. burgdorferi*.

Cefuroxime is well absorbed following oral administration and is maximized when taken with food. It is eliminated in the urine via glomerular filtration and tubular secretion. Dosage adjustment is required in renal insufficiency.

Adverse Effects/Precautions

Cefuroxime is generally well tolerated. Gastrointestinal effects including nausea, vomiting, diarrhea, and abdominal pain are the most common adverse effects associated with cefuroxime. Hypersensitivity reactions may occur infrequently (rash, urticaria, angioedema, fever, eosinophilia). Cefuroxime use should be approached cautiously in patients who have a documented history of anaphylaxis to penicillin; cross allergenicity may occur.

Pregnancy: FDA category B.

Cefuroxime Axetil (Ceftin)

Drug Interactions

Concomitant administration of probenecid with cefuroxime increases peak serum concentrations by 30% and the area under the curve by 50%.

Preparation *Rx*

Tablets	250 & 500 mg	Ceftin	
Oral suspension	125 mg/5 ml	Ceftin	100 ml
Oral suspension	250 mg/5 ml	Ceftin	50 & 100 ml

Selected References

Barnett ED, Klein JO. Use of oral cephalosporins in infants and children. Curr Clin Top Infect Dis 1997; 17: 316–33.

Marshall WF, Blair JE. The cephalosporins. Mayo Clin Proc 1999; 74: 187–95.

Morrow JD. The oral cephalosporins – a review. Am J Med Sci 1992; 303: 35–9.

Cephalexin (Keflex)

Dose and Administration

Adults: Usual adult dose is 250 to 500 mg orally every 6 hours. The maximum recommended dose is 4 g daily in divided doses.

Children: Usual pediatric dose is 25 to 50 mg/kg orally per day in divided doses every 6 hours. For otitis media, 75 to 100 mg/kg per day in divided doses should be given.

Uses

FDA-approved: Treatment of the following mild to moderate infections due to susceptible micro-organisms: respiratory tract infections caused by *Streptococcus pneumoniae* and *Streptococcus pyogenes* (e.g. pharyngitis, tonsillitis); otitis media due to *S. pneumoniae*, *Haemophilus influenzae*, staphylococci, streptococci, and *Moraxella catarrhalis*; skin and skin structure infections caused by staphylococci and/or streptococci; osteomyelitis caused by staphylococci and/or *Proteus mirabilis*; and genitourinary tract infections (e.g. cystitis, prostatitis) caused by *Escherichia coli, P. mirabilis*, and *Klebsiella pneumoniae*.

Pharmacology

Cephalexin is a β-lactam antimicrobial that is classified as a first-generation cephalosporin. The cephalosporins exert their antibacterial effects via interference with the synthesis of peptidoglycan, a major structural component of the bacterial cell wall. Defective bacterial cell walls are ultimately formed, resulting in cell lysis and bacterial death.

Cephalexin demonstrates activity primarily against aerobic gram-positive cocci, including methicillin-susceptible *Staphylococcus aureus* and *Staphylococcus epidermidis* (β-lactamase and non-β-lactamase-producing strains), *S. pyogenes, Streptococcus agalactiae*, and *S. pneumoniae*. Cephalexin has limited gram-negative activity, yet some strains of *P. mirabilis, E. coli*, and *Klebsiella* species may be susceptible.

Cephalexin is well absorbed following oral administration and may be taken with food. It is eliminated in the urine via glomerular filtration and tubular secretion. Dosage adjustment is required in renal insufficiency.

Adverse Effects/Precautions

Cephalexin is generally well tolerated. Gastrointestinal effects including nausea, vomiting, and diarrhea are the most common adverse effects associated with cephalexin. Hypersensitivity reactions (e.g. rash, urticaria, angioedema, fever, eosinophilia) may occur infrequently. Cephalexin use should be approached cautiously in patients who have a documented history of anaphylaxis to penicillin; cross allergenicity may occur.

Pregnancy: FDA category B.

Preparation *Rx*

Capsules	250 & 500 mg	Keflex
		Various generics
Tablets	500 mg	Keftab

Cephalexin (Keflex)

Oral suspension	125 mg/5 ml	Various generics	100 & 200 ml
Oral suspension	250 mg/5 ml	Various generics	100 & 200 ml

Selected References

Barnett ED, Klein JO. Use of oral cephalosporins in infants and children. Curr Clin Top Infect Dis 1997; 17: 316–33.

Marshall WF, Blair JE. The cephalosporins. Mayo Clin Proc 1999; 74: 187–95.

Morrow JD. The oral cephalosporins – a review. Am J Med Sci 1992; 303: 35–9.

Penicillin (Pen VK)

Dose and Administration

Primary, secondary or early latent syphilis: Give benzathine penicillin 2.4 million units (adults) or 50 000 units/kg (children) IM as a single dose.

Late latent, latent of unknown duration or tertiary syphilis: Give benzathine penicillin 7.2 million units (adults) or 150 000 units/kg (children) total, administered as three IM doses of 2.4 million units (adults) or 50 000 units/kg (children) each at 1-week intervals.

Neurosyphilis: Give penicillin G 18 to 24 million units a day administered as 3 to 4 million units IV every 4 hours for 10 to 14 days.

Oral therapy (Penicillin VK): For systemic infections, oral dosing ranges from 125 to 500 mg (adults & children > 12 years) or 25 to 50 mg/kg per day divided (children) every 6 to 8 hours depending on severity. For prophylaxis of pneumococcal infections or recurrent rheumatic fever, give 250 mg (adults and children > 5 years) or 125 mg (children < 5 years) orally twice a day.

Uses

Treatment of syphilis including primary, secondary, latent or tertiary, and neurologic or congenital infection; enterococcal infections including endocarditis; streptococcal infections including pharyngitis, tonsillitis, pneumonia, otitis media, skin and skin structure infections, meningitis, and septicemia; meningitis due to *Neiserria meningitidis*; skin infections due to *Clostridium perfringens* (e.g. gas gangrene, empyema); and tetanus due to *Clostridium tetani*.

Pharmacology

The penicillins are β-lactam antibiotics that inhibit bacterial cell wall synthesis via binding to penicillin proteins. The affinity for these proteins as well as their activity against different bacteria varies among the penicillin class members. Penicillin is classified as a natural penicillin and is rapidly hydrolyzed and thus inactivated by penicillinases produced by multiple organisms.

Natural penicillins generally exhibit activity against nonpenicillinase-producing strains of *Staphylococcus aureus*, *Staphylococcus epidermidis*, *Streptococcus pneumoniae*, other streptococci (groups A, B, C, G, H, K, L, and M), nonenterococcal group D streptococci, viridans streptococci, and some enterococci. Gram-negative activity includes *N. meningitidis* and most nonpenicillinase-producing strains of *Neisseria gonorrhoeae*. The natural penicillins are also active against some anaerobic bacteria including *Peptococcus*, *Peptostreptococcus*, *Fusobacterium*, and some strains of *Clostridia* and *Bacteroides*. Penicillin is also active against the spirochete *Treponema pallidum*, and is considered the drug of choice for syphilis.

Members of the natural penicillin class include benzylpenicillin (penicillin G) and phenoxymethyl penicillin (penicillin VK). Penicillin G is rapidly degraded by gastric acid following oral administration, which limits its clinical utility via the oral route. Penicillin G is preferred for intravenous administration and is also available as intramuscular repository formulations (procaine or benzathine) designed for slow release and maintenance of prolonged serum concentrations over an extended time period. Penicillin VK is the preferred product for oral administration because it is more stable in the presence of gastric acid as compared with penicillin G. Penicillin excretion occurs primarily via tubular secretion. Dosage adjustment is recommended in patients with renal insufficiency.

Adverse Effects/Precautions

Hypersensitivity reactions are common with penicillin and range from mild rash, eosinophilia, and fever to anaphylaxis, which can be fatal.

Patients who have developed hypersensitivity to a penicillin may experience cross reactivity if exposed to other β-lactam antibiotics including cephalosporins and carbapenems.

Gastrointestinal adverse effects including nausea, vomiting, abdominal pain, and diarrhea are common with oral penicillin administration.

Rare hematologic adverse effects include hemolytic anemia, transient neutropenia, leukopenia, and thrombocytopenia.

Acute interstitial nephritis has occurred rarely with intravenous penicillin. Symptoms of this reaction include fever, proteinuria, hematuria, rash, and dysuria.

Neurologic reactions including hallucinations, confusion, seizures, and encephalopathy have occurred. The majority of cases have occurred in patients with renal insufficiency receiving high doses of intravenous penicillin.

The Jarisch–Herxheimer reaction may occur when using penicillin for syphilis. The reaction presents as headache, fever, chills, sweating, sore throat, myalgia/arthralgia, tachycardia, and increased blood pressure. It generally occurs within 2 to 12 hours of the initial dose of penicillin and is due to the release of pyrogens and endotoxins from phagocytosed organisms. A flare in disease symptomatology may also occur.

Pregnancy: FDA category B.

Drug Interactions

Probenecid interferes with the tubular secretion of penicillin. The combination is used therapeutically to produce higher and prolonged serum concentrations of penicillin. Penicillin VK may decrease the efficacy of oral contraceptives.

Preparation *Rx*

Penicillin G Potassium (Aqueous)

Injection	5 & 20 million unit	Generic	

Penicillin G Sodium (Aqueous)   Generic

Injection	5 million unit		

Penicillin G Benzathine

Injection	300 000 units/ml	Bicillin L-A	10 ml
Injection	600 000 units/ml	Bicillin L-A	1, 2 & 4 ml

Penicillin G Procaine

Injection	600 000 units/ml	Generic	1 & 2 ml

Penicillin G Benzathine + Penicillin G Procaine Combined

Injection	150 000 units + 150 000 units/ml	Bicillin C-R	10 ml
Injection	300 000 units + 300 000 units/ml	Bicillin C-R	1, 2 & 4 ml

Penicillin (Pen VK)

Injection	900 000 units + 300 000 units/2 ml	Bicillin C-R 900–300	
Phenoxymethyl penicillin			
Tablets	250 & 500 mg	Pen-Vee K, Veetids Various generics	
Oral suspension	125 mg/5 ml	Veetids Various generics	100 & 200 ml
Oral suspension	250 mg/5 ml	Veetids Various generics	100 & 200 ml

Selected References

Centers for Disease Control and Prevention. Sexually transmitted diseases treatment guidelines 2002. Morbid Mortal Weekly Rep 2002; 51(no. RR-6): 1–78.

Scaglione F, Demartini G, Arcidiacono MM, et al. Optimum treatment of streptococcal pharyngitis. Drugs 1997; 53: 86–97.

Wright AJ. The penicillins. Mayo Clin Proc 1999; 74: 290–307.

Azithromycin (Zithromax)

Dose and Administration

Adults: Give 500 mg orally on day 1 followed by 250 mg once a day for a total of 5 days. For the prevention of disseminated *Mycobacterium avium* complex disease, the recommended oral dose is 1200 mg taken once weekly. For urethritis or cervicitis due to *Chlamydia trachomatis* and chancroid due to *Haemophilus ducreyi*, 1 g should be taken orally as one dose.

The IV form should be administered as 500 mg IV once daily followed by oral therapy for completion of therapy.

Pediatrics: Usual dose 10 mg/kg orally for 5 days.

Uses

FDA-approved: Treatment of mild to moderate cases of the following infections: acute bacterial exacerbation of chronic bronchitis due to *Haemophilus influenzae*, *Moraxella catarrhalis*, or *Streptococcus pneumoniae*; community-acquired pneumonia due to *S. pneumoniae* or *H. influenzae*; pharyngitis/tonsillitis due to *Streptococcus pyogenes*; acute otitis media due to *H. influenzae*, *M. catarrhalis*, or *S. pneumoniae*; uncomplicated skin and skin structure infections due to *Staphylococcus aureus*, *Streptococcus pyogenes* or *Streptococcus agalactiae*; and nongonococcal urethritis and cervicitis due to *C. trachomatis*. It is also approved for the prevention of disseminated *M. avium* complex disease in HIV-infected patients. The IV form is approved for community-acquired pneumonia due to *Chlamydia pneumoniae*, *H. influenzae*, *Legionella pneumophila*, *M. catarrhalis*, *Mycoplasma pneumoniae*, *S. aureus*, or *S. pneumoniae* and pelvic inflammatory disease due to *C. trachomatis*, *Neisseria gonorrhoeae*, or *Mycoplasma hominis* in patients who require initial intravenous therapy. Another use is chancroid.

Pharmacology

Azithromycin is a macrolide antibiotic that inhibits bacterial protein synthesis in susceptible organisms by reversibly binding to the 50S ribosomal subunit. Based on similar mechanisms of action, azithromycin should not be combined with clindamycin or chloramphenicol to prevent antibacterial antagonism. Its spectrum of activity is expanded as compared with erythromycin. It retains similar gram-positive activity (e.g. *S. pyogenes, S. pneumoniae, S. aureus*); however, it has greater gram-negative activity than erythromycin or clarithromycin. Susceptible gram-negative organisms include *Neisseria meningitidis*, *N. gonorrhoeae*, *H. ducreyi*, *H. influenzae*, *M. catarrhalis*, and *Bordetella pertussis*. Azithromycin also exerts activity against *Treponema pallidum*, *M. pneumoniae*, *L. pneumophila*, *Chlamydia* species, and *M. avium* complex.

Azithromycin is more acid stable than erythromycin. It is widely distributed throughout the body and concentrations in pulmonary macrophages, poly-morphonuclear leukocytes, and genital/pelvic tissues remain increased for several days following administration. Penetration of the cerebrospinal fluid is negligible and therefore it should not be used to treat infections of the central nervous system. Azithromycin is excreted primarily in the feces.

Azithromycin (Zithromax)

Adverse Effects/Precautions

The most common adverse effects involve the gastrointestinal tract and include nausea, vomiting, diarrhea, and abdominal pain. Serious allergic reactions have occurred rarely with azithromycin. Reversible elevations in liver function tests may occur.

Pregnancy: FDA category B.

Drug Interactions

Azithromycin does not affect the cytochrome P450 system, unlike erythromycin and clarithromycin. When combined with warfarin, however, cases of increased prothrombin times and INRs have been reported. Therefore, if azithromycin is combined with warfarin, close monitoring should be performed.

Special Considerations

Administration with food may lessen the gastrointestinal adverse effects. The oral suspension single packets should be mixed with 60 ml of water and taken immediately. The glass should be mixed with an additional 60 ml of water and ingested to ensure the entire dose is consumed.

Preparation *Rx*

Tablets	250, 500 & 600 mg tablets	Zithromax	
Tablets	500 mg	Zithromax TRI-PAK	3 tablets per pack
	250 mg	Zithromax Z-Pak	6 tablets per pack
Oral suspension	1 g packets	Zithromax	Box of 3 & 10 pkts
Oral suspension	100 mg/5 ml	Zithromax	15 ml
Oral suspension	200 mg/5 ml	Zithromax	15, 22.5 & 30 ml
Injection	500 mg	Zithromax	

Selected References

Alvarez-Elcoro S, Enzler MJ. The macrolides: erythromycin, clarithromycin, and azithromycin. Mayo Clin Proc 1999; 74: 613–34.

Centers for Disease Control and Prevention. Sexually transmitted diseases treatment guidelines 2002. Morbid Mortal Weekly Rep 2002; 51(no. RR-6): 1–78.

Zuckerman JM, Kaye KM. The newer macrolides: azithromycin and clarithromycin. Infect Dis Clin North Am 1995; 9: 731–43.

Clarithromycin (Biaxin)

Dose and Administration

Adults: Give 250 to 500 mg orally twice a day depending on the type of infection. For acute exacerbation of chronic bronchitis or sinusitis, an alternative regimen is 1 gram (as two 500 mg extended release tablets) given orally once a day.

Children: Give 15 mg/kg per day orally divided twice a day.

Uses

FDA-approved: Treatment of the following infections: pharyngitis/tonsillitis due to *Streptococcus pyogenes*; acute maxillary sinusitis due to *Haemophilus influenzae*, *Moraxella catarrhalis*, or *Streptococcus pneumoniae*; acute otitis media due to *H. influenzae*, *M. catarrhalis* or *S. pneumoniae*; acute bacterial exacerbation of chronic bronchitis due to *H. influenzae*, *Haemophilus parainfluenzae*, *M. catarrhalis*, or *S. pneumoniae*; community-acquired pneumonia due to *Mycoplasma pneumoniae*, *H. parainfluenzae*, *S. pneumoniae*, or *Chlamydia pneumoniae* (TWAR); uncomplicated skin and skin structure infections due to *Staphylococcus aureus* or *S. pyogenes*; disseminated mycobacterial infections due to *Mycobacterium avium* or *Mycobacterium intracellulare*. Clarithromycin is also indicated for *Helicobacter pylori* eradication and for prevention of disseminated *Mycobacterium avium* complex (MAC) disease in patients with advanced HIV infection.

Pharmacology

Clarithromycin is a macrolide antibiotic that inhibits bacterial protein synthesis in susceptible organisms by reversibly binding to the 50S ribosomal subunit. Based on similar mechanisms of action, clarithromycin should not be combined with clindamycin or chloramphenicol to prevent antibacterial antagonism. Clarithromycin demonstrates comparable or better *in vitro* activity against gram-positive organisms (e.g. *S. pyogenes, S. pneumoniae, S. aureus)* as compared to erythromycin; however, organisms that are resistant to erythromycin are generally cross-resistant to clarithromycin. Gram-negative activity is greater than with erythromycin but less than with azithromycin. Susceptible gram-negative organisms include *H. influenzae*, *M. catarrhalis*, and *Bordetella pertussis*. Clarithromycin also exerts activity against *M. pneumoniae*, *Legionella pneumophila*, *C. pneumoniae*, *H. pylori*, and *Mycobacterium avium* complex.

Clarithromycin is well absorbed following oral administration, and it can be taken with or without food. It undergoes rapid metabolism to produce its active metabolite, 14-hydroxyclarithromycin, which is responsible for its enhanced activity against *H. influenzae* as compared with erythromycin. It is eliminated by both renal and non-renal mechanisms. The dose should be halved or the interval doubled in patients with a creatinine clearance of < 30 ml/minute.

Adverse Effects/Precautions

The most common adverse effects are diarrhea, nausea, abnormal taste, dyspepsia, abdominal pain/discomfort, and headache.

Allergic reactions including urticaria, mild to life-threatening skin eruptions, and anaphylaxis have occurred.

Other adverse events include glossitis, stomatitis, oral moniliasis, vomiting, tongue discoloration, thrombocytopenia, leukopenia, neutropenia, reversible tooth discoloration, and dizziness.

Clarithromycin (Biaxin)

Reversible hearing loss and alterations of the sense of smell with taste perversion or taste loss have occurred.

Transient CNS events including anxiety, behavioral changes, confusional states, depersonalization, disorientation, hallucinations, insomnia, manic behavior, nightmares, psychosis, tinnitus, tremor, and vertigo have been reported during postmarketing use.

Hepatic dysfunction including increased liver enzymes, and hepatocellular and/or cholestatic hepatitis, with or without jaundice, have been infrequently reported with clarithromycin. This hepatic dysfunction may be severe and is usually reversible.

Pregnancy: FDA category C.

Drug Interactions

Clarithromycin is an inhibitor of the CYP 3A4 isoenzyme and thus has the potential to be involved in numerous drug interactions. Concomitant administration of clarithromycin with pimozide is contraindicated due to the potential for cardiac arrhythmias (QT prolongation, ventricular tachycardia, ventricular fibrillation, and torsades de pointes) due to inhibition of hepatic metabolism of pimozide. Clarithromycin can increase the serum concentrations of carbamazepine, theophylline, digoxin, cyclosporine, tacrolimus, phenytoin, and valproate. Additionally, when used concomitantly with warfarin, prothrombin times and INRs may increase. Close monitoring is recommended.

Preparation *Rx*

Tablets	250 & 500 mg	Biaxin Filmtabs	
Extended release tablets	500 mg	Biaxin XL	
Extended release tablets	500 mg	Biaxin XL Pac	14 tablets
Oral granules	125 mg/5 ml	Biaxin	50 & 100 ml
Oral granules	250 mg/5 ml	Biaxin	50 & 100 ml

Selected References

Alvarez-Elcoro S, Enzler MJ. The macrolides: erythromycin, clarithromycin, and azithromycin. Mayo Clin Proc 1999; 74: 613–34.

Sturgill MG, Rapp RP. Clarithromycin: review of a new macrolide antibiotic with improved microbiologic spectrum and favorable pharmacokinetic and adverse effect profiles. Ann Pharmacother 1992; 26: 1099–108.

Zuckerman JM, Kaye KM. The newer macrolides: azithromycin and clarithromycin. Infect Dis Clin North Am 1995; 9: 731–43.

Erythromycin (various)

Dose and Administration

Adults: The dose of all derivatives except the ethylsuccinate formulations is expressed in terms of erythromycin base and the usual recommended dose is 250 mg orally every 6 hours or 333 mg every 8 hours. The maximum recommended daily dose is 4 g in divided doses for more severe infections. For the ethylsuccinate formulation, a dose of 400 mg is considered equivalent to 250 mg of the base formulation.

Pediatrics: For all formulations, the usual dose is 30 to 50 mg/kg per day divided into four doses. For more severe infections, this dose can be doubled.

Uses

FDA-approved: Treatment of the following infections: upper and lower respiratory tract infections of mild to moderate severity caused by *Streptococcus pyogenes* or *Streptococcus pneumoniae*; listeriosis caused by *Listeria monocytogenes*; respiratory tract infections due to *Mycoplasma pneumoniae*; skin and skin structure infections of mild to moderate severity caused by *S. pyogenes* or *Staphylococcus aureus*; pertussis (whooping cough) caused by *Bordetella pertussis*; diphtheria due to *Corynebacterium diphtheriae*; erythrasma due to *Corynebacterium minutissimum*; conjunctivitis of the newborn, pneumonia of infancy, and urogenital infections during pregnancy due to *Chlamydia trachomatis* when tetracyclines are contraindicated or not tolerated; nongonococcal urethritis caused by *Ureaplasma urealyticum*; Legionnaires' disease caused by *Legionella pneumophila*.

Pharmacology

Erythromycin is a macrolide antibiotic that inhibits bacterial protein synthesis in susceptible organisms by reversibly binding to the 50S ribosomal subunit. Based on similar mechanisms of action, erythromycin should not be combined with clindamycin or chloramphenicol to prevent antibacterial antagonism. It demonstrates activity generally against most streptococci including *S. pyogenes* and *S. pneumoniae*; however, penicillin-resistant strains of *S. pneumoniae* are usually resistant to erythromycin. Methicillin-sensitive strains of *S. aureus* are generally susceptible. Activity against gram-negative organisms is variable but *Neisseria meningitidis*, *Neisseria gonorrhoeae* and *B. pertussis* are usually susceptible. Erythromycin also exerts activity against *Treponema pallidum*, *M. pneumoniae*, *L. pneumophila*, *Chlamydia* species, *Campylobacter jejuni* and some strains of *Rickettsia*.

Erythromycin is available as several different derivatives and formulations with varying bioavailabilities following oral administration. The estolate salt is the least susceptible to acid degradation and the best absorbed salt as compared with the base, stearate, and ethylsuccinate formulations. To maximize absorption most erythromycin formulations should be taken on an empty stomach. The estolate salt, however, has improved absorption in the presence of food. Erythromycin is extensively metabolized in the liver and is excreted primarily in the bile. Penetration of the cerebrospinal fluid is negligible and therefore erythromycin should not be used to treat infections of the central nervous system.

Erythromycin (various)

Adverse Effects/Precautions

Gastrointestinal adverse effects are common and include nausea, vomiting, diarrhea, and abdominal cramps. Allergic reactions may occur with all salt formulations but are thought to be more common with the estolate salt. Reversible cholestatic hepatitis rarely occurs with the estolate derivative and is associated with more than 10 days of therapy. Erythromycin can prolong the QT interval and its use should be avoided in patients at risk of QT prolongation. The estolate derivative is contraindicated in patients with hepatic dysfunction, while all other derivatives should be used cautiously in this patient population.

Pregnancy: FDA category B.

Drug Interactions

Erythromycin is a CYP 3A4 inhibitor and is involved in numerous drug interactions. Increased serum concentrations of theophylline, warfarin, phenytoin, carbamazepine, disopyramide, and cyclosporine can occur when used concomitantly with erythromycin. Erythromycin should not be co-administered with the HMGCoA reductase inhibitors (e.g. atorvastatin, lovastatin, simvastatin), owing to an increased risk of myopathy.

Special Considerations

Although erythromycin should generally be taken on an empty stomach, patients may need to take it with food to minimize gastrointestinal upset.

Preparation *Rx*

Erythromycin base

Enteric coated tablets	250 & 500 mg	Ery-Tab	
		Various generics	
Enteric coated capsules	250 mg	ERYC	
		Various generics	
Coated particles, tablets	333 & 500 mg	PCE Dispertab	

Erythromycin estolate

Oral suspension	125 mg/5 ml	Various generics	200 ml
Oral suspension	250 mg/5 ml	Various generics	150 & 200 ml
Erythromycin ethylsuccinate	400 mg	Erythromycin ES E.E.S. 400 Various generics	
Oral drops	100 mg/2.5 ml	EryPed	50 ml
Oral suspension	200 mg/5 ml	EryPed 200 E.E.S. Granules Various generics	100 & 200 ml
Oral suspension	400 mg/5 ml	EryPed 400 Various generics	100 & 200 ml

Erythrocin lactobionate

Injection	500 & 1000 mg	Erythrocin	

Erythromycin (various)

Erythromycin stearate

| Tablets | 250 & 500 mg | Erythrocin stearate |
| | | Various generics |

Selected References

Alvarez-Elcoro S, Enzler MJ. The macrolides: erythromycin, clarithromycin, and azithromycin. Mayo Clin Proc 1999; 74: 613–34.

Preston DA. Microbiological aspects of erythromycin. Pediatr Infect Dis 1986; 5: 120–3.

Washington JA, Wilson WR. Erythromycin: a microbial and clinical perspective after 30 years of clinical use (first of two parts). Mayo Clin Proc 1985; 60: 189–203.

Ciprofloxacin (Cipro)

Dose and Administration

The usual oral dose is 250 to 750 mg orally twice a day depending on the indication and infection severity. For uncomplicated urinary tract infections, 100 to 250 mg twice daily can be administered for 3 days. Uncomplicated gonorrhea can be treated with a single dose of 500 mg. For chancroid, give 500 mg twice daily for 3 days.

Intravenous dosing ranges from 200 to 400 mg twice a day with transition to oral therapy when clinically feasible.

Uses

FDA-approved: Treatment of sinusitis, lower respiratory tract infections (e.g. nosocomial pneumonia, acute exacerbation of chronic bronchitis), urinary tract infections (e.g. cystitis, pyelonephritis), chronic bacterial prostatitis, intra-abdominal infections in combination with metronidazole, skin and skin structure infections, bone and joint infections, infectious diarrhea, typhoid fever, and uncomplicated cervical and urethral gonorrhea. Ciprofloxacin is also indicated when combined with piperacillin for prophylaxis of infection in febrile neutropenia.

Pharmacology

Ciprofloxacin is a fluoroquinolone antibacterial agent. It inhibits DNA gyrase (topoisomerase II), a key enzyme involved in bacterial DNA synthesis. Ciprofloxacin has *in vitro* activity against both gram-positive and gram-negative organisms; however, due to emergence of resistance among gram-positive organisms (e.g. *Staphylococcus aureus*, *Streptococcus pneumoniae*) it is most reliable for the treatment of gram-negative infections. Activity against staphylococci is better than that against streptococci. It has limited clinical utility for respiratory tract infections where *S. pneumoniae* is expected to be a likely pathogen, and should be avoided for empiric treatment of these infections. Use for infections due to gram-positive organisms should be guided by the results of susceptibility testing.

Gram-negative organisms that are generally susceptible include the Enterobacteriaceae, *Pseudomonas aeruginosa*, *Neisseria gonorrhoeae*, *Haemophilus influenzae*, and *Campylobacter jejuni*. Ciprofloxacin also has some activity against *Chlamydia* species and mycobacteria.

Ciprofloxacin is well absorbed following oral administration, and it can be administered with or without food. It is widely distributed throughout the body and has good penetration in multiple tissues. Excretion occurs primarily via the kidney, and dose adjustment is required in patients with renal insufficiency.

Adverse Effects/Precautions

The most common adverse effects are nausea, diarrhea, vomiting, abdominal pain, headache, and rash.

Administration to immature animals has resulted in permanent damage to cartilage of the weight-bearing joints. Additionally, reports exist of Achilles tendon rupture having occurred in adults. Patients should be instructed to discontinue therapy if pain, inflammation or other signs of tendon rupture are noted. Use in pediatric patients is discouraged unless the benefit of using ciprofloxacin (e.g. organism resistant to other antibacterials) outweighs any potential risk.

Severe hypersensitivity reactions have occurred. These include anaphylaxis, rash, fever, eosinophilia, jaundice, and hepatic necrosis. Some of these reactions have been fatal and have occurred following administration of a single dose.

Ciprofloxacin (Cipro)

Convulsions, increased intracranial pressure, and toxic psychosis have occurred rarely with ciprofloxacin. Avoid use in patients with a predisposition for these events. Pregnancy: FDA category C.

Drug Interactions

Concurrent administration with products containing multivalent cations such as iron, calcium, zinc, magnesium or aluminum can significantly impair the absorption of ciprofloxacin. Thus these products (e.g. antacids, multivitamins, sucralfate) should be administered 6 hours before or 2 hours after ciprofloxacin. Concomitant administration with theophylline can significantly increase theophylline concentrations; thus serum concentration monitoring and appropriate dose adjustment should be performed. Co-administration with warfarin may increase prothrombin times. Close monitoring is advised.

Preparation *Rx*

Tablets	100 mg	Cipro Cystitis Pack	#6
Tablets	250, 500 & 750 mg	Cipro	
Oral suspension	250 mg & 500 mg/5 ml	Cipro	100 ml
Solution for injection	200 & 400 mg	Cipro	

Selected References

Centers for Disease Control and Prevention. Sexually transmitted diseases treatment guidelines 2002. Morbid Mortal Weekly Rep 2002; 51(no. RR-6): 1–78.

Gentry LO, Ramirez-Ronda CH, Rodriguez-Noriega F., et al. Oral ciprofloxacin vs. parenteral cefotaxime in the treatment of difficult skin and skin structure infections. A multicenter trial. Arch Intern Med 1989; 149: 2579–83.

Walker RC. The fluoroquinolones. Mayo Clin Proc 1999; 74: 1030–7.

Ofloxacin (Floxin)

Dose and Administration

The usual dose is 200 to 400 mg by mouth or intravenously twice a day depending on the indication and infection severity. For uncomplicated urinary tract infections, 200 mg orally twice daily can be administered for 3 days. Uncomplicated gonorrhea can be treated with a single oral dose of 400 mg.

Uses

FDA-approved: Treatment of lower respiratory infections (e.g. community-acquired pneumonia, acute exacerbation of chronic bronchitis), urinary tract infections (e.g. cystitis, pyelonephritis), chronic bacterial prostatitis, uncomplicated skin and skin structure infections, uncomplicated cervical and urethral gonorrhea, nongonoccal urethritis and cervicitis, and mixed infections of the urethra and cervix (e.g. pelvic inflammatory disease).

Pharmacology

Ofloxacin is a fluoroquinolone antibacterial agent. It inhibits DNA gyrase (topoisomerase II), a key enzyme involved in bacterial DNA synthesis. Ofloxacin has *in vitro* activity against both gram-positive and gram-negative organisms. Compared to ciprofloxacin it has similar gram-positive but slightly less gram-negative activity. Activity against staphylococci is better than that against streptococci. Gram-negative organisms that are generally susceptible include the Enterobacteriaceae *Pseudomonas aeruginosa*, *Neisseria gonorrhoeae*, *Haemophilus influenzae*, and *Moraxella catarrhalis*. Ofloxacin also has good activity against atypical organisms, including *Chlamydia* species, *Mycoplasma* species, and *Legionella pneumophila*. Mycobacteria may also be susceptible.

Owing to emergence of resistance among gram-positive organisms (e.g. *Staphylococcus aureus*, *Streptococcus pneumoniae*) it is most reliable for the treatment of gram-negative and atypical infections. It has limited clinical utility for respiratory tract infections where *S. pneumoniae* is expected to be a likely pathogen and should be avoided for empiric treatment of these infections. Use for infections due to gram-positive organisms should be guided by the results of susceptibility testing.

Ofloxacin is well absorbed following oral administration, and it can be administered with or without food. It is widely distributed throughout the body and has good penetration in multiple tissues. Excretion occurs primarily via the kidney, and dose adjustment is required in patients with renal insufficiency.

Adverse Effects/Precautions

The most common adverse effects are nausea, diarrhea, insomnia, headache, dizziness, and vaginitis.

Transient visual disturbances including photophobia and decreased visual acuity have been reported with ofloxacin.

Administration to immature animals has resulted in permanent damage to cartilage of the weight-bearing joints. Additionally, reports exist of Achilles tendon rupture having occurred in adults. Patients should be instructed to discontinue therapy if pain, inflammation or other signs of tendon rupture are noted. Use in pediatric patients is discouraged unless the benefit of using ofloxacin (e.g. organism resistant to other antibacterials) outweighs any potential risk.

Severe hypersensitivity reactions have occurred. These include anaphylaxis, rash, fever, eosinophilia, jaundice, and hepatic necrosis. Some of these reactions have been fatal and have occurred following administration of a single dose.

Convulsions, increased intracranial pressure, and toxic psychosis have occurred rarely with ofloxacin. Avoid use in patients with a predisposition for these events.

Pregnancy: FDA category C.

Drug Interactions

Concurrent administration with products containing multivalent cations such as iron, calcium, zinc, magnesium or aluminum can significantly impair the absorption of ofloxacin. Therefore, these products (e.g. antacids, multivitamins, sucralfate) should be administered 2 hours before or after ofloxacin.

Preparation *Rx*

Tablets	200, 300 & 400 mg	Floxin

Selected References

Centers for Disease Control and Prevention. Sexually transmitted diseases treatment guidelines 2002. Morbid Mortal Weekly Rep 2002; 51(no. RR-6): 1–78.

Todd PA, Faulds D. Ofloxacin. A reappraisal of its antimicrobial activity, pharmacology and therapeutic use. Drugs 1991; 42: 825–76.

Walker RC. The fluoroquinolones. Mayo Clin Proc 1999; 74: 1030–7.

Doxycycline (Vibramycin)

Dose and Administration

Acne vulgaris: Give 100 mg orally twice a day.

Lymphogranuloma venereum: Give 100 mg orally twice a day for 21 days.

Nongonoccal nonchlamydial urethritis: Give 100 mg orally twice a day for 7 days.

Chlamydia trachomatis infection: Give 100 mg orally twice a day for 7 days.

Epididymitis: Give 100 mg orally twice a day for 10 days.

Sexually transmitted gastrointestinal syndromes (proctitis, proctocolitis, enteritis): Give 100 mg orally twice a day for 7 days.

Primary or secondary syphilis in penicillin-allergic patients: Give 100 mg orally twice a day for 14 days.

Latent syphilis in penicillin-allergic patients: Give 100 mg orally twice a day. If the duration of infection is less than 1 year, administer for 14 days. If duration of infection is unknown or greater than 1 year, administer for 4 weeks.

Other infections due to susceptible organisms (e.g. *Rickettsia*, *Chlamydia, Mycoplasma* species): Give 100 mg orally or intravenously every 12 hours.

Uses

FDA-approved: Treatment of acne vulgaris; rickettsial infections such as Rocky Mountain spotted fever, typhus, and Q fever; respiratory tract infections caused by *Mycoplasma pneumoniae*; lymphogranuloma venereum, uncomplicated urethritis, endocervical or rectal infections, and inclusion conjunctivitis caused by *Chlamydia trachomatis*; psittacosis caused by *Chlamydia psittaci;* nongonococcal urethritis caused by *Ureaplasma urealyticum*; infections secondary to *Borrelia recurrentis* and *burgdorferi* (Lyme disease); and cholera caused by *Vibrio cholerae*.

Pharmacology

The exact mechanism of action for doxycycline in acne is unknown but is thought to be related to its antibacterial activity. Doxycycline inhibits protein synthesis in susceptible organisms through reversible binding to the 30S ribosomal subunit. Growth of *Propionibacterium acnes* on the skin surface and free fatty acid concentrations in sebum are decreased. These actions result in decreased inflammation and microcomedo formation. Doxycycline exhibits good antimicrobial activity against *Rickettsia*, *Chlamydia*, *Borrelia,* and *Mycoplasma* species.

Absorption is approximately 90 to 100% when administered on an empty stomach. Administration with food or milk may decrease absorption up to 20%. To maximize absorption, doxycycline should generally be taken on an empty stomach; however, administration with food may be required to minimize gastrointestinal upset. Doxycycline is eliminated equally in the urine and feces in patients with normal renal function. The dose does not require adjustment in patients with renal impairment.

Adverse Effects/Precautions

Gastrointestinal effects are common (nausea, vomiting, diarrhea, abdominal pain, epigastric burning, anorexia).

The risk of pseudotumor cerebri is increased with the combination of doxycycline and isotretinoin.

Doxycycline (Vibramycin)

Photosensitivity may occur in individuals when exposed to sunlight, including sunlamps.

Permanent yellow-gray-brown discoloration of the teeth can develop in children less than or equal to 8 years of age who ingest doxycycline or when ingested by the mother during pregnancy.

Superinfection with nonsusceptible organisms can occur with doxycycline therapy, including oral and anogenital candidiasis.

Pregnancy: FDA category D.

Drug Interactions

Doxycycline absorption is impaired by concomitant administration of dairy products, fluoroquinolones, sucralfate, or any product containing iron, zinc, calcium, aluminum, magnesium, or bismuth. Administration should be separated by at least 1 to 2 hours.

Use of doxycycline with oral contraceptives may decrease the efficacy of the contraceptive; therefore alternative methods of contraception should be recommended during doxycycline therapy.

Concomitant administration of doxycycline and warfarin may cause elevated prothrombin times.

Special Considerations

Doxycycline should be taken with an adequate amount of fluid to reduce the risk of esophageal irritation and ulceration. If gastric irritation occurs, doxycycline may be given with food.

Preparation *Rx*

Capsules	50 & 100 mg	Vibramycin Hyclate (100 mg capsule only)	
		Various generics	
Tablets	100 mg	Vibra-Tabs	
		Various generics	
Oral syrup	25 mg/5 ml	Vibramycin Monohydrate	60 ml
Oral syrup	50 mg/5 ml	Vibramycin Calcium	480 ml
Injection	100 mg	Doxy 100	
		Generic	

Selected References

Centers for Disease Control and Prevention. Sexually transmitted diseases treatment guidelines 2002. Morbid Mortal Weekly Rep 2002; 51(no. RR-6): 1–78.

Schachner L. The treatment of acne: a contemporary review. Pediatr Clin North Am 1983; 30: 501–10.

Smilack JD. The tetracyclines. Mayo Clin Proc 1999; 74: 727–9.

Minocycline (Minocin)

Dose and Administration

Acne vulgaris: Give 50 mg orally one to three times a day.

Infections due to susceptible organisms: Give 200 mg by mouth or intravenously as an initial dose followed by 100 mg every 12 hours.

Uses

FDA-approved: Treatment of moderate to severe inflammatory acne vulgaris. Minocycline can also be used to treat infections secondary to rickettsiae, chlamydiae, and mycoplasma; however, doxycycline is generally used as the preferred tetracycline for these infections.

Pharmacology

The exact mechanism of action for minocycline in acne is unknown but is probably related to its antibacterial activity. Minocycline inhibits protein synthesis in susceptible organisms through reversible binding to the 30S ribosomal subunit. Growth of *Propionibacterium acnes* on the skin surface and free fatty acid concentrations in sebum are decreased. These actions result in decreased inflammation and microcomedo formation. Minocycline exhibits good antimicrobial activity against *Rickettsia*, *Chlamydia*, and *Mycoplasma* species. Minocycline also displays activity against *Staphylococcus aureus* resistant to other tetracyclines. Although it also has activity against a variety of other gram-positive and gram-negative organisms, resistance rates have been increasing nationwide and thus local susceptibility patterns and patient-specific culture data should guide decisions regarding minocycline use.

Absorption is approximately 90 to 100% when administered on an empty stomach. Administration with food, including dairy products, may decrease absorption up to 20%. To maximize absorption, minocycline should generally be taken on an empty stomach; however, administration with food may be required to minimize gastrointestinal upset. Minocycline is eliminated primarily via the hepatobiliary system.

Adverse Effects/Precautions

Gastrointestinal effects are common (nausea, vomiting, diarrhea, abdominal pain, epigastric burning, anorexia).

Reversible vestibular adverse effects (dizziness, ataxia, vertigo) may occur with minocycline. These effects are generally dose-related and are more common in women.

Minocycline has been associated with rare cases of reversible systemic lupus erythematosus (SLE).

The risk of pseudotumor cerebri is increased with the combination of minocycline and isotretinoin.

Skin and mucous membrane pigmentation have been associated with minocycline.

Photosensitivity may occur in individuals when exposed to sunlight, including sunlamps. There is some evidence that photosensitivity may be less with minocycline as compared with other tetracyclines; however, caution should still be exercised.

Minocycline (Minocin)

Permanent yellow-gray-brown discoloration of the teeth can develop in children less than or equal to 8 years of age who ingest minocycline or when ingested by the mother during pregnancy.

Superinfection with nonsusceptible organisms can occur with minocycline therapy, including oral and anogenital candidiasis.

Pregnancy: FDA category D.

Drug Interactions

Minocycline absorption is impaired by concomitant administration of sucralfate or any product containing iron, zinc, calcium, aluminum, magnesium, or bismuth. Administration should be separated by at least 1 to 2 hours with minocycline.

Use of minocycline with oral contraceptives may decrease the efficacy of the contraceptive; therefore alternative methods of contraception should be recommended during minocycline therapy. Concomitant administration of minocycline and warfarin may cause elevated prothrombin times.

Special Considerations

Minocycline may be effective in patients with acne unresponsive to tetracycline or erythromycin. The drug should be taken with an adequate amount of fluid to reduce the risk of esophageal irritation and ulceration.

Preparation *Rx*

Capsules	50 & 100 mg	Minocin
		Various generics
Capsules	50, 75 & 100 mg	Dynacin
		Various generics
Injection	100 mg	Minocin

Selected References

Freeman K. Therapeutic focus. Minocycline in the treatment of acne. Br J Clin Pract 1989; 43: 112–15.

Schachner L. The treatment of acne: a contemporary review. Pediatr Clin North Am 1983; 30: 501–10.

Smilack JD. The tetracyclines. Mayo Clin Proc 1999; 74: 727–9.

Tetracycline (Sumycin)

Dose and Administration

Acne vulgaris: 500 to 1000 mg orally divided four times daily for 1 to 2 weeks or until clinical improvement is noted. The dosage can then be decreased to 125 to 500 mg daily or to the lowest dose that suppresses lesions. Prolonged therapy may be necessary to control acne symptoms.

Primary or secondary syphilis: 500 mg orally four times a day for 2 weeks.

Latent syphilis: 500 mg orally four times a day. If the duration of infection is less than 1 year, administer for 2 weeks. If duration of infection is unknown or greater than 1 year, administer for 4 weeks.

Uses

FDA-approved: Treatment of acne vulgaris. Primary, secondary, or latent syphilis in nonpregnant patients with a documented penicillin allergy is another indication.

Pharmacology

The exact mechanism of action for tetracycline in acne is unknown but is thought to be related to its antibacterial activity. Tetracycline inhibits protein synthesis in susceptible organisms through reversible binding to the 30S ribosomal subunit. Growth of *Propionibacterium acnes* on the skin surface and free fatty acid concentrations in sebum are decreased. These actions result in decreased inflammation and microcomedo formation.

Absorption is approximately 60 to 80% when administered on an empty stomach. Administration with food or milk decreases absorption by 50% or greater. Tetracycline is eliminated primarily as unchanged drug in the urine; therefore the dose should be adjusted according to the severity of renal impairment.

Adverse Effects/Precautions

Gastrointestinal effects are common (nausea, vomiting, diarrhea, abdominal pain, epigastric burning, anorexia).

Other adverse effects include maculopapular and erythematous rashes, hypersensitivity reactions, hemolytic anemia, thrombocytopenia, neutropenia, and eosinophilia.

Photosensitivity may occur in individuals when exposed to sunlight, including sunlamps.

Tetracycline may precipitate renal failure (azotemia, hyperphosphatemia, and acidosis) in patients with underlying renal dysfunction. Subsequent drug accumulation and liver toxicity may occur.

Permanent yellow-gray-brown discoloration of the teeth can develop in children less than or equal to 8 years of age who ingest tetracycline or when ingested by the mother during pregnancy.

Superinfection with nonsusceptible organisms can occur with tetracycline therapy, including oral and anogenital candidiasis.

Pregnancy: FDA category D.

Tetracycline (Sumycin)

Drug Interactions

Tetracycline absorption is impaired by concomitant administration of dairy products, fluoroquinolones, sucralfate, or any product containing iron, zinc, calcium, aluminum, magnesium, or bismuth. Administration should be separated by at least 4 hours.

Use of tetracycline with oral contraceptives may decrease the efficacy of the contraceptive; therefore alternative methods of contraception should be recommended during tetracycline therapy.

Concomitant administration of tetracycline and warfarin may cause elevated prothrombin times.

Special Considerations

Administration of outdated or degraded tetracycline has resulted in a reversible adverse event similar to Fanconi syndrome characterized by nausea, vomiting, polyuria, polydipsia, proteinuria, acidosis, glycosuria, and gross aminoaciduria. Patients should be instructed to discard any unused tetracycline after therapy to avoid this reaction.

Preparation *Rx*

Tablet	250 & 500 mg	Sumycin	
		Various generics	
Capsule	250 & 500 mg	Brodspec	
		Sumycin	
		Tetracon	
		Various generics	
Suspension	125 mg/ml	Sumycin	473 ml

Selected References

Budden MG. Topical and oral tetracycline in the treatment of acne vulgaris. Practitioner 1988; 232: 669–74.

Centers for Disease Control and Prevention. Sexually transmitted diseases treatment guidelines 2002. Morbid Mortal Weekly Rep 2002; 51(no. RR-6): 1–78.

Schachner L. The treatment of acne: a contemporary review. Pediatr Clin North Am 1983; 30: 501–10.

Dapsone

Dose and Administration

Leprosy: Give 50 to 100 mg orally once a day as part of a multidrug regimen.

Dermatitis herpetiformis: Give 50 mg orally once a day as initial therapy and titrate based on resolution of pruritus and lesions. The dose should then be lowered to the smallest dose that controls symptoms. Maintenance doses generally range from 25 to 400 mg.

Uses

Treatment of leprosy as a component of multiple drug therapy, dermatitis herpetiformis, eruptions (e.g. bullous or mucocutaneous) of systemic and discoid lupus erythematosus, bullous pemphigoid, and pemphigus vulgaris. It is also used for multiple inflammatory and pustular dermatoses.

Monitoring

The manufacturer recommends monitoring complete blood counts weekly for the initial month of therapy, monthly for the next 6 months, and periodically thereafter. Liver function tests should also be regularly monitored. Patients of Asian, African-American, and Mediterranean descent should be screened for glucose-6-phosphate dehydrogenase (G-6-PD) deficiency prior to initiating dapsone therapy.

Pharmacology

Dapsone is a sulfone antibacterial. Its exact mechanism of action has not been fully characterized. It is thought, however, that it has a similar mechanism to sulfonamides and thus inhibits synthesis of bacterial folic acid. Dapsone may have an immuno-modulatory effect, which may explain its activity in the treatment of dermatologic diseases. Dapsone displays activity against mycobacteria, including *Mycobacterium leprae* and *Mycobacterium tuberculosis*. It also displays some activity against *Pneumocystis carinii* and *Plasmodium*.

Absorption is good following oral administration. It undergoes extensive acetylation in the liver and is excreted in the urine.

Adverse Effects/Precautions

Dose-related hemolysis and methemoglobinemia are common adverse effects. Hemolysis generally occurs in patients taking doses greater than 200 mg per day. Changes in hematologic indices include a decrease in hemoglobin by 1 to 2 g/dl, an increase in reticulocytes by 2 to 12%, a shortened erythrocyte life span, and increased methemoglobin. These changes do not necessitate dapsone discontinuation unless severe symptoms occur (e.g. hypoxia, cyanosis). Patients with G-6-PD deficiency suffer more severe adverse hematologic effects. Cutaneous hypersensitivity manifested as exfoliative dermatitis, erythema multiforme, toxic epidermal necrolysis, urticaria, and erythema nodosum may occur. Peripheral neuropathy and loss of motor function may occur rarely. Adverse hepatic effects include toxic hepatitis and cholestatic jaundice. Leprosy reactional states may result following initiation of therapy.

Pregnancy: FDA category C.

Dapsone

Drug Interactions

Some protease inhibitors (e.g. amprenavir, saquinavir, ritonavir) may increase dapsone concentrations and therefore cause increased hematologic toxicity. Combination of dapsone with other medications known to cause bone marrow suppression should be approached with caution.

Preparation *Rx*

Tablets   25 & 100 mg   Generic

Selected References

Uetrecht J. Dapsone and sulfapyridine. Clin Dermatol 1989; 7: 111–20.

Wolf R, Tuzun B, Tuzun Y. Dapsone: unapproved uses or indications. Clin Dermatol 2000; 18: 37–53.

Trimethoprim–Sulfamethoxazole (Bactrim, Septra)

Dose and Administration

Dosage forms of TMP-SMX are provided as a ratio of trimethoprim 1 mg to sulfamethoxazole 5 mg.

Oral: Usual oral dose is one TMP-SMX 160/800 mg tablet twice a day. Cystitis can be treated with 3 days of therapy whereas other indications require longer durations.

Intravenous: Usual IV dose is 8 to 20 mg/kg of the trimethoprim component daily divided into two to four doses depending on the infection severity.

Uses

FDA-approved: Treatment of urinary tract infections (e.g. cystitis, pyelonephritis), acute otitis media, acute bacterial exacerbations of chronic bronchitis, enteritis (Shigellosis), *Pneumocystis carinii* pneumonia (treatment and prophylaxis), and traveler's diarrhea. Other uses include *Nocardia* infections, sinusitis, prophylaxis of urinary tract infections, granuloma inguinale (donovanosis), and toxoplasmosis.

Pharmacology

The combination of trimethoprim and sulfamethoxazole (TMP-SMX) results in a synergistic bactericidal effect against gram-positive and gram-negative organisms via inhibition of several steps in bacterial folic acid synthesis. Sulfamethoxazole is a sulfonamide antibacterial that competitively antagonizes the formation of dihydrofolic acid from *para*-aminobenzoic acid (PABA) via competitive inhibition of dihydropteroate synthetase. Trimethoprim inhibits the bacterial enzyme dihydrofolate reductase, which is responsible for the formation of tetrahydrofolic acid from dihydrofolic acid. These combined actions ultimately result in decreased formation of bacterial DNA and bacterial death.

TMP-SMX generally displays activity against *Streptococcus pneumoniae* (penicillin-susceptible), *Streptococcus pyogenes*, *Staphylococcus aureus*, *Haemophilus influenzae*, *Moraxella catarrhalis*, *Nocardia* species, *Stenotrophomonas maltophilia*, and most Enterobacteriaceae. It is also active against *P. carinii*. The combination is not effective against enterococci, *Pseudomonas aeruginosa* or most anaerobes.

It should be noted that increased TMP-SMX resistance has been seen with *H. influenzae*, gram-negative uropathogens (e.g. *E. coli*), staphylococci, and streptococci. Owing to its unreliability, TMP-SMX should not be used for treatment of group A β-hemolytic *S. pyogenes* pharyngitis and may not be appropriate for initial empiric therapy of skin and soft-tissue infections secondary to staphylococci or streptococci. Local susceptibility patterns should be consulted for empiric use.

TMP-SMX is well absorbed following oral administration. It is excreted primarily in the urine and requires dose adjustment in renal insufficiency.

Adverse Effects/Precautions

Common adverse effects include nausea, vomiting, anorexia, skin rash, and urticaria. Serious hypersensitivity reactions of the skin include Stevens–Johnson syndrome, toxic epidermal necrolysis, erythema multiforme, and exfoliative dermatitis. Rashes usually present within 7 to 14 days of therapy and are generally erythematous, maculopapular, morbilliform, and pruritic. Other serious but rare adverse effects include agranulocytosis, aplastic or hemolytic anemia, and fulminant hepatic necrosis. Patients who are folate-depleted at baseline may be at increased risk of hematologic adverse effects. Folic acid can be administered without altering the efficacy of TMP-SMX.

Trimethoprim–Sulfamethoxazole (Bactrim, Septra)

The incidence of the aforementioned dermatologic and hematologic reactions is considered rare in the general population but is much greater in patients who are infected with the human immunodeficiency virus (HIV). Desensitization may be required if continued therapy is necessary.

TMP-SMX can cause crystalluria, and therefore patients should be instructed to drink plenty of fluids to prevent kidney stone formation.

Pregnancy: FDA category C.

Drug Interactions

TMP-SMX can potentiate the hypoprothrombinemic effects of warfarin. Prothrombin times and INRs should be monitored closely and warfarin doses decreased as warranted. When combined with sulfonylureas (e.g. glyburide, glipizide), hypoglycemia may occur secondary to displacement of the sulfonylurea from protein binding sites. Additionally, concomitant administration with methotrexate can lead to methotrexate displacement from protein as well as competition for renal tubular excretion. As a result, bone marrow suppression may occur. TMP-SMX should be combined cautiously with other medications, including methotrexate, which can cause bone marrow suppression.

Preparation *Rx*

Tablets	160/800 mg	Bactrim DS
		Septra DS
		Generic
Tablets	80/400 mg	Bactrim
		Septra
		Generic
Oral suspension	40–200 mg/5 ml	Septra Suspension
Injection	16–80 mg/ml	Generic

Selected References

Epstein ME, Amodio-Groton M, Sadick NS. Antimicrobial agents for the dermatologist. II. Macrolides, fluoroquinolones, rifamycins, tetracyclines, trimethoprim–sulfamethoxazole, and clindamycin. J Am Acad Dermatol 1997; 37: 365–83.

Gregg CR. Drug interactions with antiinfective therapies. Am J Med 1999; 106: 227–37.

Smilack JD. Trimethoprim–sulfamethoxazole. Mayo Clin Proc 1999; 74: 730–4.

Clindamycin Phosphate (Cleocin)

Dose and Administration

Acne vulgaris: Give 150 mg orally twice a day.

Bacterial vaginosis: Give 300 mg orally twice a day for 7 days.

Serious infections in adults: Give 150 to 450 mg orally every 6 hours. For IV/IM administration, give 600 to 2700 mg/day (maximum 4.8 g/day) divided into two or four doses depending on the type and severity of infection. The maximum dose for a single IM injection is 600 mg.

Serious infections in children: Give 8 to 25 mg/kg per day orally divided into three or four doses. For IV/IM administration, give 15 to 20 mg/kg per day (< 1 month) or 15 to 40 mg/kg per day (> 1 month) in three or four divided doses.

Prophylaxis of bacterial endocarditis in penicillin-allergic patients: 600 mg (adults) or 20 mg/kg (children) orally or intravenously as a single dose 1 hour (by mouth) or 30 minutes (IV) prior to the procedure.

Uses

FDA-approved: Clindamycin is indicated in the treatment of serious infections caused by susceptible anaerobic bacteria, and susceptible strains of streptococci and staphylococci when penicillin is not an appropriate option. These include lower respiratory tract infections (e.g. pneumonia, empyema), skin and soft-tissue infections, intra-abdominal infections (e.g. peritonitis, abscesses), septicemia, and gynecologic infections (e.g. endometritis, pelvic inflammatory disease, pelvic cellulitus, and bacterial vaginosis). Other uses include, but are not limited to, acne vulgaris, and as an alternative to penicillin for bone and joint infections, prophylaxis of neonatal group B streptococcal disease, and endocarditis prophylaxis of patients with cardiac risk factors who are undergoing high-risk procedures.

Pharmacology

Clindamycin is a derivative of the lincosamide antibiotic, lincomycin. It inhibits bacterial protein synthesis in susceptible organisms by reversibly binding to the 50S ribosomal subunit. Because macrolides and chloramphenicol have a similar mechanism of action, concomitant use with clindamycin should be avoided to prevent antibacterial antagonism. Clindamycin demonstrates reliable activity against most anaerobes except for some *Clostridium* species, including *Clostridium difficile*. In addition, resistance to *Bacteroides fragilis* has increased throughout the USA and local susceptibility patterns should be consulted. Clindamycin is also active against gram-positive aerobic organisms, including pneumococci and other streptococci and methicillin-susceptible staphylococci. It does not have reliable activity, however, against enterococci or gram-negative aerobic organisms. Therefore, clindamycin should be used concomitantly with other appropriate antibiotics when gram-negative aerobes may be present (e.g. intra-abdominal infection).

Clindamycin is well absorbed following oral administration. It can be administered with food. Clindamycin does not penetrate the cerebrospinal fluid to an appreciable extent and should not be used for treating infections of the central nervous system. Clindamycin is extensively metabolized in the liver with subsequent excretion in the urine.

Clindamycin Phosphate (Cleocin)

Adverse Effects/Precautions

Gastrointestinal upset manifested as diarrhea, abdominal pain, esophagitis, nausea, and vomiting is common.

Mild to life-threatening antibiotic-associated pseudomembranous colitis (PMC) due to *C. difficile* infection can develop. Symptoms usually include severe diarrhea and abdominal pain, which may be associated with blood or mucus in the stool. If PMC is suspected, clindamycin should be discontinued.

Urticaria and mild to moderate rashes (e.g. morbilliform, maculopapular) are common with clindamycin. Erythema multiforme and Stevens–Johnson syndrome have also been rarely reported.

Transient elevation of liver enzymes may occur.

Transient leukopenia, thrombocytopenia, and neutropenia may also occur.

Pregnancy: FDA category B.

Special Considerations

Clindamycin capsules should be taken with a full glass of water to avoid potential esophageal irritation.

Preparation *Rx*

Capsules	75, 150 & 300 mg	Cleocin HCL	
Capsules	150 & 300 mg	Various generics	
Oral suspension	75 mg/5 ml	Cleocin Pediatric	100 g
Injection	150 mg/ml	Cleocin Phosphate	2, 4, 6 & 60 ml

Selected References

Centers for Disease Control and Prevention. Sexually transmitted diseases treatment guidelines 2002. Morbid Mortal Weekly Rep 2002; 51(no. RR-6): 1–78.

Falagas ME, Gorbach SL. Clindamycin and metronidazole. Med Clin North Am 1995; 79: 845–7.

Kasten MJ. Clindamycin, metronidazole, and chloramphenicol. Mayo Clin Proc 1999; 74: 825–33.

Clofazimine (Lamprene)

Dose and Administration

Multibacillary leprosy: Give 50 mg orally per day (plus an additional 300 mg dose once per month) as part of a multidrug regimen with dapsone and rifampin.

Dermatologic indications: 100 to 400 mg per day depending on the indication.

Uses

Its primary role is for treatment of multibacillary leprosy as a component of multiple drug therapy. Other uses include erythema nodosum leprosum, *Mycobacterium avium* complex infections, pyoderma gangrenosum, psittacosis, psoriasis, and discoid lupus erythematosus.

Pharmacology

Clofazimine is a phenazine dye that has antimycobacterial, anti-inflammatory, and immunosuppressive activity. It is primarily active against *Mycobacterium leprae*, *Mycobacterium tuberculosis*, *Mycobacterium bovis*, *Mycobacterium fortuitum*, and *M. avium* complex (MAC). It exerts its activity by inhibiting replication and growth via binding to mycobacterial DNA. Although the precise mechanism in dermatologic disorders is unknown, it is probably related to its enhancement of neutrophil and macrophage phagocytosis.

Clofazimine is erratically absorbed and should be taken with a meal to maximize absorption. It is widely distributed throughout the tissues and remains in the body for prolonged periods. Clofazimine is primarily excreted in the feces.

Adverse Effects/Precautions

Dose-related gastrointestinal complaints including anorexia, nausea, diarrhea, and abdominal pain are the most common adverse effects. If severe symptoms develop, clofazimine should be discontinued to prevent bowel obstruction. Fatal gastro-intestinal events (e.g. splenic infarction, bowel obstruction) have been reported. Pink, red, brown or black skin discoloration may occur. Additionally, the cornea, conjunctiva, and body fluids (e.g. lacrimal fluid, semen, urine, sweat, feces) may become discolored. Other dermatologic adverse effects include dry skin, ichthyosis, pruritus, follicular and papular rashes, and seborrheic dermatitis.

Pregnancy: FDA category C.

Preparation *Rx*

Capsules   50 mg   Lamprene

Selected References

Arbiser JL, Moschella SL. Clofazimine: a review of its medical uses and mechanisms of action. J Am Acad Dermatol 1995; 32: 241–7.

Landow RK. New drugs for dermatologic diseases. Derm Clin 1988; 6: 575–84.

Mensing H. Clofazimine in dermatitis ulcerosa (pyoderma gangrenosum). Dermatologica 1988; 177: 232–6.

Mupirocin (Bactroban)

Dose and Administration

Cream/ointment: Apply to the affected area three times daily for 10 days. The area may be covered with gauze dressing if necessary.

Nasal ointment: Apply half of the ointment from the single-use tube into one nostril and the remaining amount in the second nostril twice daily for 5 days. The nostrils should be pressed together and released repetitively for approximately 1 minute after application to facilitate spread throughout the nares.

Uses

The cream formulation is indicated for the treatment of secondarily infected traumatic skin lesions (up to 10 cm in length or 100 cm^2 in area) due to susceptible strains of *Staphylococcus aureus* and *Streptococcus pyogenes*. The regular ointment is indicated for impetigo due to *S. aureus* and *S. pyogenes*, whereas the nasal ointment is indicated for the eradication of nasal colonization with methicillin-resistant *S. aureus* in adult patients and health-care workers.

Pharmacology

Mupirocin, also known as pseudomonic acid A, is an antibacterial agent that primarily exerts its activity against gram-positive organisms. Susceptible organisms include *S. aureus* (methicillin-susceptible and -resistant), β-hemolytic streptococci and *S. pyogenes*. Some strains of *Staphylococcus epidermidis* and *Staphylococcus saprophyticus* are also inhibited by mupirocin. Although its mechanism of action has not been fully determined, it inhibits bacterial protein synthesis via binding to isoleucyl transfer RNA synthetase. Systemic absorption is less than 1% following topical application.

Adverse Effects/Precautions

Mupirocin is fairly well tolerated and the majority of adverse effects are local in nature.

Pregnancy: FDA category B.

Special Considerations

Patients not showing a clinical response within 3 to 5 days of application should be re-evaluated.

Preparation *Rx*

Cream	2%	Bactroban	15 & 30 g
Ointment	2%	Bactroban	22 g
Nasal ointment	2%	Bactroban	1 g tubes, #10 per carton

Selected References

Bass JW, Chan DS, Creamer KM, et al. Comparison of oral cephalexin, topical mupirocin, and topical bacitracin for treatment of impetigo. Pediatr Infect Dis 1997; 16: 708–10.

Dux PH, Fields L, Pollock D. 2% topical mupirocin versus systemic erythromycin and cloxacillin in primary and secondary skin infections. Curr Ther Res 1986; 40: 933–40.

Goldfarb J, Crenshaw D, O'Horo J, et al. Randomized clinical trial of topical mupirocin versus oral erythromycin for impetigo. Antimicrob Agents Chemother 1988; 32: 1780–3.

Polymyxin B Sulfate/Bacitracin Zinc/Neomycin Sulfate (Neosporin)

Dose and Administration

Apply to cleansed affected area one to three times per day. A sterile bandage may be used to cover the wound.

Uses

Prevention of bacterial infection in minor skin cuts, abrasions, and burns. It is also used to prevent wound infection following minor surgical procedures and for treatment of secondarily infected skin disorders.

Pharmacology

Polymyxin B is a bactericidal antibiotic that is a cationic surface-active agent (detergent). It interferes with phospholipids of the bacterial plasma membrane. Diminished membrane integrity leads to leakage of intracellular components and subsequent cell death. Spectrum of activity is limited to gram-negative organisms and primarily includes *Pseudomonas aeruginosa*, *Escherichia coli*, *Klebsiella* species, and *Enterobacter*.

Bacitracin interferes with the incorporation of amino acids into the bacterial cell wall. It is primarily active against gram-positive organisms, including staphylococci, streptococci, anaerobic cocci, corynebacteria, and clostridia.

Neomycin is an aminoglycoside antibiotic (bactericidal). It binds to the 30S subunit of the microbial ribosome, altering mRNA function. The defective proteins formed are incorporated into the bacterial cell wall but do not function appropriately, allowing leakage into the cell and subsequent cell death. Neomycin is primarily active against gram-negative organisms (except *P. aeruginosa*), but does have some activity against gram-positive bacteria (*Staphylococcus aureus*). All streptococci, gram-positive bacilli, and anaerobes are resistant.

Systemic absorption of Neosporin is minimal when applied to intact skin. Absorption may occur, however, when applied to denuded or abraded skin.

Adverse Effects/Precautions

Neomycin can cause contact dermatitis in approximately 10% of patients. Hypersensitivity may be more common with prolonged and repetitive use. Reactions may include rash, erythema, pruritus, and burning. Rare anaphylactoid reactions can also occur with topical application.

Significant systemic absorption can occur when used for large skin ulcers or denuded skin areas, granulating wounds, and burns. Subsequent systemic sequelae have included ototoxicity, nephrotoxicity, and neuromuscular blockade. These events appear to occur most commonly in patients with underlying renal dysfunction.

Preparation OTC

Polymyxin B sulfate 5000 units, bacitracin zinc 400 units, & neomycin 3.5 mg/g

Ointment	Neosporin	15 & 30 g
		0.9 g, #10 packets

Selected References

MacDonald RH, Beck M. Neomycin: a review with particular reference to dermatological usage. Clin Exp Dermatol 1983; 8: 249–58.

Maddox JS, Ware JC, Dillon HC Jr. The natural history of streptococcal skin infection: prevention with topical antibiotics. J Am Acad Dermatol 1985; 13: 207–12.

Wilkson RD, Carey WD. Topical mupirocin versus topical Neosporin in the treatment of cutaneous infections. Int J Dermatol 1988; 27: 514–15.

Polymyxin B Sulfate/Bacitracin Zinc (Polysporin)

Dose and Administration

Apply to cleansed affected area one to three times per day. A sterile bandage may be used to cover the wound.

Uses

Prevention of bacterial infection in minor skin cuts, abrasions, and burns. It is also used to decrease the risk of wound infection following minor surgical procedures and for treatment of secondarily infected skin disorders.

Pharmacology

Polymyxin B is a bactericidal antibiotic that is a cationic surface-active agent (detergent). It interferes with phospholipids of the bacterial plasma membrane. Diminished membrane integrity leads to leakage of intracellular components and subsequent cell death. Spectrum of activity is limited to gram-negative organisms and primarily includes *Pseudomonas aeruginosa*, *Escherichia coli*, *Klebsiella* species, and *Enterobacter*.

Bacitracin interferes with the incorporation of amino acids into the bacterial cell wall. It is primarily active against gram-positive organisms, including staphylococci, streptococci, anaerobic cocci, corynebacteria, and clostridia.

Systemic absorption of Polysporin when applied to intact or denuded skin is minimal.

Adverse Effects/Precautions

Polysporin is fairly well tolerated, and the majority of adverse effects are local in nature. Hypersensitivity reactions ranging in symptomatology may occur rarely.

Preparation *OTC*

Polymyxin B sulfate 10 000 units & bacitracin zinc 500 units/g

Ointment	Polysporin	15 & 30 g
		0.9 g packets
Powder	Polysporin	10 g

Selected References

Knowles SR, Shear NH. Anaphylaxis from bacitracin and polymixin B (Polysporin) ointment. Int J Dermatol 1995; 34: 572–3.

Maddox JS, Ware JC, Dillon HC Jr. The natural history of streptococcal skin infection: prevention with topical antibiotics. J Am Acad Dermatol 1985; 13: 207–12.

Walton MA, Carino E, Herndon DN, Heggers JP. The efficacy of Polysporin First Aid Antibiotic Spray (polymixin B sulfate and bacitracin zinc) against clinical burn wound isolates. J Burn Care Rehab 1991; 12: 116–19.

Anticancer and Immunosuppressant Drugs

Adalimumab (Humira)

Dose and Administration

Psoriasis: 80 mg loading dose, 40 mg every other week; or 80 mg for two loading doses, then 40 mg weekly.

Rheumatoid arthritis: 40 mg SC every other week.

Uses

FDA-approved: Rheumatoid arthritis.

Other: Psoriasis (and other severe inflammatory skin diseases) and psoriatic arthritis.

Monitoring

Tuberculin skin test before initiation of treatment to rule out latent tuberculosis.

Pharmacology

Adalimumab is a recombinant IgG_1 monoclonal antibody that binds to tumor necrosis factor (TNF)α. Adalimumab also lyses surface TNF-expressing cells *in vitro* in the presence of complement. TNFα is a cytokine that mediates chronic inflammation when overexpressed. It up-regulates other cytokines, chemokines, adhesion molecules and tissue factor, activates neutrophils, and induces proliferation.

Contraindications

Patients with active infections, including chronic or localized infections. Do not administer live vaccines in patients receiving adalimumab. Nursing mothers.

Adverse Effects/Precautions

Increased risk of infection and lymphoma. New onset or exacerbation of demyelinating disorders. Lupus-like syndrome. Injection site allergic reaction. Anaphylaxis.

Pregnancy: FDA category B.

Drug Interactions

No adjustment in dosing known when taking adalimumab and methotrexate concurrently.

Preparation *Rx*

Single-use vial 40 mg

References

Chew Al, Bennett A, Smith CH, et al. Successful treatment of severe psoriasis and psoriatic arthritis. Br J Dermatol 2004; 151: 492–6.

Patel T, Gordon KB. Adalimumab: efficacy and safety in psoriasis & rheumatoid arthritis. Dermatol Ther 2004; 17: 2427–31.

Alefacept (Amevive)

Dose and Administration

Intramuscular injections: 15 mg given once weekly.

Intravenous bolus administration: 7.5 mg administered once weekly (the IV dosing form was discontinued by the manufacturer).

The recommended regimen is a course of 12 weekly injections.

An additional 12-week cycle of weekly injections may be started as long as the CD4 lymphocyte counts are within normal limits and at least a 12-week interval has passed since the prior course of therapy. There is not significant literature on treatment beyond two courses with alefacept.

Use

For the treatment of adults (over age 18 years) with chronic moderate to severe plaque psoriasis who are candidates for systemic therapy or phototherapy.

Pharmacology

Alefacept is an immunosuppressant that is created through recombinant DNA technology. It is a dimeric fusion protein that is made of the extracellular CD2-binding portion of the human leukocyte function antigen-3 (LFA- 3) linked to the Fc portion of human IgG_1. It interferes with leukocyte activation because it binds to the lymphocyte antigen CD2, inhibiting the interaction of LFA-3 on antigen-presenting cells and CD2 on T lymphocytes.

Adverse Effects/Precautions

Alefacept may cause immunosuppression due to the reduction in circulating CD4 and CD8 lymphocytes. Therefore, the risk of infection, malignancy, and the reactivation of latent infections is increased.

Do not initiate alefacept therapy in patients with suppressed CD4 lymphocyte counts. CD4 lymphocyte counts should be monitored weekly during the 12-dose regimen and used to guide dosing (withhold dosing if CD4 lymphocyte counts fall below 250 cells/µl). Discontinue if CD4 counts remain < 250 cells/µl for 1 month.

There have been reports of liver injury (e.g. asymptomatic transaminases, fatty infiltration of the liver, hepatitis, decompensation of cirrhosis with liver failure, and acute liver failure). Evaluate any patient on alefacept with indications of liver injury (e.g. persistent nausea, anorexia, fatigue, vomiting, abdominal pain, jaundice, easy bruising, dark urine or pale stools).

Frequently reported adverse effects include pharyngitis, dizziness, increased cough, nausea, pruritus, myalgias, chills, injection site pain, and injection site inflammation.

Alefacept is contraindicated in patients with a known hypersensitivity to alefacept or any of its components. It should not be given to patients with clinically significant infections. Discontinue alefacept if serious infection, malignancy, or clinically significant signs of liver injury occur.

Pregnancy: FDA category B.

Alefacept (Amevive)

Drug Interactions

Drug interaction studies have not been performed at this time. Caution should be used if considering live or live-attenuated vaccines.

Preparation *Rx*

Both the intravenous and intramuscular forms are available in cartons of four dose packs, or a carton with one dose pack. Store at 36–46°F (2–8°C) and protect from light. Each dose pack includes sterile water as the diluent, two #23 gauge needles, and a syringe. The reconstituted alefacept should be stored at room temperature and used either immediately or within 4 hours.

IM administration: 15 mg powder for IM injection should be reconstituted with 0.6 ml of sterile water. 0.5 ml of the reconstituted solution contains 15 mg of alefacept.

IV administration: 7.5 mg powder for IV administration should be reconstituted with 0.6 ml of sterile water. 0.5 ml of the reconstituted solution contains 7.5 mg of alefacept.

Selected Reference

Bos JD, Hagenaars C, Das PK, et al. Predominance of 'memory' T cells (CD4+, CDw29+) over 'naïve' T cells (CD4+, CD45R+) in both normal and diseased human skin. Arch Dermatol Res 1989; 281: 24–30.

Ellis C, Krueger GG. Treatment of chronic plaque psoriasis by selective targeting of memory effector T lymphocytes. N Engl J Med 2001; 345: 248–55.

Alitretinoin Gel (Panretin)

Dose and Administration

Gel should be applied generously to all lesions with care to avoid normal skin and mucosal surfaces. Starting frequency is two times daily then gradually increased to four times daily, if tolerated. Reduce application frequency or discontinue drug for a few days if severe irritation occurs. Responses were noted as early as 2 weeks, but usually between 4 and 14 weeks, after initiation of therapy.

Allow gel to dry for 3 to 5 minutes before covering with clothing. Do not use occlusive dressings with the gel. Continue indefinitely if lesions are responsive.

Uses

For the topical treatment of cutaneous, AIDS-related Kaposi's sarcoma (KS) lesions. Alitretinoin gel is not indicated when systemic anti-KS treatment is needed (e.g. symptomatic visceral involvement, lymphedema, > 10 new KS lesions in prior month) and will not prevent new lesions. Limited information on use with liposomal doxorubicin.

Pharmacology

A naturally occurring, endogenous retinoid, alitretinoin binds to and activates all known intracellular retinoid receptor subtypes. Once activated, these receptors function as transcription factors that regulate the expression of genes that control differentiation and proliferation in all cells. Alitretinoin was shown to inhibit growth of KS cells *in vivo*. Systemic absorption of alitretinoin gel is insignificant, and plasma concentrations in patients were similar to those in nontreated subjects.

Adverse Effects/Precautions

Adverse effects occur almost exclusively at the site of application. Dermal toxicity typically begins as erythema and may worsen and progress to edema with erythema. Dermal toxicity may be dose-limiting, with intense erythema, edema, and vesiculation. Severe local adversities occurred in approximately 10% of patients.

Pregnancy: FDA category D.

Minimize sun exposure to treated areas, and do not use sun lamps while using alitretinoin (to reduce the risk of photosensitivity).

Drug–Drug Interactions

Alitretinoin gel should not be used with DEET (N,*N*-diethyl-*m*-toluamide)-containing products, such as insect repellent.

No studies of interactions with systemic antiretroviral agents, macrolide antibiotics, or azole antifungals have been conducted.

Preparation *Rx*

Gel   0.1%   Panretin   60 g

Selected References

Duvic M, Friedman-Kien AE, Looney DJ, et al. Topical treatment of cutaneous lesions of acquired immunodeficiency syndrome-related Kaposi sarcoma using alitretinoin gel: results of phase 1 and 2 trials. Arch Dermatol 2000; 136: 1461–9.

Stevens VJ, LaMarca A, Miller R, et al. The combination of topical alitretinoin gel plus liposomal doxorubicin appears safe and effective as treatment for AIDS-related cutaneous Kaposi's sarcoma (abstract). Presented at the 60th Annual Meeting of the American Academy of Dermatology, New Orleans, LA, February 2002.

Walmsley S, Northfelt DW, Melosky B, et al. Treatment of AIDS-related cutaneous Kaposi's sarcoma with topical alitretinoin (9-*cis*-retinoic acid) gel. J AIDS 1999; 22: 235–46.

Aminolevulinic Acid (Levulan Kerastick)

Dose and Administration

Apply 20% aminolevulinic acid topical solution to scalp or face lesions using the enclosed applicator. A second application may be applied after the first has dried. Patients must be told to keep the treated actinic keratoses dry and out of bright light during the time period before the blue light treatment.

Photoactivation of the aminolevulinic acid is performed with blue-light illumination (BLU-U Blue Light Photodynamic Therapy Illuminator) 14 to 18 hours later. Photoactivation is applied for 1000 seconds in order to achieve a therapeutic dose of 10 J/cm^2. This treatment may be repeated in 8 weeks.

Uses

FDA-approved dermatologic uses: Non-hyperkeratotic actinic keratosis of the face and scalp.

Other uses: Superficial and nodular basal cell carcinomas.

Pharmacology

Aminolevulinic acid is an endogenous substance produced in the rate-limiting initial step of the heme synthetic pathway. Application results in production of excess protoporphyrin IX, a photosensitizing agent. It is thought that protoporphyrin IX preferentially accumulates in malignant cells due to their inherent decreased activity of ferrochelatase, an enzyme that converts protoporphyrin IX to heme. When phototherapy is applied to the treated region, the photosensitization of the protoporphyrin IX causes the production of oxygen free radicals that destroy the cell membrane.

Topical aminolevulinic acid reaches its peak within the lesion approximately 11 hours after application. The half-life within the lesion is 30 hours.

Adverse Effects/Precautions

Topical aminolevulinic acid is contraindicated in patients with skin photosensitivity disorders at wavelengths of 400 to 450 nanometers, porphyria, or porphyrin hypersensitivity.

The most common dermatologic adverse effect is phototoxicity; other adverse effects include edema, erythema, pruritus, burning, hyperpigmentation, hypopigmentation, erosion, and skin irritation.

Patients should be advised to avoid sunlight or bright light exposure up to 40 hours after topical application. Patients should be advised to wear a wide-brimmed hat or similar head covering to protect themselves from the sunlight. Sunscreens will not protect the patient against the photosensitization of visible light.

Pregnancy: FDA category C.

Drug Interactions

It is possible that concomitant use of other drugs that cause photosensitization (e.g. tetracyclines, phenothiazides, sulfonylureas, thiazide diuretics, and griseofulvin) will increase the photosensitivity reaction of actinic keratoses treated with aminolevulinic acid.

Preparation *Rx*

Topical solution   20%   Levulan Kerastick   #4, 6 & 12

Selected Reference

Peng Q, Warlow T, Berg K, et al. 5-Aminolevulinic acid-based photodynamic therapy. Cancer 1997; 79: 2282–308.

Azathioprine (Imuran)

Dose and Administration

Initial dose of 1 mg/kg per day by mouth (either once or twice daily dosing). The dose may be increased at increments of 0.5 mg/kg per day up to a maximum dose of 2.5 mg/kg per day.

Uses

FDA-approved: Prevention of rejection in renal transplant patients and for the management of severe, active rheumatoid arthritis unresponsive to nonsteroidal anti-inflammatory drugs. Other uses include vasculitis and systemic lupus erythematosus.

Monitoring

Periodic measurement of serum transaminases, including alkaline phosphatase, and bilirubin is indicated for early detection of hepatotoxicity, and neutrophil and platelet counts for early detection of leukopenia and/or thrombocytopenia. Consider screening for malignancies where clinically indicated.

Pharmacology

Azathioprine is a purine analog that is cleaved *in vivo* to 6-mercaptopurine. It interferes with purine nucleotide synthesis and metabolism, and alters the synthesis and function of RNA. It also suppresses delayed cell-mediated hypersensitivity and produces variable alterations in antibody production. Specifically, it suppresses T-cell activity more than B-cell activity and has potent anti-inflammatory properties.

Azathioprine is well absorbed following oral administration and is rapidly cleaved *in vivo* to mercaptopurine. Blood concentrations are not predictive of therapeutic efficacy as the magnitude and duration of clinical effects correlate with thiopurine nucleotide concentrations in tissues rather than with plasma concentrations.

Adverse Effects/Precautions

The principle serious toxic effects are hematologic and gastrointestinal.

Leukopenia and/or thrombocytopenia are dose dependant and can occur late in the course of therapy. Dose reduction or temporary withdrawal allows reversal of these toxicities. Bone marrow toxicity and leukopenia are more commonly seen when azathioprine is used for suppression of graft rejection than when used for rheumatoid arthritis. There are rare individuals with inherited deficiency of the enzyme thiopurine methyltransferase who may be unusually sensitive to the myelosuppressive effect of azathioprine and who may develop rapid bone marrow suppression following initiation of treatment. Because of chronic immuno-suppression, patients should be informed of the risk of malignancy.

Intestinal hypersensitivity characterized by severe nausea and vomiting has been reported and may be accompanied by diarrhea, rash, fever, malaise, myalgias, elevations in liver enzymes, and occasionally hypotension. It is reversible on discontinuation of the drug. Secondary infection and neoplasia are also significant risks.

Other adverse effects of low frequency include skin rashes, alopecia, fever, arthralgias, steatorrhea, negative nitrogen balance, and reversible interstitial pneumonitis.

Azathioprine (Imuran)

Pregnancy: FDA category D.

Patients previously treated with alkylating agents may have a prohibiting risk of neoplasia if treated with azathioprine.

Drug Interactions

Allopurinol increases azathioprine concentrations requiring a reduction of azathioprine to approximately 25–30% of usual doses. Concomitant use with angiotensin converting enzyme inhibitors has been reported to induce anemia and severe leukopenia. Azathioprine may inhibit the anticoagulant effect of warfarin.

Preparation *Rx*

Tablets	50 mg	Imuran
Injection	100 mg vial	Imuran

Selected References

Dutz JP, Ho VC. Immunosuppressive agents in dermatology. An update. Dermatol Clin 1998; 16: 235–51.

Flores F, Kerdel F. Other novel immunosuppressants. Dermatol Clin 2000; 18: 475–83.

Tan BB, Lear JT, Gawkrodger DJ, English JS. Azathioprine in dermatology: a survey of current practice in the UK. Br J Dermatol 1997; 136: 351–5.

Bexarotene (Targretin) Systemic

Dose and Administration

$300\,mg/m^2$ per day by mouth with food is the recommended starting dose. If a patient does not show any response after 8 weeks of therapy, the dose may be increased to $400\,mg/m^2$ per day.

No more than a 1-month supply should be prescribed at one time so that the results of the monthly pregnancy test can be assessed.

Uses

For the treatment of cutaneous manifestations of cutaneous T-cell lymphoma (CTCL) in patients who are refractory to at least one prior systemic therapy. Targretin has also shown promise in the treatment of moderate to severe plaque psoriasis. A topical preparation has shown efficacy in Kaposi's sarcoma and early-stage CTCL.

Monitoring

Pregnancy test, as above.

Baseline fasting lipid profile, LFTs, thyroid function tests, and CBC with differential should be obtained. Lipids and LFTs should be monitored weekly for at least 4 weeks followed by monitoring every 8 weeks. CBC counts and thyroid function tests should be monitored periodically throughout treatment. Antitriglyceride therapy should be initiated to maintain fasting triglycerides below $400\,mg/dl$.

Pharmacology

Bexarotene selectively binds and activates retinoid X receptor (RXR) subtypes. Binding of the drug to retinoic acid receptors is minimal. Once activated, RXR receptors function as transcription factors that regulate the expression of genes that control cellular differentiation and proliferation. Bexarotene inhibits the *in vitro* growth of some tumor cell lines of hematopoietic and squamous cell origin. It has less toxicity as compared with other retinoids in clinical use.

Bexarotene is highly protein bound (> 99%) and < 1% of the drug is excreted in urine. Renal impairment can significantly alter protein binding. Elimination half-life is 7 hours. Hepatic insufficiency can significantly alter drug elimination.

Adverse Effects/Precautions

WARNING: Bexarotene can cause severe birth defects. It is contraindicated in women who are pregnant or considering pregnancy. A negative pregnancy test is necessary 1 week prior to initiating therapy and monthly during therapy. Women of childbearing age who receive bexarotene should use at least two forms of reliable contraception 1 month prior to the first dose, during treatment, and for 1 month after the last dose of bexarotene.

Pregnancy: FDA category X.

Hypertriglyceridemia, decreased HDL, and hypercholesterolemia occur in a majority of patients; the incidence of adverse effects increases with higher doses. Lipid effects are usually reversible with cessation of therapy and may be tempered by dose reduction or concomitant antilipid therapy. Pancreatitis secondary to elevated triglycerides has been reported.

Elevations in LFTs have been reported. Discontinuation of therapy should be considered if LFTs are greater than three times the upper limit of normal.

Clinical hypothyroidism caused by bexarotene therapy can be treated by concomitant thyroid hormone replacement. Hypothyroidism may be reversed on cessation of therapy.

Leukopenia (dose-related), headache, myalgias, rash, dry skin and mucous membranes, and cataracts have also been reported.

Eczema, exfoliative dermatitis, and local pain have been reported.

Drug Interactions

Bexarotene oxidative metabolites appear to be formed by the cytochrome P450 3A4 isoenzyme. Therefore, ketoconazole, itraconazole, erythromycin, gemfibrozil, grapefruit juice, and other inhibitors of cytochrome P450 3A4 would be expected to lead to an increase in plasma bexarotene concentrations. Furthermore, rifampin, phenytoin, phenobarbital, and other inducers of cytochrome P450 may reduce plasma bexarotene concentrations.

Concomitant administration of gemfibrozil resulted in substantial increases in plasma concentrations of bexarotene; therefore gemfibrozil should not be used concomitantly.

Preparation *Rx*

Capsules   75 mg   Targretin

Selected References

Duvic M, Martin AG, Kim Y, et al. Phase 2 and 3 clinical trial of oral bexarotene (targretin capsules) for the treatment of refractory or persistent early-stage cutaneous T-cell lymphoma. Arch Dermatol 2001; 137: 581–93.

Smit JV, de Jong EMGJ, van Hooijdonk CAEM, et al. Systemic bexarotene significantly inhibits proliferation and inflammation and improves normal differentiation in moderate to severe plaque psoriasis: an immunohistochemical study. 2nd International Congress of 'Psoriasis: from Gene to Clinic', London, 2–4 December 1999.

Bexarotene (Targretin) Topical

Dose and Administration

Gel should be applied generously to all lesions with care to avoid normal skin and mucosal surfaces. Starting frequency is once every other day for 1 week, then increased to once daily for 1 week, then two times a day for 1 week, then up to four times a day, if tolerated. Responses were noted at twice daily to four times daily dosing with the earliest response seen at 4 weeks after initiation of therapy. Allow gel to dry completely before covering with clothing. Do not use occlusive dressings with the gel. Gel should be continued indefinitely if lesions are responsive.

Uses

FDA-approved for the topical treatment of early-stage cutaneous T-cell lymphoma (CTCL), particularly stages IA and IIB unresponsive or intolerant to other therapies.

Monitoring

Pregnancy test, as above.

Pharmacology

Bexarotene selectively binds and activates retinoid X receptor (RXR) subtypes; binding of the drug to retinoic acid receptors is minimal. Once activated, RXR receptors function as transcription factors that regulate the expression of genes that control cellular differentiation and proliferation. Bexarotene inhibits the *in vitro* growth of some tumor cell lines of hematopoietic and squamous cell origin, and in some *in vivo* animal models it induces tumor regression. It may have less toxicity as compared with other retinoids in clinical use.

In patients applying only low to moderate doses of the gel, there is minimal potential for significant plasma concentrations of bexarotene to be achieved. It is highly protein bound (> 99%), and < 1% of the drug is excreted in the urine. Metabolism is via cytochrome P450; therefore, hepatic insufficiency may result in decreased drug clearance. Renal impairment can significantly alter protein binding thus altering the pharmacokinetics of this drug.

Adverse Effects/Precautions

WARNING: Bexarotene can cause severe birth defects. It is contraindicated in women who are pregnant or considering pregnancy. A negative pregnancy test is necessary 1 week prior to initiating therapy and monthly during therapy. Women of childbearing age who receive bexarotene should use at least two forms of reliable contraception 1 month prior to the first dose, during treatment, and for 1 month after the last dose of bexarotene.

Pregnancy: FDA category X.

Most common adverse events at the application site are rash, pain, skin disorder, and pruritus. Dose-limiting adverse effects include rash, contact dermatitis, and pruritus.

Advise patients to minimize exposure to sunlight and artificial UV light during use, due to the drug's photosensitizing potential.

Drug–Drug Interactions

Concomitant use of ketoconazole, itraconazole, erythromycin, and grapefruit juice could increase bexarotene plasma concentrations, but due to insignificant drug plasma concentrations with low to moderate gel use, these interactions are unlikely to cause any adverse effects. Bexarotene gel should not be used with DEET (*N,N*-diethyl-*m*-toluamide)-containing products, such as insect repellent.

Preparation *Rx*

Gel	1%	Targretin Gel	60 g

Colchicine

Dose and Administration

Adults: Usual adult dose is 0.5 to 1.2 mg.

Gout: In acute gouty arthritis give 0.5 to 1.2 mg orally every 1 to 2 hours until pain relief or unacceptable adverse effects, or 2 mg IV over 2 to 5 minutes followed by 0.5 mg IV every 6 hours. Maximum 8 mg/day orally or 4 mg/day IV. For gout prophylaxis give 0.5 to 1 mg orally once to three times daily depending on severity.

Behçet's syndrome: Adults: 0.5 mg orally three times daily.

Administer with food to minimize gastrointestinal irritation.

Uses

FDA approved for use in acute gout and for gout prophylaxis. Other uses include amyloidosis, Behçet's syndrome, dermatitis herpetiformis, familial Mediterranean fever, idiopathic thrombocytopenic purpura, necrotizing vasculitis, palmoplantar pustulosis, psoriasis, pyoderma gangrenosum, and scleroderma.

Pharmacology

Colchicine has anti-inflammatory effects mediated by inhibition of neutrophil migration. Colchicine also has antimitotic actions, which may cause many of the adverse side-effects on proliferating tissues such as the skin, hair, and bone marrow. Other pharmacologic actions include decreasing body temperature, suppressing the respiratory center, and vasomotor stimulation leading to hypertension.

Oral colchicine is rapidly absorbed, with the peak anti-inflammatory effect occurring within 24 to 48 hours. Enterohepatic recirculation occurs to a large extent and can lead to adverse gastrointestinal effects with larger dosages. Colchicine distributes to the kidney, liver, spleen, and intestinal tissues and concentrates primarily in the leukocytes for up to 10 days after administration.

The liver, kidneys, and other tissues metabolize colchicine. Dosage adjustment is required in renal insufficiency. It is not recommended for routine use in patients with a creatinine clearance of less than 50 ml/minute. Colchicine and its metabolites are excreted primarily in the feces. Renal elimination may increase in patients with hepatic disease.

Adverse Effects/Precautions

Adverse gastrointestinal effects are very common and include nausea, vomiting, diarrhea, abdominal pain, anorexia, and adynamic ileus. These adverse reactions may indicate colchicine toxicity, and the drug should be discontinued until symptoms resolve (usually 24 to 48 hours).

Chronic administration of colchicine can induce bone marrow suppression, including aplastic anemia, pancytopenia, thrombocytopenia, leukopenia, or agranulocytosis.

Elevated plasma concentrations of colchicine have been associated with myopathy, peripheral neuropathy, and nephrotoxicity.

An injection site reaction characterized by erythema, swelling, and pain at the injection site can occur, resulting in skin necrosis and tissue necrosis if the drug is

Colchicine

injected intramuscularly or subcutaneously. Cardiac arrhythmias have been reported with rapid intravenous administration.

Hypersensitivity reactions, urticaria and angioedema, occur rarely as does nonthrombocytopenic purpura, prostration, hypothyroidism, alopecia, stomatitis, and bladder spasm.

Acute overdoses of colchicine can be fatal with multiple organ failure. Intravenous use of colchicine should be avoided if possible. Adjustment of dosages should be made in patients with renal failure as indicated above.

Preparation *Rx*

Tablets	0.5 & 0.6 mg
Solution for injection	0.5 mg/ml, 2 ml

Selected References

Aram H. Colchicine in dermatologic therapy. Int J Dermatol 1983; 22: 566–9.

Famaey JP. Colchicine in therapy. State of the art and new perspectives for an old drug. Clin Exp Rheumatol 1988; 6: 305–17.

Ghate JV, Jorizzo JL. Behçet's disease and complex aphthosis. J Am Acad Dermatol 1999; 40: 1–18.

Cyclophosphamide (Cytoxan)

Dose and Administration

For dermatologic indications, cyclophosphamide dosing is usually in the range of 1 to 5 mg/kg orally per day.

Uses

FDA-approved: Treatment of malignant disease (lymphoma, leukemia, myeloma, mycosis fungoides, and other malignancies) and steroid-unresponsive nephrotic syndrome in children. Other uses include refractory, inflammatory skin diseases, sometimes as a steroid-sparing agent, including systemic lupus erythematosus, sarcoidosis, and vasculitis.

Monitoring

Hematologic tests (neutrophils and platelets) should be monitored regularly to determine the degree of hematologic suppression. Urine should be examined for red cells, which may precede hemorrhagic cystitis.

Pharmacology

Cyclophosphamide is converted in the liver to active alkylating metabolites that are thought to act by cross-linking DNA. The drug half-life is 3 to 12 hours.

Adverse Effects/Precautions

Secondary malignancies have developed in some patients treated with cyclophosphamide. It interferes with oogenesis in spermatogenesis and may cause sterility in both sexes. Hemorrhagic cystitis may develop and can be severe and even fatal; forced fluid intake helps prevent cystitis. Cardiac toxicity has been reported. Serious, sometimes fatal, infections may develop, owing to immunosuppression. Alopecia can occur with cyclophosphamide therapy, but hair can be expected to grow back after treatment is discontinued. Very rare reports of Stevens–Johnson syndrome and toxic epidermal necrolysis have been reported; a causal relationship has not been established.

Pregnancy: FDA category D.

Drug Interactions

The leukopenic activity of cyclophosphamide may be increased by high doses of phenobarbital. Cyclophosphamide may cause marked and persistent inhibition of cholinesterase activity; if a patient has been treated with cyclophosphamide within 10 days of general anesthesia, the anesthesiologist should be alerted.

Special attention to the possible development of the toxicity should be exercised in patients with leukopenia, thrombocytopenia, tumor cell infiltration of bone marrow, previous X-ray therapy, previous therapy with other cytotoxic agents, and impaired hepatic or renal function. Cyclophosphamide may interfere with normal wound healing.

Preparation Rx

| Tablets | Cytoxan | 25 & 50 mg |
| Injection | Cytoxan | 100, 200, 500, 1000 & 2000 mg |

Selected References

Dutz JP, Ho VC. Immunosuppressive agents in dermatology. An update. Dermatol Clin 1998; 16: 235–51.

Frangogiannis NG, Boridy I, Mazhar M, et al. Cyclophosphamide in the treatment of toxic epidermal necrolysis. South Med J 1996; 89: 1001–3.

Werth VP. Pulse intravenous cyclophosphamide for treatment of autoimmune blistering disease. Is there an advantage over oral routes? Arch Dermatol 1997; 33: 229–30.

Cyclosporine (Neoral, Sandimmune)

Dose and Administration

The recommended starting dose for treatment of psoriasis will depend on the severity of the patient's condition. The initial dose is usually 2.5 mg/kg per day orally divided twice daily and slowly increased if necessary. The maximum dermatologic dose is 5 mg/kg per day.

Uses

FDA-approved for severe rheumatoid arthritis and prophylaxis of organ rejection. Also approved for adult, nonimmunocompromised patients with severe, recalcitrant, plaque psoriasis who have failed to respond to at least one systemic therapy (e.g. psoralen plus ultraviolet A (PUVA), retinoids, methotrexate) or in patients for whom other systemic therapies are contraindicated or cannot be tolerated.

Other uses include atopic dermatitis, pyoderma gangrenosum, lichen planus, granuloma annulare, Behçet's disease, bullous pemphigoid, pemphigus vulgaris, epidermolysis bullosa acquisita, Hailey–Hailey disease, systemic lupus erythematosus, scleroderma, dermatomyositis, graft-versus-host disease, chronic urticaria, vitiligo, photodermatosis, chronic pigmented purpura, pityriasis lichenoides chronica, annular elastolytic giant cell granuloma, and hidradenitis suppurativa.

Monitoring

Periodic monitoring of electrolytes, creatinine, blood urea nitrogen, uric acid, liver function tests, and complete blood counts should be performed. Blood pressure and cyclosporine drug concentrations should be closely monitored as well.

Pharmacology

Cyclosporine is a potent immunosuppressive agent that acts by suppressing cell-mediated and, to a lesser extent, humoral immunity. Cyclosporine preferentially and reversibly inhibits immunocompetent T-helper lymphocytes. T-suppressor cells may also be suppressed. Cyclosporine also inhibits lymphokine production and release. Cyclosporine is 90% protein bound. Elimination is primarily hepatic, and the half-life is approximately 19 hours.

Adverse Effects/Precautions

Adverse effects are dose-related and can be serious; therefore, the lowest possible maintenance dose should be used. Early in the course of therapy, nausea, headache, fatigue, or myalgias may occur. At increased doses, physicians should inquire about tremor in the hands, paresthesias, and sensitivity to hot and cold in the distal extremities.

Hypertrichosis, gingival hyperplasia, hypertension, renal insufficiency, elevated cholesterol and triglycerides, and elevated bilirubin may occur. Uric acid may increase but rarely requires anti-gout therapy. Serum magnesium may decrease; replacement is indicated.

Antihypertensive therapy during cyclosporine treatment can treat hypertension that may develop. Reducing the dose of cyclosporine may also be warranted.

Cyclosporine (Neoral, Sandimmune)

Cyclosporine should be used with extreme caution in patients with pre-existing renal or hepatic disease. Cyclosporine is contraindicated during pregnancy or lactation and should not be used in patients in whom immunosuppression would be unacceptable.

Pregnancy: FDA category C.

Drug Interactions

Cyclosporine is a CYP450 3A4 substrate and thus has the potential to be involved in numerous drug interactions. Drugs that may potentiate renal dysfunction with cyclosporine include aminoglycosides, vancomycin, trimethoprim–sulfamethoxazole, melphalan, nonsteroidal anti-inflammatory drugs, amphotericin B, ketoconazole, and tacrolimus.

Drugs that increase cyclosporine concentrations include diltiazem, nicardipine, verapamil, fluconazole, itraconazole, ketoconazole, cimetidine, clarithromycin, erythromycin, quinupristin/dalfopristin, colchicine, amiodarone, methylprednisolone, allopurinol, bromocriptine, danazol, and metoclopramide.

Drugs that decrease cyclosporine concentrations include nafcillin, rifampin, carbamazepine, phenobarbital, phenytoin, octreotide, orlistat, ticlopidine. St John's wort may also decrease concentrations.

Avoid use of live attenuated vaccines with concomitant use of cyclosporine.

Special Considerations

Neoral and Gengraf are not bioequivalent to Sandimmune and thus conversion from either product to Sandimmune on a mg-to-mg basis may result in lower cyclosporine blood concentrations. When switching between products, increased serum concentration monitoring should be performed to avoid the potential of under- or overdosing.

Preparation *Rx*

Microemulsion oral solution	100 mg/ml	Neoral (generic = Gengraf)
Microemulsion soft gelatin capsules	25 & 100 mg	Neoral (generic = Gengraf)
Gelatin capsule	25 & 100 mg	Sandimmune
Oral solution	100 mg/ml	Sandimmune
Solution for injection	50 mg/ml	Sandimmune

Selected References

Fivenson DP. Nonsteroidal treatment of autoimmune skin diseases. Dermatol Clin 1997; 15: 695–705.

Flores F, Kerdel F. Other novel immunosuppressants. Dermatol Clin 2000; 18: 475–83.

Koo J. Duration of remission of psoriasis therapies. J Am Acad Dermatol 1999; 41: 51–9.

Lebwohl M, Ellis C, Gottlieb A, et al. Cyclosporine consensus conference: with emphasis on the treatment of psoriasis. J Am Acad Dermatol 1998; 39: 464–75.

Denileukin Diftitox (Ontak)

Dose and Administration

The recommended treatment cycle is 9 or 18 micrograms per kg per day administered IV over at least 15 minutes for 5 consecutive days every 21 days. If infusional adverse reactions occur, the infusion should be discontinued or the rate should be reduced depending on the severity of the reaction. Most patients respond within three treatment cycles. Safe and effective dosing in psoriasis has not been established.

Uses

FDA-approved for use in recurrent or refractory cutaneous T-cell lymphoma in patients whose malignant cells express the CD25 component of the interleukin-2 (IL-2) receptor. It has also been used in the treatment of moderate-to-severe psoriasis.

Monitoring

Prior to initiating therapy and periodically throughout therapy for cutaneous T-cell lymphoma the following should be assessed: malignant cells testing for CD25 expression, CBC, blood chemistry panel, LFTs, renal function tests, serum albumin, and antibody titers to denileukin, diphtheria toxin, and IL-2.

Pharmacology

Denileukin diftitox is an IL-2 receptor-specific diphtheria toxin fusion protein that directs the toxin to cells that express the IL-2 receptor. It interacts with the high-affinity IL-2 receptor (CD25/CD122/CD132) on the cell surface and inhibits cellular protein synthesis, resulting in cell death within hours.

Accumulation does not occur with repeat doses. The elimination half-life is 70 to 80 minutes. Development of antibodies to denileukin diftitox does impact clearance rates.

Adverse Effects/Precautions

Acute hypersensitivity reactions occur in a majority of patients during or within 24 hours of infusion. Symptoms (in decreasing order of frequency) include hypotension, back pain, dyspnea, vasodilatation, rash, chest pain or tightness, tachycardia, dysphagia or laryngismus, syncope, and anaphylaxis. Resuscitative drugs and equipment should be readily available during administration.

Vascular leak syndrome is characterized by two of the following three symptoms: hypotension, edema, and hypoalbuminemia. The onset of symptoms is usually delayed and may persist or worsen after cessation of treatment. Special caution should be taken in patients with pre-existing cardiovascular disease prior to starting therapy.

Other possible adverse effects include hypotension, asthenia, dizziness, confusion, amnesia, and paresthesias. Nausea, vomiting, and diarrhea are frequent during or after infusion and are most common and severe during initial treatment cycles.

Increases in serum creatinine and abnormal urinalysis findings are non-dose-limiting adverse effects. Reversible transaminase elevations may occur.

Fever, chills, arthralgias, myalgias, and headaches are more common adverse effects.

Pregnancy: FDA category C.

Denileukin Diftitox (Ontak)

Preparation Rx

Solution for injection   150 micrograms per ml, 2 ml   Ontak

Selected References

Bagel J, Garland WT, Breneman D, et al. Administration of $DAB_{389}IL-2$ to patients with recalcitrant psoriasis: a double-blind, phase II multicenter trial. J Am Acad Dermatol 1998; 38: 938–44.

Gottlieb SL, Gilleaudeau P, Johnson R, et al. Response of psoriasis to a lymphocyte-selective toxin ($DAB_{389}IL-2$) suggests a primary immune, but not keratinocyte, pathogenic basis. Nat Med 1995; 1: 442–7.

Talpur R, Apisarnthanarax N, Ward S, Duvic M. Treatment of refractory peripheral T-cell lymphoma with denileukin diftitox (ONTAK). Leuk Lymphoma 2002; 43: 121–6.

Efalizumab (Raptiva)

Dose and Administration

Adult: Single dose of 0.7 mg/kg SC, followed by weekly SC doses of 1 mg/kg (maximum single dose not to exceed a total of 200 mg).

Use

FDA-approved: Treatment of adults (over age 18 years) with chronic moderate to severe plaque psoriasis who are candidates for systemic therapy or phototherapy.

Pharmacology

Efalizumab binds to CD11a (the α-subunit of leukocyte function antigen-1, LFA-1) and blocks the interaction between LFA-1 and intercellular adhesion molecule-1 (ICAM-1). Thus, the adhesion of leukocytes to other cell types (e.g. keratinocytes) is inhibited, resulting in the blockade of T lymphocyte activation and trafficking. The blockade of this pathway extends to psoriatic skin where ICAM-1 expression is up-regulated, consequently interfering with the pathophysiology of psoriasis.

Adverse Effects/Precautions

May cause immunosuppression due to the drug's effect on T lymphocyte activation and migration, and thus increases the risk of infection or malignancy. Reactivation of latent infections is also possible. Serious infections reported include, but are not limited to, pneumonia, sepsis, and aseptic meningitis. If a patient develops a serious infection, efalizumab should be discontinued.

May cause thrombocytopenia, and monitoring of platelet counts during therapy is recommended monthly for the first 3 months, then every 3 months with continued treatment. Hemolytic anemia has also been reported, with a usual onset of 4 to 6 months after initiation. Discontinue efalizumab if thrombocytopenia or hemolytic anemia develop.

Other frequently reported adverse effects include headache, fever, chills, nausea, and myalgias. Though rare, it has been reported that efalizumab has been associated with worsening or new forms of psoriasis.

Should not be given to patients with clinically significant infections. Discontinue efalizumab if a serious infection, malignancy, or thrombocytopenia occur.

Pregnancy: FDA category C.

Drug Interactions

Live, live-attenuated, and acellular vaccines should not be given concurrently. Patients receiving other immunosuppressants should not receive efalizumab.

Preparation Rx

Four trays/carton: Each tray contains a 125 mg single-use vial of powder (must be refrigerated at 36–46°F (2–8°C)) for injection with a single-use pre-filled diluent syringe of sterile water (1.3 ml) for injection. Two #25 gauge needles and alcohol swabs are also provided. The reconstituted efalizumab must be stored at room temperature and be used within 8 hours. Protect stored product from light.

Selected Reference

Werther WA, Gonzalez TN, O'Connor SJ, et al. Humanization of an anti-lymphocyte function-associated antigen (LFA)-1 monoclonal antibody and reengineering of the humanized antibody for binding to rhesus LFA-1. J Immunol 1996; 157: 4986–95.

Etanercept (Enbrel)

Dose and Administration

Psoriatic arthritis: 50 mg subcutaneously weekly.

Plaque psoriasis: 50 mg subcutaneously twice weekly for 3 months, followed by a maintenance dose of 50 mg weekly.

Rotate sites for injection (thigh, abdomen, upper arm). Do not inject in areas where skin is tender, bruised, red, or hard.

Uses

FDA-approved for treatment of adult patients with chronic moderate to severe plaque psoriasis and psoriatic arthritis. Other FDA-approved indications include ankylosing spondylitis, polyarticular-course juvenile rheumatoid arthritis, and moderate to severe rheumatoid arthritis.

Other uses include toxic epidermal necrolysis, neutrophilic dermatitis, bullous dermatitis, cicatricial pemphigoid, and other severe inflammatory skin diseases.

Pharmacology

Etanercept is a dimeric fusion protein that binds to the human p75 TNF receptor and blocks interactions with cell-surface TNF receptors. TNF is involved in inflammatory and immune responses. Etanercept can also modulate biologic responses regulated by TNF.

Contraindications

Etanercept should not be administered to patients with sepsis or with known hypersensitivity to etanercept or any of its components.

Adverse Effects/Precautions

Increased risk of infection and malignancy. Central nervous system demyelinating disorders such as transverse myelitis, optic neuritis, multiple sclerosis, and seizure disorder have been associated with etanercept. Rare cases of pancytopenia including aplastic anemia have been reported. The needle cover of the syringe contains natural rubber (latex) which may cause an allergic reaction in individuals sensitive to natural rubber. Mild to moderate injection site reactions. There have been reports of new onset and worsening congestive heart failure while on etanercept. Treatment with etanercept has been associated with development of antinuclear antibodies and rarely can be associated with a lupus-like syndrome.

Pregnancy: FDA Category B.

Drug Interactions

Concurrent therapy with anakinra is not recommended, owing to increased risk of neutropenia. Patients should not receive live vaccinations while on etanercept.

Methotrexate administration is not altered when used concurrently with etanercept.

Preparation *Rx*

Prefilled syringe: 50 mg/ml single-use prefilled syringe for subcutaneous injection. Store prefilled syringes in the refrigerator at 36–46°F (2–8°C). Supplied in a carton containing four dose trays. Each dose tray contains one prefilled syringe with a #27 gauge needle.

Multiple-use vials: 25 mg vials of powder to be reconstituted with 1 ml of sterile water (supplied). The powder must be refrigerated at 36–46°F. The reconstituted solution must be used within 14 days and refrigerated at 36–46°F. The multiple-use vials are supplied in a carton containing four dose trays. Each dose tray contains a single vial of powder (25 mg etanercept), one syringe for diluent containing 1 ml of sterile water for injection, one #27 gauge needle, one vial adapter, one plunger, and two alcohol swabs.

References

Mahe E, Descamps V. Anti-TNF alpha in dermatology. Ann Dermatol Venerol 2002; 129: 1374–9.

Papp KA. Etanercept in psoriasis. Expert Opin Pharmacother 2004;5:2139–46.

Williams JD, Griffiths CE. Cytokine blocking agents in dermatology. Clin Exp Dermatol 2002; 27: 585–90.

Yamauchi PS, Gindi V, Lowe NJ. The treatment of psoriasis and psoriatic arthritis with etanercept: practical considerations on monotherapy, combination therapy, and safety. Dermatol Clin 2004; 22: 449–59.

Fluorouracil (Efudex)

Uses, Dose and Administration

Actinic or solar keratoses: Apply cream or solution twice daily to entire region of affected areas until the inflammatory response reaches the erosion, necrosis, and ulceration stage. Usual duration of therapy is 2 to 4 weeks. Complete healing of lesions may not be evident for 1 to 2 months following cessation of therapy. Carac product labeling is limited to the face and anterior scalp.

Superficial basal cell carcinomas: only the 5% strength is recommended. Apply cream or solution twice daily in an amount sufficient to cover the lesions. Therapy should continue for at least 3 to 6 weeks and may continue for 10 to 12 weeks. Patients should be followed for a reasonable period of time to determine whether a cure has been achieved.

Note: Efudex should be applied with a nonmetal applicator or suitably gloved hand. If applied with the fingers, the hands should be washed thoroughly immediately afterwards. In addition, great care should be taken not to apply in the eyes, nose, or mouth area.

Pharmacology

Antineoplastic agent that blocks the methylation of deoxyuridylic acid to thymidylic acid, thereby interfering with DNA synthesis. It essentially creates a thymine deficiency, resulting in unbalanced cell growth and eventual cell death. Effects are most significant on rapidly growing cells. Cure rates of 93% for actinic keratosis and superficial basal cell carcinoma have been reported for patients compliant with this regimen until the proper endpoint. Systemic absorption of topical fluorouracil is approximately 5 to 6 mg per total daily dose of 100 mg. Negligible amounts of labeled material were found in plasma, urine, and expired CO_2 after 3 days of treatment with ^{14}C-labeled Efudex.

Adverse Effects/Precautions

Pregnancy: FDA category X.

Absence of dipyrimidine dehydrogenase activity (DPD; catabolic enzyme) listed as contraindication to Carac. A case of life-threatening systemic toxicity was reported with the topical use of fluorouracil 5% in a patient with DPD enzyme deficiency. Symptoms included severe abdominal pain, bloody diarrhea, vomiting, fever, and chills. Physical examination revealed stomatitis, erythematous skin rash, neutropenia, thrombocytopenia, inflammation of the esophagus, stomach, and small bowel. Although this case was observed with 5% fluorouracil cream, it is unknown whether patients with profound DPD enzyme deficiency would develop systemic toxicity with lower concentrations of topically applied fluorouracil.

Expected effects of treatment include pain, pruritus, and burning at the site of application. Patients should be advised to avoid exposure to sunlight during and immediately following treatment, as the intensity of the inflammatory reaction may increase. Patients undergoing successful treatment exhibit erythema, inflammation, and erosions at the sites of application. Dryness may also occur. Treated areas may be unsightly during and after therapy for a period of a few weeks. To foster compliance, it is imperative to adequately counsel and encourage patients during treatment.

Fluorouracil (Efudex)

Topical fluorouracil may exacerbate other dermatologic conditions such as melasma and rosacea.

Preparation *Rx*

Solution	2% & 5%	Efudex	10 ml
	1%	Fluoroplex	30 ml
Cream	5%	Efudex	25 g
	1%	Fluoroplex	30 g
	0.5%	Carac	30 g

Selected References

Barnaby JW, Styles AR, Cockerell CJ. Actinic keratoses. Differential diagnosis and treatment. Drugs Aging 1997; 11: 186–205.

Dinehart SM. Actinic keratoses: scientific evaluation and public health implications. J Am Acad Dermatol 2000; 42: S25–S28.

Schwartz RA. Therapeutic perspectives in actinic and other keratoses. Int J Dermatol 1996; 35: 533–8.

Hydroxychloroquine Sulfate (Plaquenil)

Uses, Dose and Administration

Rheumatoid arthritis: Initial dose is 400 to 600 mg (310 to 465 mg base) daily. Maintenance dose (after approximately 4 to 12 weeks) is usually 200 to 400 mg (155 to 310 mg base) daily. Maximal efficacy may not occur until after 1 to 4 months of therapy.

Lupus erythematosus, discoid or systemic: Initial dose is 400 mg (310 mg base) once or twice daily, followed by maintenance doses of 200 to 400 mg (155 to 310 mg base) daily. Response onset may be several weeks.

Porphyria cutanea tarda (PCT) in patients who have not responded to less toxic therapies: Low doses (e.g. 200 mg twice weekly) have been used as an alternative or adjunct to phlebotomy. A lower 'test' dose of 50 mg/week may be used initially.

Other FDA-approved uses: Malaria (suppressive and acute attacks), extraintestinal amebiasis, lupus erythematosus, discoid or systemic, and rheumatoid arthritis.

Monitoring

Ophthalmologic examinations (e.g. visual acuity, slit lamp, funduscopic, visual field tests), particularly with long-term therapy, should be performed at baseline and every 3 months. Hepatic function and complete blood counts should be monitored periodically.

Pharmacology

Hydroxychloroquine is a 4-aminoquinoline compound. Its mechanism of antimalarial action is unclear, but is believed to interfere with nucleic acid synthesis. Its mechanism of action for other approved indications is also unknown, although it appears to possess anti-inflammatory activity. In mild rheumatoid arthritis, it has been used as an initial disease-modifying antirheumatic drug (DMARD) and as add-on therapy with methotrexate, with or without sulfasalazine or another DMARD. It also mobilizes tissue porphyrins, promoting renal porphyrin excretion.

Adverse Effects/Precautions

Dermatologic reactions include pruritus, lichen planus-like eruptions, pleomorphic skin eruptions (including Stevens–Johnson syndrome and acute generalized exanthematous pustulosis), skin and mucosal pigmentary changes, bleaching of hair, alopecia, and photosensitivity.

Ocular toxicity (e.g. irreversible retinal damage, visual disturbances) has occurred with use of high doses or extended duration of therapy.

Gastrointestinal discomfort (e.g. nausea, vomiting, epigastric distress, abdominal cramps, diarrhea) may be minimized by administration with food or milk.

Isolated cases of abnormal liver function and fulminant hepatic failure have occurred. Caution is advised in patients with hepatic impairment, alcoholism, or receiving concurrent hepatotoxic medications.

Other adverse effects include muscular weakness, headache, mild CNS stimulation, nerve deafness, and retinal or visual field abnormalities.

May exacerbate psoriasis.

Pediatric ingestion of as little as 0.75 g of chloroquine base has resulted in fatality, therefore use caution in this population (including households with children).

Pregnancy: FDA category C.

Preparation *Rx*

Tablets	200 mg as sulfate	Plaquenil
	(155 mg hydroxychloroquine base)	

Selected References

Cainelli T, Di Padova C, Marchesi L, et al. Hydroxychloroquine versus phlebotomy in the treatment of porphyria cutanea tarda. Br J Dermatol 1983; 108: 593–600.

Isaacson D, Elgart M, Turner ML. Antimalarials in dermatology. Int J Dermatol 1982; 21: 379–95.

Marchesi L, Di Padova C, Cainelli T, et al. A comparative trial of desferrioxamine and hydroxychloroquine for treatment of porphyria cutanea tarda in alcoholic patients. Photodermatology 1984; 1: 286-92.

O'Dell JR, Haire CE, Erikson N. Treatment of rheumatoid arthritis with methotrexate alone, sulfasalazine and hydroxychloroquine, or a combination of all three medications. N Engl J Med 1996; 334: 1287–91.

Wallace DJ. Antimalarial agents and lupus. Rheum Dis Clin North Am 1994;20:243–63.

Hydroxyurea (Hydrea, Droxia)

Dose and Administration

All doses are based on patient actual or ideal weight, whichever is less. Although protocols vary, for most solid tumors, chronic myelogenous leukemia (CML), and melanoma, doses range from 20 to 30 mg/kg orally once daily or 80 mg/kg as a single dose every third day. The intermittent regimen may be preferred, as toxicity requiring discontinuation is rare.

For psoriasis, dosing is 1.5 g orally divided into three daily doses for 1 month with a maintenance dose of 500 mg twice daily.

Uses

FDA-approved: Head and neck cancers, CML, melanoma (both adult and pediatric use), ovarian carcinoma, and sickle cell anemia.

Other uses include brain carcinoma, breast carcinoma, cervical carcinoma, gastrointestinal carcinoma, HIV infections (to decrease viral load), idiopathic hypereosinophilic syndrome, non-Hodgkin's lymphoma, polycythemia vera, psoriasis, renal calculi or chronic urinary tract infections, thalassemia, essential thrombocythemia, and uterine sarcoma.

Pharmacology

Hydroxyurea has a dual mechanism of action. It inhibits conversion of DNA bases by inhibiting RNA reductase. It also has antiretroviral activity, potentiating the activity of reverse transcriptase inhibitors (e.g. zidovudine, didanosine, lamivudine). For psoriasis, hydroxyurea may be effective as a second-line agent in patients who are unresponsive or intolerant to methotrexate. The maximum therapeutic response to hydroxyurea is within 4 to 8 weeks with possible relapse in less than 4 weeks.

Hydroxyurea is metabolized by the liver and excreted in the urine as urea and unchanged drug. The drug half-life is 2 to 4.5 hours.

Adverse Effects/Precautions

The most common adverse reaction is myelosuppression, especially leucopenia, but also thrombocytopenia and anemia; therefore, blood counts should be closely monitored. If the white blood cell (WBC) count is less than 2500, or platelets are less than 100 000, hydroxyurea should be held for 3 days. When the CBC improves, therapy can be resumed.

Gastrointestinal disturbances occur in about 25% of patients and include nausea, vomiting, diarrhea, constipation, and anorexia.

Other adverse effects include macrocytosis (recommend prophylactic folic acid supplementation), temporary renal tubular dysfunction, and various dermatologic effects. Hydroxyurea is associated with maculopapular eruptions, skin ulcers, and facial erythema. Ulcerative lichen planus-like dermatitis has been noted in both acute and long-term hydroxyurea therapy. Symptoms include facial erythema, erosive buccal mucosal lesions, palmar erythematous scaling, and ulcers on plantar feet and dorsal hand.

Rare incidences of dermatomyositis and dermatomyositis-like eruptions have been reported in less than 0.1% of patients on long-term therapy, and most resolve with treatment withdrawal.

Hydroxyurea (Hydrea, Droxia)

Although rare, leg ulcerations may develop. Predisposing factors include underlying disease states, circulatory deficiencies, and pedal edema. Although there is no consistent correlation between dose and duration of therapy, most patients developing this adversity have received therapy for at least 2 to 4 years.

Rare incidence of nail changes such as melanonychia (longitudinal pigmented nail bands) require only reassurance. Additional rare dermatologic effects include alopecia and acral erythema.

Other rare adverse reactions include CNS effects (drowsiness, dizziness, disorientation, hallucinations, convulsions, and headaches), mucositis, aphthous ulcers, cystitis, hepatitis, pulmonary reactions, lupus erythematosus, and fever.

Pregnancy: FDA category D.

Preparation *Rx*

Capsules	200, 300 & 400 mg	Droxia
	500 mg	Hydrea

Selected References

Farber EM, Pearlman D, Abel EA. An appraisal of current systemic chemotherapy for psoriasis. Arch Dermatol 1976; 112: 1679–88.

Rotstein H, Baker C. The treatment of psoriasis. Med J Aust 1990; 152: 153–4.

Taveira LM, Goncalves C, Paiva A, et al. Efficacy of hydroxyurea in the treatment of a patient with erythrodermic psoriasis and chronic myelogenous leukemia. J Eur Acad Derm Venereol 1997; 9: 266–8.

Infliximab (Remicade)

Dose and Administration

Administer infusion over 2 hours. Patients should be observed for side-effects for at least 1 hour after infusion. Medications for hypersensitivity reactions (acetaminophen, antihistamine, corticosteroid, and epinephrine) should be available. In the event of an infusion-related reaction (see Adverse Effects), administer medication as appropriate and slow the infusion. If the reaction is severe or does not resolve, discontinue the infusion.

Psoriasis and psoriatic arthritis: 3–5 mg/kg IV at 0, 2, and 6 weeks, then every 6 to 8 weeks.

Rheumatoid arthritis: 3 mg/kg IV at 0, 2, and 6 weeks, then every 8 weeks. For patients with suboptimal response, may use 10 mg/kg or administer every 4 weeks.

Ankylosing spondylitis: 5 mg/kg IV at 0, 2, and 6 weeks, then every 8 weeks.

Crohn's disease: 5 mg/kg IV at 0, 2, and 6 weeks, then every 8 weeks. For fistulas, if patient does not respond after three doses, no additional infliximab should be given. Doses up to 10 mg/kg may be used for maintenance.

Uses

FDA-approved: Rheumatoid arthritis (in combination with methotrexate), Crohn's disease (reducing signs/symptoms and for fistulizing disease) and psoriatic arthritis.

Other: Psoriasis (and other severe inflammatory skin diseases), ankylosing spondylitis.

Monitoring

Prior to treatment, patients should be evaluated for latent tuberculosis infection with a tuberculin skin test. Treatment for latent tuberculosis infection should be initiated prior to therapy with infliximab.

Pharmacology

Infliximab is a chimeric human–murine monoclonal antibody that binds to TNFα, preventing binding to its receptors. TNFα is a cytokine that mediates chronic inflammation when overexpressed. It potentiates other cytokines, chemokines, adhesion molecules and tissue factor; activates neutrophils; and induces proliferation and increased synthesis of IL-6 and metalloproteinases by fibroblasts.

Contraindications

History of hypersensitivity to infliximab or other murine proteins, or any excipients of the product. Patients with moderate or severe heart failure (NYHA class III/IV) should not receive doses > 5 mg/kg.

Warnings

Serious infections, including re-activation of latent tuberculosis. Should not be given to patients with clinically important, active infection. Concurrent administration with anakinra (interleukin-1 antagonist) is not recommended.

Infliximab (Remicade)

Adverse Effects/Precautions

Increased risk of infection.

Associated with infusion-related reactions (20%), most occurring within 2 hours of infusion. Reactions include urticaria, dyspnea, and/or hypotension; however, serum sickness-like reactions have occurred in Crohn's disease patients 3 to 12 days after therapy was reinstituted following an extended period without Remicade treatment. Symptoms associated with these reactions include fever, rash, headache, sore throat, myalgias, polyarthralgias, hand and facial edema, and/or dysphagia.

For ankylosing spondylitis, safety of re-administration other than every 6 to 8 weeks is not known.

Lupus-like syndrome.

Optic neuritis, seizure, demyelinating disorders including multiple sclerosis.

Reports of leukopenia, neutropenia, thrombocytopenia, pancytopenia (causality not established).

Breastfeeding should be discontinued for at least 6 months after infliximab treatment.

Pregnancy: FDA category B.

Drug Interactions

Formation of antibodies to infliximab is reduced when used concurrently with methotrexate, azathioprine, or 6-mercaptopurine. It is recommended that live vaccines not be given concurrently.

Preparation *Rx*

Intravenous injection   100 mg   Remicade

Selected References

Gottelieb AB, Evans RE, Li S, et al. Infliximab induction therapy for patients with severe plaque-type psoriasis: a randomized double-blind, placebo-controlled trial. J Am Acad Dermatol 2004; 51: 534–42.

Winterfield L, Menter A. Psoriasis and its treatment with infliximab-mediated tumor necrosis factor alpha blockade. Dermatol Clin 2004; 22: 437–43.

Winterfield L, Menter A. Infliximab. Dermatol Ther 2004; 17: 409–26.

Interferon α-2a (Roferon-A)

Uses, Dose and Administration

FDA-approved dermatology use: AIDS-related Kaposi's sarcoma:

Induction: 36 million IU daily (SC or IM) for 10 to 12 weeks. (Alternative induction regimen: day 1, 3 million IU; day 2, 9 million IU; day 3, 18 million IU; then 36 million IU daily for the remainder of the 10 to 12 week induction.)

Maintenance: 36 million IU three times weekly.

Should intolerable adversities develop, the dose should be reduced by 50% or the drug discontinued until adversities resolve.

Other FDA-approved uses include chronic hepatitis C, hairy cell leukemia, and chronic myelogenous leukemia (chronic phase, Philadelphia chromosome positive). Other dermatology (unapproved) uses have included Behçet's disease and cutaneous T-cell lymphoma.

Monitoring

Prior to and periodically during therapy: CBC with differential, hemoglobin, thyroid stimulating hormone (in patients with pre-existing thyroid abnormalities, every 3 months), serum chemistry, blood glucose (especially with pre-existing diabetes mellitus), liver and renal function tests, ECG (with pre-existing cardiac abnormalities), and ophthalmologic examination (in patients with visual changes).

Pharmacology

Endogenous interferons (IFNs) are proteins or glycoproteins produced primarily from leukocytes (IFNα), fibroblasts (IFNβ), and immune cells (IFNγ). Biologic action occurs via IFN binding to specific cell-surface receptors, subsequently affecting intracellular processes. Actions include antiviral, immunomodulatory, and antiproliferative effects. Commercially available IFNα-2a and IFNα-2b are of recombinant DNA origin (using genetically engineered *Escherichia coli*) and differ at only one position in the amino acid sequence. Although FDA-labeled for different uses, evidence is lacking to suggest significant differences in clinical actions between the available IFNαs. In the treatment of AIDS-related Kaposi's sarcoma, greater response is observed in patients otherwise asymptomatic, with no prior opportunistic infection, and a baseline CD4 lymphocyte count > 200 cells/mm^3.

Adverse Effects/Precautions

Interferon α-2a can cause and/or aggravate fatal or life-threatening neuropsychiatric, autoimmune, ischemic, and infectious disorders. Patients should be monitored closely with periodic clinical and laboratory evaluations. Patients with persistently severe or worsening signs or symptoms of these conditions should be withdrawn from therapy. Use caution or avoid treatment in patients with pre-existing debilitating conditions such as cardiac disease, pulmonary disease, diabetes mellitus, autoimmune diseases, immunosuppression, decompensated liver disease, myelosuppression, and thyroid abnormalities.

Depression and suicidal ideation have occurred. CNS effects include somnolence, agitation, seizure disorders, and psychotic disturbances.

Most common: flu-like illness (e.g. fever, chills, myalgia, fatigue), gastrointestinal distress, weight loss, taste disturbances, dizziness, decreased mental status, coughing, alopecia, and rash.

Interferon α-2a (Roferon-A)

Less common: cardiac adversities (e.g. palpitations, arrhythmia), neutropenia/thrombocytopenia, peripheral neuropathy, renal failure (rare), hepatic transaminase elevations, retinal toxicity, and exacerbation of psoriasis.

Pregnancy: FDA category C.

Drug Interactions

Myelosuppressive agents (additive toxicity); hepatic elimination of theophylline reduced (and potentially other drugs metabolized by CYP450); CNS depressants (additive toxicity); interleukin-2 (potential renal failure).

Special Considerations

Consider subcutaneous administration (instead of intramuscular) in patients with thrombocytopenia. Store vials and syringes under refrigeration. Product contains benzyl alcohol.

Preparation *Rx*

Roferon-A (interferon α-2a, recombinant)

Single-use injectable solution

    3 million IU/1 ml vial

    6 million IU/1 ml vial

    9 million IU/0.9 ml vial (also may be used as a multidose vial)

    36 million IU/1 ml vial

Single-use prefilled syringes

    3 million IU/0.5 ml syringe

    6 million IU/0.5 ml syringe

    9 million IU/0.5 ml syringe

Multidose injectable solution

    9 million IU/0.9 ml vial (also may be used as a single-dose vial)

    18 million IU/3 ml vial

Selected References

Hurd DS, Conte ET. Practical uses of the interferons in dermatology. Int J Dermatol 1998; 37: 881–96.

Shaart FM, Bratzke B, Ruszczak ZB, et al. Long term therapy of HIV associated Kaposi's sarcoma with recombinant interferon alpha 2a. Br J Dermatol 1991; 124: 62–8.

Stadler R. Interferons in dermatology: present-day standard. Dermatol Clin 1998; 16: 377–98.

Interferon α-2b (Intron A)

Uses, Dose and Administration

FDA-approved dermatology uses:

AIDS-related Kaposi's sarcoma: 30 million IU/m^2 three times weekly (subcutaneously or intramuscularly). Should intolerable adversities develop, the dose should be reduced by 50% or the drug discontinued until adversities resolve. After an initial response is observed, continue until disease progression or there is a maximal response after 16 weeks.

Malignant melanoma:

Induction: 20 million IU/m^2, 5 days per week for 4 consecutive weeks (all doses intravenous; add dose to 100 ml normal saline and administer over 20 minutes).

Maintenance: 10 million IU/m^2, three times weekly for 48 weeks (subcutaneously). Temporarily discontinue for development of the following: granulocytes $< 500/mm^3$, AST/ALT elevation > 5 times the upper limit of normal. Once resolved, reinstate therapy at 50% of the previous dose. Should granulocytes decrease to $< 250/mm^3$ or AST/ALT increase to > 10 times the upper limit of normal, discontinue therapy.

Condylomata acuminata:

Provider-administered regimen: 1 million IU into each lesion three times weekly (alternate days) for 3 weeks. Maximum response usually observed within 4 to 8 weeks. A second course may be initiated if outcomes are unsatisfactory after 12 to 16 weeks. A maximum of five lesions may be treated during a course of therapy.

Must administer as a 1 million IU/0.1 ml concentration. Use a Tuberculin-type syringe and a 25- to 30-gauge needle. Inject intralesionally, directing the needle at the center of the wart base, at an angle almost parallel to the skin. Use care not to inject subcutaneously. A small wheal should be expected to appear at the injection site.

Other FDA-approved uses include hairy cell leukemia, follicular lymphoma, chronic hepatitis C, and chronic hepatitis B. Other dermatology (unapproved) uses have included Behçet's disease, basal cell carcinoma, and squamous cell carcinoma.

Monitoring

Prior to and periodically during therapy: CBC with differential, hemoglobin, TSH (in patients with pre-existing thyroid abnormalities, every 3 months), serum chemistry, blood glucose (especially with pre-existing diabetes mellitus), liver and renal function tests, ECG (with pre-existing cardiac abnormalities), and ophthalmologic examination (in patients with visual changes).

Specifically for malignant melanoma patients, it is recommended to monitor WBC with differential and liver function tests weekly during the initiation phase and monthly for the remainder of therapy.

Pharmacology

Endogenous interferons (IFNs) are proteins or glycoproteins produced primarily from leukocytes (IFNα), fibroblasts (IFNβ), and immune cells (IFNγ). Biologic

Interferon α-2b (Intron A)

action occurs via IFN binding to specific cell-surface receptors, subsequently affecting intracellular processes. Actions include antiviral, immunomodulatory, and antiproliferative effects. Commercially available IFNα-2a and IFNα-2b are of recombinant DNA origin (using genetically engineered *Escherichia coli*) and differ at only one position in the amino acid sequence. Although FDA-labeled for different uses, evidence is lacking to suggest significant differences in clinical actions between the available IFNαs.

In the treatment of AIDS-related Kaposi's sarcoma, greater response is observed in patients otherwise asymptomatic, with no prior opportunistic infection, and a baseline CD4 lymphocyte count of > 200 cells/mm^3.

Adverse Effects/Precautions

IFNα-2b can cause and/or aggravate fatal or life-threatening neuropsychiatric, autoimmune, ischemic, and infectious disorders. Patients should be monitored closely with periodic clinical and laboratory evaluations. Patients with persistently severe or worsening signs or symptoms of these conditions should be withdrawn from therapy. Use caution or avoid treatment in patients with pre-existing debilitating conditions such as cardiac disease, pulmonary disease, diabetes mellitus, autoimmune diseases, immunosuppression, decompensated liver disease, myelosuppression, and thyroid abnormalities.

Most common: flu-like illness (e.g. fever, chills, myalgia, fatigue), gastrointestinal distress, weight loss, taste disturbances, dizziness, decreased mental status, coughing, alopecia, and rash.

Less common: cardiac adversities (e.g. palpitations, arrhythmia), neutropenia/thrombocytopenia, peripheral neuropathy, renal failure (rare), hepatic transaminase elevations, retinal toxicity, and exacerbation of psoriasis.

Depression and suicidal ideation have occurred. CNS effects include somnolence, agitation, seizure disorders, and psychotic disturbances.

Use caution or avoid treatment in patients with pre-existing debilitating conditions such as cardiac disease, pulmonary disease, diabetes mellitus, autoimmune diseases, immunosuppression, decompensated liver disease, myelosuppression, and thyroid abnormalities. Avoid use in AIDS patients with rapidly progressive visceral disease.

Pregnancy: FDA category C.

Drug Interactions

Myelosuppressive agents (additive toxicity); reduced hepatic elimination of theophylline (and potentially other drugs metabolized by CYP450); CNS depressants (additive toxicity); interleukin-2 (potential renal failure).

Special Considerations

Consider subcutaneous administration (instead of intramuscular) in patients with thrombocytopenia. Store product under refrigeration. After powder is reconstituted, the resultant solution is stable under refrigeration for 1 month. Diluent contains benzyl alcohol.

Interferon α-2b (Intron A)

Preparation *Rx*

Intron A select product availability.

Powder for injection, with 1 ml diluent vial (bacteriostatic water for injection): 10 million IU, 18 million IU, 50 million IU.

Solution for injection: Multidose pens (each box contains disposable needles and alcohol swabs):

Six doses of 3 million IU (18 million IU) multidose pen (22.5 million IU per 1.5 ml per pen)

Six doses of 5 million IU (30 million IU) multidose pen (37.5 million IU per 1.5 ml per pen)

Six doses of 10 million IU (60 million IU) multidose pen (75 million IU per 1.5 ml per pen)

Kits:

Pak-3, containing six vials, 3 million IU per vial; six syringes, six alcohol swabs

Pak-5, containing six vials, 5 million IU per vial; six syringes, six alcohol swabs

Pak-10, containing six vials, 10 million IU per vial; six syringes, six alcohol swabs

Multidose vials:

18 million IU multidose vial (22.8 million IU per 3.8 ml per vial)

25 million IU multidose vial (32 million IU per 3.2 ml per vial)

Selected References

Beutner KR, Ferenczy A. Therapeutic approaches to genital warts. Am J Med 1997; 102: 28–37.

Centers for Disease Control and Prevention. 1998 Guidelines for treatment of sexually transmitted diseases. Morbid Mortal Weekly Rep 1998; 47: 88–98.

Hurd DS, Conte ET. Practical uses of the interferons in dermatology. Int J Dermatol 1998; 37: 881–96.

Stadler R. Interferons in dermatology: present-day standard. Dermatol Clin 1998; 16: 377–98.

Leflunomide (Arava)

Dose and Administration

Loading dose: 100 mg by mouth daily for 3 days.

Maintenance therapy: 20 mg by mouth daily, reduce to 10 mg/day if not tolerated.

Uses

FDA-approved: Rheumatoid arthritis. Other uses: Severe, treatment-resistant psoriasis.

Monitoring

Monitoring of serum hepatic enzymes is recommended at baseline monthly for the first 6 months. If stable, they may be extended to every 6 to 8 weeks thereafter.

Additionally, a baseline and monthly platelet count, white blood cell count, and hemoglobin and hematocrit should be drawn for the first 6 months, then every 6 to 8 weeks thereafter.

Pharmacology

Leflunomide is an immunomodulatory agent that inhibits the mitochondrial enzyme dihydroorotate dehydrogenase which is involved in *de novo* pyrimidine synthesis and has antiproliferative activity. Rheumatologic benefits of leflunomide are evident within 4 weeks, and efficacy is maintained for durations up to 24 months.

Adverse Effects/Precautions

WARNING: Pregnancy must be excluded before the start of treatment with leflunomide. It is contraindicated in pregnant women, or women of childbearing potential who are not using reliable contraception.

Pregnancy: FDA category X.

The most common adverse effects include diarrhea, respiratory infections, nausea, headache, rash, increased serum hepatic aminotransferases, dyspepsia, alopecia, and weight loss.

Leflunomide is not recommended in patients with severe immunodeficiencies, bone marrow dysplasias, evidence of infection with hepatitis B or C, or uncontrolled infections (because of its immunosuppression potential).

Special Considerations

Toxicity to leflunomide and its metabolites may persist long after discontinuation of the drug due to its prolonged half-life (14 days). The manufacturer recommends a drug-elimination protocol to achieve undetectable plasma concentrations after stopping leflunomide. This protocol involves administration of cholestyramine (8 g three times daily for 11 days) to expedite the excretion of leflunomide.

Preparation *Rx*

Tablets   10, 20 & 100 mg   Arava

Selected References

Affolter VK, Moore PF. Canine cutaneous and systemic histiocytosis: reactive histiocytosis of dermal dendritic cells. Am J Dermatopathol 2000; 22: 40–8.

Jarman ER, Kuba A, Montermann E, et al. Inhibition of murine IgE and immediate cutaneous hypersensitivity responses to ovalbumin by the immunomodulatory agent leflunomide. Clin Exp Immunol 1999; 115: 221–8.

Prakash A, Jarvis B. Leflunomide: a review of its use in active rheumatoid arthritis. Drugs 1999; 58: 1137–64.

Schuna AA, Megeff C. New drugs for the treatment of rheumatoid arthritis. Am J Health Syst Pharm 2000; 57: 225–34.

Leucovorin Calcium

Dose and Administration

Methotrexate rescue: Start leucovorin 24 hours after the beginning of the methotrexate infusion at a dose of 15 mg (approximately 10 mg/m^2) orally every 6 hours for 10 doses.

Megaloblastic anemia due to folic acid deficiency: Up to 1 mg orally daily.

Uses

Leucovorin is commonly used to rescue cells exposed to folate antagonists, to treat folate-deficient megaloblastic anemias, and for the prevention of methotrexate-induced toxicity following high-dose therapy or overdose.

Monitoring

Serum creatinine and methotrexate concentrations should be determined at least once daily. Leucovorin administration, hydration, and urinary alkalinization (pH of 7.0 or greater) should be continued until the methotrexate level is below 5 x 10^{-8} mol/l (0.05 micromolar). The leucovorin dose should be adjusted or leucovorin rescue extended, based on the above guidelines.

Pharmacology

Leucovorin, also referred to as folinic acid, is a racemic mixture of the isomers of the fully reduced form of folic acid. The administered L-isomer of leucovorin is rapidly metabolized to other reduced folates, which replete folate and continue the folic acid cycle. Unlike folic acid, leucovorin can bypass methotrexate-induced inhibition of folate metabolism. Thus, leucovorin (and not folic acid) should be used for the treatment of acute methotrexate overdose.

Adverse Effects/Precautions

Leucovorin is well tolerated, and adverse reactions are rare. Hypersensitivity to leucovorin or benzyl alcohol can result in urticaria and anaphylaxis. High intravenous doses have been associated with nausea/vomiting.

Pregnancy: FDA category C.

Drug Interactions

Significant drug interactions include interference with the activity of anticonvulsants such as phenytoin, phenobarbital, primidone, or other barbiturates as well as with capecitabine, fluorouracil, methotrexate, pyrimethamine, sulfamethoxazole–trimethoprim, trimethoprim, and trimetrexate.

Preparation *Rx*

Generics (former brand name, Wellcovorin)
Tablets   5, 10, 15 & 25 mg
Powder for injection   50, 100, 200, 300 & 350 mg

Mechlorethamine, Topical (Nitrogen mustard; Mustargen)

Use, Dose and Administration

Mycosis fungoides: Ointment (0.01%): Apply in an amount sufficient to cover the lesion one to four times daily for 6 to 12 months or until the lesions disappear. Continue application every 2 to 7 days if the lesions do not recur (maintenance therapy). Maintenance therapy is usually discontinued after 3 years if lesions have not recurred. Using protective gloves, the solution or ointment can be applied to the entire body surface with minimal application to the perineum, axillary, inguinal, and inframammary areas.

Monitoring

Leukocyte and platelet counts and uric acid concentrations should be monitored closely during mechlorethamine therapy.

Pharmacology

Mechlorethamine exerts its chemotherapeutic effects by substituting alkyl groups for hydrogen ions. Mechlorethamine reacts readily with phosphate, amino, hydroxyl, sulfhydryl, carboxyl, and imidazole groups on amino acids. This reaction leads to DNA–DNA interstrand and DNA–protein cross-linking, DNA strand breakage and interference in DNA replication, transcription of RNA, and nucleic acid function. Nitrogen mustard impairs protein synthesis and glycolysis and is mutagenic and radiomimetic.

Metabolites of the drug are excreted in the urine.

Adverse Effects/Precautions

WARNING: This drug is highly toxic and must be handled and administered with care. Avoid inhalation of dust or vapors and contact with skin or mucous membranes.

Pregnancy: FDA category D.

Mechlorethamine should be used cautiously in patients who have had previous myelosuppressive therapy. Severe bone marrow suppression, including neutropenia and thrombocytopenia, is a relative contraindication to mechlorethamine depending on the disease. Any active infection should be treated prior to receiving mechlorethamine, and there is increased risk of infections and/or reactivation of latent infections with treatment. Intramuscular administration and subcutaneous administration of mechlorethamine are contraindicated due to severe skin and tissue necrosis that may occur.

Dental work should be performed prior to initiating mechlorethamine therapy or deferred until blood counts return to normal, and patients should be instructed on proper oral hygiene.

Allergic and irritant dermatitis are common with topical application. Avoid vaccination and close contact with those receiving live vaccinations.

Mechlorethamine, Topical (Nitrogen mustard; Mustargen)

Drug Interactions

Owing to the thrombocytopenic effects of mechlorethamine, an additive risk of bleeding may be seen in patients receiving anticoagulants, NSAIDs, aspirin, strontium-89 chloride, and thrombolytic agents. Sargramostim, GM-CSF, and filgrastim, G-CSF, are contraindicated for use in patients within 24 hours of treatment with antineoplastic agents. Enhanced respiratory depression from succinylcholine has been reported during mechlorethamine use.

Preparation *Rx*

Powder for injection   10 mg/vial used to prepare 0.01% ointment

Selected References

Apisarnthanarax N, Talpur R, Duvic M. Treatment of cutaneous T cell lymphoma: current status and future directions. Am J Clin Dermatol 2002; 3: 193–215.

Kim YH. Management with topical nitrogen mustard in mycosis fungoides. Dermatol Ther 2003; 16: 288–98.

Muche JM, Gellrich S, Sterry W. Treatment of cutaneous T-cell lymphomas. Semin Cutan Med Surg 2000; 19: 142–8.

Zackheim HS. Cutaneous T-cell lymphoma: update of treatment. Dermatology 1999; 199: 102–5.

Methotrexate (Rheumatrex)

Dose and Administration

Weekly single oral or IM dose: Start with 2.5 to 5 mg/week test dose, then 10 to 25 mg/week until adequate response is achieved.

Divided oral dose schedule: 2.5 mg at 12-hour intervals for three doses. Gradually adjust dose to achieve optimal clinical response, not to exceed 30 mg/week.

Once the optimal response is achieved, reduce dosage to the lowest possible amount and longest possible rest period. Supplement with folic acid 1 mg daily.

Uses

FDA-approved: Severe, recalcitrant, disabling psoriasis not controlled by other therapies (only when the diagnosis is firmly established by biopsy or dermatologic consultation), rheumatoid arthritis, and multiple neoplastic diseases. Other uses include mycosis fungoides, sarcoidosis, vasculitis, systemic lupus erythematosus, and other severe, refractory inflammatory diseases.

Monitoring

Baseline assessment should include a complete blood count with differential and platelet counts, hepatic enzymes, renal function tests, and a chest X-ray. During therapy of rheumatoid arthritis and psoriasis, monitoring of these parameters is recommended: hematology at least monthly, renal function and liver function every 1 to 2 months. More frequent monitoring is indicated when changing the dose and during periods of increased risk of elevated methotrexate concentrations (e.g. dehydration).

Pharmacology

Methotrexate inhibits dihydrofolate reductase interfering with DNA synthesis and repair. Actively proliferating tissues (malignant cells, bone marrow, fetal cells, and mucosal cells) are generally more sensitive to this effect. Use in psoriasis is based on the rapid growth of psoriasis epithelium, but the effectiveness may be due to an anti-inflammatory effect.

The half-life is 3 to 10 hours in patients receiving doses commonly used in psoriasis. 80 to 90% of the drug is excreted in the urine within 24 hours. Elimination is reduced in patients with impaired renal function.

Adverse Effects/Precautions

In the event of toxicity/overdosage, leucovorin is indicated to diminish the toxicity and counteract the effects.

Most reactions are reversible if detected early; the dose should be reduced or stopped, and leucovorin used if necessary.

Hematologic: Severe anemia, leukopenia and/or thrombocytopenia.

Gastrointestinal: Acute or chronic hepatotoxicity may occur. Chronic hepatotoxicity may be life-threatening, is related to total cumulative doses, is not always detected by liver function tests, and may require liver biopsy for detection. Diarrhea and ulcerative stomatitis require interruption of therapy; otherwise, hemorrhagic enteritis and death from intestinal perforation could occur.

Methotrexate (Rheumatrex)

Pulmonary: Pulmonary symptoms/pneumonitis may occur and may require discontinuation of treatment and evaluation for possible infectious etiology.

Skin: Radiation dermatitis and sunburn may be 'recalled'. May cause hair loss. Mouth sores may occur and may be reduced by folate supplementation.

Other frequently reported adverse reactions include oral ulceration, leukopenia, nausea, abdominal distress, malaise, fatigue, chills, fever, dizziness, and decreased resistance to infection.

Pregnancy: FDA category X. Pregnancy should be avoided if either partner is using methotrexate (during and for a minimum of 3 months after therapy for males and during and for at least one ovulatory cycle after therapy for females).

Drug Interactions

Increased methotrexate toxicity

Penicillins and probenecid (reduced renal tubular secretion).

Sulfonamides and trimethoprim (additive effect on folate inhibition).

Salicylates, phenylbutazone, phenytoin, and sulfonamides (displacement from albumin). Nonsteroidal anti-inflammatory drugs may be used in combination with methotrexate; however, unexpectedly severe bone marrow suppression and gastrointestinal toxicity have been reported.

Increased hepatotoxicity with acitretin (or other retinoids) and alcohol.

Increased risk of infection when used in combination with live vaccines.

Preparation *Rx*

Rheumatrex:
Tablets	2.5 mg
Solution for injection	50, 100, 200 & 250 mg

Selected References

Baughman RP. Methotrexate for sarcoidosis. Sarcoidosis Vasculitis Diffuse Lung Dis 1998; 15: 147–9.

Passo MH, Hashkes PJ. Use of methotrexate in children. Bull Rheum Dis 1998; 47: 1–5.

Roenigk HH Jr, Auerbach R, Maibach H, et al. Methotrexate in psoriasis: consensus conference. J Am Acad Dermatol 1998; 38: 478–85.

Shiroky JB. The use of folates concomitantly with low-dose pulse methotrexate. Rheum Dis Clin North Am 1997; 23: 969–80.

Wilke WS. Methotrexate use in miscellaneous inflammatory diseases. Rheum Dis Clin North Am 1997; 23: 855–82.

Methyl Aminolevulinate (Metvix)

Dose and Administration

WARNING: This cream has demonstrated a high rate of contact sensitization. Nitrile gloves should be worn (not vinyl or latex).

This product is not intended for application by patients or unqualified medical personnel and is therefore only dispensed to physicians.

Photodynamic therapy for non-hyperkeratotic actinic keratosis with methyl aminolevulinate is a multi-stage process. Two treatment sessions 7 days apart should be conducted. Not more than 1 g (1/2 tube) should be applied per treatment session. One session consists of:

Lesion debriding: Before applying the cream, the surface of the lesions should be prepared with a small dermal curette to remove scales and crusts and roughen the surface of the lesion. This is to facilitate access of the cream and light to all parts of the lesion. Only nitrile gloves should be worn during this and subsequent steps and Universal Precautions should be taken. Vinyl and latex gloves do not provide adequate protection when using this product.

Application of cream: Using a spatula, apply a layer of cream about 1 mm thick to the lesion and the surrounding 5 mm of normal skin. Do not apply more than 1 g of cream for each patient per treatment session. The area to which the cream has been applied should then be covered with an occlusive, non-absorbent dressing for 3 hours. Multiple lesions may be treated during the same treatment session. Each treatment field is limited to a diameter of 55 mm. Only nitrile gloves should be worn by the qualified health-care provider in order to avoid skin contact with the cream.

Wait for 3 hours (at least 2.5, no more than 4 hours). After application, patients should avoid exposure of the photosensitive sites to sunlight or bright indoor light during the period prior to red light treatment (may result in stinging or burning and may cause erythema and/or edema of lesions).

Removal of dressing and rinsing off excess cream: Following removal of the occlusive dressing, clean the area with saline and gauze. Nitrile gloves should be worn at this step by the trained physician.

Illumination of the treated lesion: Ensure the correct light dose is administered. The light intensity at the lesion surface should not be higher than $200 \, mW/cm^2$. Patient and operator should adhere to safety instructions and Universal Precautions provided with the lamp. The patient and operator should wear protective goggles during illumination. Patients should be advised that transient stinging and/or burning at the target lesion sites may occur during the period of light exposure.

The CureLight BroadBand Model CureLight 01 lamp is approved for use with PDT with methyl aminolevulinate. The lamp should be carefully calibrated so that dosing is accurate and immediately thereafter the lesion should be exposed to red light with a continuous spectrum of 570 to 670 nm and a total light dose of $75 \, J/cm^2$. Use disposable protective plastic sleeves on the positioning device and on the light measuring probe and discard each sleeve after each patient treatment. Use of the cream without subsequent red light illumination is not recommended.

Lesion response should be assessed 3 months after treatment.

Methyl Aminolevulinate (Metvix)

Uses

FDA-approved: Non-hyperkeratotic actinic keratosis of the face and scalp in immunocompetent patients when used in conjunction with lesion preparation (debridement using a sharp dermal curette) in the physician's office, when other therapies are unacceptable or considered less appropriate.

Other uses: Superficial and nodular basal cell carcinomas.

Pharmacology

Photosensitization occurs through metabolic conversion of methyl aminolevulinate (prodrug) to photoactive porphyrins that accumulate in the skin lesions to which the cream has been applied. When phototherapy is applied to the treated region, the accumulated photoactive porphyrins produce a photodynamic reaction, resulting in a cytotoxic process dependent on the simultaneous presence of oxygen. The absorption of light results in an excited state of porphyrin molecules, and subsequent spin transfer from photoactive porphyrins to molecular oxygen generates singlet oxygen, which can further react to form superoxide and hydroxyl radicals.

Three hours after application of the cream, the fluorescence in the treated lesions was significantly greater than that seen in both treated and untreated normal skin, and after application of vehicle cream to normal skin. After application for 28 hours and subsequent illumination (as approved), complete photobleaching of Protoporphyrin IX occurred with levels of Protoporphyrin IX, returning to pretreatment values within 1 hour after illumination.

Contraindications

Cutaneous photosensitivity, known allergies to porphyrins, peanut and almond oil.

Adverse Effects/Precautions

During the period prior to red light treatment, patients should avoid exposure of the treatment sites to sunlight or bright indoor light (may result in stinging and/or burning or erythema and/or edema). After illumination, patients should keep the area covered and take light exposure precautions for at least 48 hours (e.g. wide-brimmed hat, opaque clothing). Sunscreen will not provide protection.

The patient, operator, and other persons should wear protective goggles during the red light treatment.

Methyl aminolevulinate is an irritant and sensitizer. The most common dermatologic adverse effect is phototoxicity; other adverse effects include erythema, burning, stinging, pain in the skin, local erythema, crusting, skin edema, skin peeling, blisters, and pruritus. Nitrile gloves should be worn during application.

Pregnancy: FDA category C.

Drug Interactions

It is possible that concomitant use of other drugs that cause photosensitization (e.g. tetracyclines, phenothiazides, sulfonylureas, thiazide diuretics, and griseofulvin) will increase the photosensitivity reaction.

Methyl Aminolevulinate (Metvix)

Preparation

Cream   16.8%   Metvix   2 g

Selected References

Foley P. Clinical efficacy of methyl aminolevulinate (Metvix) photodynamic therapy. J Dermatol Treat 2003; 14 (Suppl 3):15–22.

Freeman M, Vinciullo C, Francis D, et al. A comparison of photodynamic therapy using topical methyl aminolevulinate (Metvix) with single cycle cryotherapy in patients with actinic keratosis: a prospective, randomized study. J Dermatol Treat 2003; 14: 99–106.

Horn M, Wolf P, Wulf HC, et al. Topical methyl aminolaevulinate photodynamic therapy in patients with basal cell carcinoma prone to complications and poor cosmetic outcome with conventional treatment. Br J Dermatol 2003; 149: 1242–9.

Pariser DM, Lowe NJ, Stewart DM, et al. Photodynamic therapy with topical methyl aminolevulinate for actinic keratosis: results of a prospective randomized multicenter trial. J Am Acad Dermatol 2003; 48: 227–32.

Rhodes LE, de Rie M, Enstrom Y, et al. Photodynamic therapy using topical methyl aminolevulinate vs. surgery for nodular basal cell carcinoma: results of a multicenter randomized prospective trial. Arch Dermatol 2004; 140: 17–23.

Siddiqui MA, Petty CM, Scott LJ. Topical methyl aminolevulinate. Am J Clin Dermatol 2004; 5: 127–37.

Mycophenolate Mofetil (CellCept) and Mycophenolic Acid (Myfortic)

Dose and Administration

Psoriasis: Initial dose, 1 g orally twice daily, may increase to 1.5 g twice daily if needed. Doses of up to 4 or 5 g/day have been used.

Uses

FDA approved: In combination with cyclosporine and corticosteroids to prevent rejection in patients receiving renal and cardiac transplants.

Other indications include psoriasis and other inflammatory skin diseases.

Monitoring

Complete blood count weekly during the first month, twice monthly for the second and third months of treatment, then monthly through the first year.

Pharmacology

Mycophenolate mofetil is rapidly absorbed and converted to the active metabolite mycophenolate acid (MPA). MPA is a potent inhibitor of inosine monophosphate dehydrogenase, inhibiting formation of guanosine nucleotides. Because T and B lymphocytes are critically dependent on synthesis of purines, MPA has potent cytostatic effects on lymphocytes. The half-life following oral administration is 18 hours.

Adverse Effects/Precautions

Principle adverse reactions include diarrhea, vomiting, leukopenia, and sepsis.

Up to 2% of patients develop severe neutropenia. Opportunistic infections may occur, particulary herpes simplex, herpes zoster, and cytomegalovirus infections. Lymphoproliferative disorders have also been observed.

Pregnancy: FDA category C. Women of childbearing potential should have a negative pregnancy test within 1 week prior to beginning therapy and effective contraception should be used before beginning therapy, during therapy and for 6 weeks following discontinuation of therapy.

Drug Interactions

Antacids and cholestyramine inhibit absorption. Probenecid (and probably other inhibitors of renal tubular secretion) reduces renal clearance of the drug. Administration of live vaccines is not recommended.

Preparation *Rx*

Mycophenolate mofetil (CellCept)

Capsules	250 mg
Tablets	500 mg
Oral suspension	200 mg/ml, 225 ml
Injection	500 mg

Mycophenolic acid (Myfortic)

Tablets, enteric coated/delayed release	180 & 360 mg

Selected References

Grundmann-Kollmann M, Korting HC, Behrens S, et al. Mycophenolate mofetil: a new therapeutic option in the treatment of blistering autoimmune diseases. J Am Acad Dermatol 1999; 40: 957–60.

Haufs MG, Beissert S, Grabbe B, et al. Psoriasis vulgaris treated successfully with mycophenolate mofetil. Br J Dermatol 1998; 138: 179–81.

Tong DW, Walder BK. Widespread plaque psoriasis responsive to mycophenolate mofetil. Aust J Dermatol 1999; 40: 135–7.

Pimecrolimus (Elidel)

Dose and Administration

Apply a thin layer of cream twice daily as long as signs/symptoms persist. May use on all skin surfaces. Re-evaluate patient if symptoms persist longer than 6 weeks. Do not use with occlusive dressings.

Use

FDA-approved: Mild-to-moderate atopic dermatitis (short-term and intermittent long-term), in nonimmunocompromised patients 2 years of age and older in whom the use of alternative, conventional therapies are inadvisable due to potential risks, inadequate response, or intolerance.

Other: Limited data on efficacy in plaque psoriasis (when used under occlusion), allergic contact dermatitis, seborrheic dermatitis, lichen planus, and vitiligo.

Pharmacology

Immunomodulator that presumably inhibits T-cell activation by inhibiting calcineurin.

Adverse Effects/Precautions

No information with use in clinically infected atopic dermatitis; allow infections to clear. Predisposition to superficial skin infection such as varicella zoster virus, herpes simplex virus, or eczema herpeticum.

Evaluate etiology of any treatment-emergent lymphadenopathy.

Patients should minimize or avoid exposure to artificial or natural sunlight.

Local symptoms, such as burning or pruritus, may occur but usually resolve as lesions heal.

Pregnancy: FDA category C.

Drug Interactions

Unlikely, based on minimal absorption, but use caution with drugs that inhibit or induce the CYP3A hepatic microsomal enzyme system.

Preparation *Rx*

Cream	1%	Elidel	30, 60 & 100 g

Selected References

Brownell I, Quan LT, Hsu S. Topical pimecrolimus in the treatment of seborrheic dermatitis. Dermatol Online J 2003; 9: 13.

Eichenfield LF, Lucky AW, Boguniewicz M, et al. 1% pimecrolimus cream for atopic dermatitis. Arch Dermatol 2003; 139: 1369–70.

Griffiths CE. Ascomycin: an advance in the management of atopic dermatitis. Br J Dermatol 2001; 144: 679–81.

Hebert AA, Warken KA, Cherill R. Pimecrolimus cream 1%: A new development in nonsteroid topical treatment of inflammatory skin diseases. Semin Cutan Med Surg 2001; 20: 260–7.

Ho VC, Gupta A, Kaufmann R, et al. Safety and efficacy of nonsteroid pimecrolimus cream 1% in the treatment of atopic dermatitis in infants. J Pediatr 2003; 142: 155–62.

Mayoral FA, Gonzalez C, Shah NS, Arciniegas C. Repigmentation of vitiligo with pimecrolimus cream: a case report. Dermatology 2003; 207: 322–3.

Wellington K, Spencer CM. SDZ ASM 981. BioDrugs 2000; 14: 409–16.

Wolff K, Stuetz A. Pimecrolimus for the treatment of inflammatory skin disease. Expert Opin Pharmacother 2004; 5: 643–55.

Quinacrine (formerly Atabrine)

Use, Dose, and Administration

Dermatology Use

Lupus erythematosus: 100 mg orally daily. After maximal response is achieved (allow up to 6 months), taper by 1 day per week every 2 months. Maintenance dose is one to three tablets per week.

Pharmacology

Historically used as treatment for and suppression of malaria and certain intestinal cestodes (e.g. giardiasis). Has fallen out of favor for anti-infective indications. Possesses a variety of actions and appears to work in lupus erythematosus by inhibiting DNA and RNA polymerase and binding to nucleoproteins, resulting in inhibition of lupus erythematosus cell factor.

Adverse Effects/Precautions

May precipitate or exacerbate porphyria or psoriasis. Aplastic anemia is rare but warrants monitoring of CBC. Ocular effects have included corneal deposits and retinopathy. Seizures have been reported but may be potentiated by concomitant corticosteroids. Hepatitis (rare).

More frequently has caused headache, dizziness, central nervous system irritability, and toxic psychosis. Also frequently causes gastrointestinal distress (e.g. nausea, vomiting, abdominal cramps, diarrhea). Associated with discoloration of urine.

Dermatologic effects include skin discoloration (yellow), eczematous eruptions, lichenoid exfoliative type reactions. Although urine and skin may turn yellow, evaluate patient for liver effects if eyes turn yellow.

Special Considerations/Preparations

Commercially available product (Atabrine) discontinued in the 1990s. Oral dosage form must be compounded using quinacrine powder. Caution in that certain Internet sites offer quinacrine, typically as part of a female sterilization kit; these products and use are not approved by the FDA and pose a consumer health hazard. Has been prepared in capsules or powder envelopes. The powder has a bitter taste, which may be masked by administration in applesauce, jelly, etc. Is not stable as a solution.

Selected References

Clark SK. Cutaneous lupus erythematosus. Postgrad Med 1986; 795: 195–203.

Wallace DJ. The use of quinacrine (Atabrine) in rheumatic diseases: a reexamination. Semin Arthritis Rheum 1989; 18: 282–97.

Werth V, Franks JR. Treatment of discoid skin lesions with azathioprine. Arch Dermatol 1986; 122: 746–7.

Sulfapyridine

Dose and Administration

Dermatitis herpetiformis: Give 250 to 1000 mg orally four times daily initially until improvement occurs. The dose should then be decreased to the lowest effective dose to minimize toxicity. Usually 1 to 4 g/day are needed for disease control.

Uses

Used as an alternative to dapsone for dermatitis herpetiformis, pyoderma gangrenosum, pemphigus vulgaris, and subcorneal pustular dermatosis.

Monitoring

Complete blood counts and liver function tests should be obtained at baseline and monitored periodically throughout therapy. Patients of Asian, African-American and Mediterranean descent should be screened for glucose-6-phosphate dehydrogenase (G-6-PD) deficiency prior to initiating sulfapyridine therapy.

Pharmacology

Sulfapyridine is a sulfonamide antibacterial that competitively antagonizes the formation of dihydrofolic acid from *para*-aminobenzoic acid (PABA) via competitive inhibition of dihydropteroate synthetase. It is no longer used, however, as an antibacterial because less toxic agents are available. Its main use is for dermatologic conditions such as dermatitis herpetiformis. Although its mechanism of action in dermatologic diseases is unknown, it may alter the protein content of glycosaminoglycans, which decreases tissue viscosity and edema that precede the formation of vesicles or bullae. These effects are thought to contribute to its efficacy in a variety of skin disorders that are characterized by granulocytic inflammation and bulla formation.

Sulfapyridine is slowly and incompletely absorbed from the gastrointestinal tract. It is extensively metabolized in the liver and subsequently excreted in the urine.

Adverse Effects/Precautions

Nausea, vomiting, and diarrhea are common adverse effects. Hematologic adverse effects include leukopenia, thrombocytopenia, agranulocytosis, and aplastic anemia. Patients with G-6-PD deficiency suffer more severe adverse hematologic effects and should not receive sulfapyridine. Cutaneous hypersensitivity manifested as exfoliative dermatitis, erythema multiforme, toxic epidermal necrolysis, Stevens–Johnson syndrome, urticaria, and erythema nodosum has been reported. Sulfapyridine should not be used in patients who have experienced hypersensitivity reactions with sulfonamides. Toxic hepatitis and fulminant hepatic necrosis may occur rarely. Patients are at risk for kidney stones secondary to crystalluria. They should be instructed to drink plenty of fluids to prevent kidney stone formation.

Drug Interactions

Sulfapyridine can potentiate the hypoprothrombinemic effects of warfarin. Prothrombin times and INRs should be monitored closely and warfarin doses decreased as warranted. When combined with sulfonylureas (e.g. glyburide, glipizide), hypoglycemia may occur secondary to displacement of the sulfonylurea

Sulfapyridine

from protein binding sites. Additionally, concomitant administration with methotrexate can lead to methotrexate displacement from protein. As a result, bone marrow suppression may occur. Sulfapyridine should be combined cautiously with other medications, including methotrexate, which can cause bone marrow suppression.

Special Considerations

Currently sulfapyridine is not commercially available in the United States; however, it can be obtained on a limited basis for dermatologic indications as part of an investigational phase III compassionate use program. To obtain the product, contact Jacobus Pharmaceutical Company, Inc. (609-921-7447). The product will be supplied to registered physicians at no cost who can then dispense the drug to qualifying patients. Patients must agree to provide informed consent. The product is currently awaiting reapproval from the Food and Drug Administration for marketing in the United States.

Preparation

Tablets   500 mg

Selected References

Fry L. Fine points in the management of dermatitis herpetiformis. Semin Dermatol 1988; 7: 206–11.

Stone OJ. Sulfapyride and sulfones decrease glycosaminoglycan viscosity in dermatitis herpetiformis, ulcerative colitis, and pyoderma gangrenosum. Med Hypotheses 1990; 31: 99–103.

Uetrecht J. Dapsone and sulfapyridine. Clin Dermatol 1989; 7: 111–20.

Sulfasalazine (Azulfidine)

Dose and Administration

Ulcerative colitis: Initiate therapy as 1 to 2 g orally per day in divided doses to minimize gastrointestinal upset. Usual maintenance doses are between 3 and 4 g/day. Daily doses of 12 g should not be exceeded.

Rheumatoid arthritis: Usual dose is 2 g/day given in divided doses.

Dermatologic indications: Doses ranging from 1 to 6 g/day may be required depending on the indication. Once improvement occurs, the dose should then be decreased to the lowest effective dose to minimize toxicity.

Uses

FDA-approved: Treatment of ulcerative colitis and rheumatoid arthritis. Also used for Crohn's disease, psoriatic arthritis, ankylosing spondylitis, dermatitis herpetiformis, discoid lupus erythematosus, and pyoderma gangrenosum.

Monitoring

Complete blood counts and liver function tests should be obtained at baseline and monitored periodically throughout therapy. Patients of Asian, African-American and Mediterranean descent should be screened for glucose-6-phosphate dehydrogenase (G-6-PD) deficiency prior to initiating sulfasalazine therapy.

Pharmacology

Sulfasalazine is a sulfonamide derivative that is cleaved to 5-aminosalicyclic acid (mesalamine) and sulfapyridine once ingested. Although its mechanism of action in dermatologic diseases is unknown, several hypotheses have been formed. These include inhibition of the cyclo-oxygenase and lipoxygenase pathways of the arachidonic acid cascade with subsequent inhibition of prostaglandin and leukotriene formation, a decrease in lymphocyte activation, and inhibition of folate metabolism. Sulfasalazine is generally reserved as an alternative to other dermatologic agents secondary to its adverse effect profile. Approximately 15% of sulfasalazine is absorbed in the small intestine, whereas 85% is cleaved by intestinal flora in the colon to sulfapyridine and 5-aminosalicylic acid. Subsequent excretion occurs in the urine.

Adverse Effects/Precautions

Nausea, vomiting, diarrhea, and anorexia are common adverse effects. Adverse central nervous system effects include headache, dizziness, malaise, and confusion. Hematologic adverse effects include leukopenia, thrombocytopenia, agranulocytosis, and aplastic anemia. Patients with G-6-PD deficiency should not receive sulfasalazine. Cutaneous hypersensitivity manifested as exfoliative dermatitis, erythema multiforme, toxic epidermal necrolysis, Stevens–Johnson syndrome, urticaria, and erythema nodosum has been reported. May cause body fluids, contact lenses, or skin to turn yellow-orange. Sulfasalazine should not be used in patients who have experienced hypersensitivity reactions with sulfonamides. Toxic hepatitis and fulminant hepatic necrosis may occur rarely. Patients are at risk for kidney stones secondary to crystalluria. They should be instructed to drink plenty of fluids to

Sulfasalazine (Azulfidine)

prevent kidney stone formation. Oligospermia and infertility have been observed in men treated with sulfasalazine.

Pregnancy: FDA category B.

Drug Interactions

Sulfasalazine can potentiate the hypoprothrombinemic effects of warfarin. Prothrombin times and INRs should be monitored closely and warfarin doses decreased as warranted. When combined with sulfonylureas (e.g. glyburide, glipizide), hypoglycemia may occur secondary to displacement of the sulfonylurea from protein binding sites. Additionally, concomitant administration with methotrexate can lead to methotrexate displacement from protein. As a result, bone marrow suppression may occur. Sulfasalazine should be combined cautiously with other medications, including methotrexate, which can cause bone marrow suppression.

Preparation *Rx*

Tablets	500 mg	Azulfidine
		Various generics
Enteric-coated extended-release tablets	500 mg	Azulfidine EN-tabs

Selected References

Clegg DO, Reda DJ, Mejias E, et al. Comparison of sulfasalazine and placebo in the treatment of psoriatic arthritis. A Department of Veterans Affairs Cooperative Study. Arthritis Rheum 1996; 39: 2013–20.

Hoult JRS. Pharmacological and biochemical actions of sulphasalazine. Drugs 1986; 32(Suppl 1): 18–26.

Newman ED, Perruquet JL, Harrington TM. Sulfasalazine therapy in psoriatic arthritis: clinical and immunologic response. J Rheumatol 1991; 18: 1379–82.

Tacrolimus, Systemic (Prograf)

Uses, Dose and Administration

Systemic tacrolimus can be administered orally and intravenously. Dose and administration vary depending on which condition is being treated.

Psoriasis: An initial dose for psoriasis of 0.05 mg/kg per day has been used, and, in cases of insufficient efficacy, has been increased to 0.10 and 0.15 mg/kg per day at the end of weeks 3 and 6, respectively.

Other: Other FDA-approved uses include prophylaxis in liver and kidney allograft recipients, as well as liver and kidney allograft rejections resistant to conventional immunosuppressive drugs.

Monitoring

Monitoring of tacrolimus plasma concentrations is recommended, particularly if any of the hepatic enzyme-inducing or -inhibiting agents are used concurrently with tacrolimus. Monitoring is also necessary to evaluate rejection (for transplant patients), toxicity, dosage, and compliance. Two methods are used for the assay of tacrolimus that use the same monoclonal antibody, enzyme-linked immunosorbent assay (ELISA) and a microparticle enzyme immunoassay (MEIA). Therapeutic concentrations for organ transplant patients range from 7 ng/ml to 20 ng/ml.

Pharmacology

Tacrolimus is a macrolide lactone isolated from *Streptomyces tsukubaensis*. Tacrolimus inhibits a calcium/calmodulin-dependent phosphatase enzyme, calcineurin, which is important in T-cell proliferation. Tacrolimus binds to cytoplasmic enzymes called FK-binding proteins. This complex then inhibits calcineurin, which inhibits the T-cell activators IL-2, IL-3, IL-4, GM-CSF, TNF-α, and γ-interferon. Reduction of T-cell activators results in the inhibition of T-cell proliferative responses to antigens and mitogens.

Metabolism of tacrolimus is mainly by the hepatic cytochrome P450 enzyme system. The elimination half-life in liver transplant patients is about 12 hours, compared with 21 hours in healthy volunteers. Tacrolimus is 100 times more potent than cyclosporine, and clinical improvement has been seen in rejection status, prolonged graft survival, and reduced need for steroid therapy.

Adverse Effects/Precautions

The most common adverse effects reported are tremors, headache, insomnia, diarrhea, nausea, anemia, alopecia, and renal impairment. Mild to moderate hypertension may develop; antihypertensive therapy may be required (consider drug interactions).

Tacrolimus has been shown to cause diabetes mellitus. Patients who show classical signs such as polydipsia or polyuria should consult their physician.

High doses may cause nephrotoxicity and neurotoxicity.

May cause hyperkalemia, therefore the use of potassium-sparing diuretics should be avoided.

Tacrolimus, Systemic (Prograf)

Tacrolimus has been shown to cause myocardial hypertrophy in infants, children, and adults. The condition appears to be reversible with dose reduction or discontinuance of therapy.

Increased risk for acquiring infections and possible development of lymphoma, due to the immunosuppressive nature of the drug.

Pregnancy: FDA category C.

Drug Interactions

Tacrolimus is metabolized by the hepatic CYP3A enzyme. Drugs that inhibit or induce this system may increase or decrease tacrolimus concentrations in the blood. Consult product labeling for complete information.

Drugs that may *increase* tacrolimus concentrations include calcium channel blockers, ketoconazole, itraconazole, clarithromycin, erythromycin, protease inhibitors, cimetidine, and metoclopramide.

Drugs that may *decrease* tacrolimus concentrations include carbamazepine, phenobarbital, phenytoin, rifampin, and rifabutin.

Tacrolimus should not be given with food, especially foods with moderate to high fat content. Tacrolimus should not be used concurrently with cyclosporine.

The administration of live vaccines is not recommended.

Preparation *Rx*

Capsules	0.5, 1 & 5 mg
Injection	5 mg/ml

Selected References

Anonymous. Systemic tacrolimus (FK 506) is effective for the treatment of psoriasis in a double-blind, placebo-controlled study. The European FK 506 Multicentre Psoriasis Study Group. Arch Dermatol 1996; 132: 419–23.

Assmann T, Homey B, Ruzicka T. Applications of tacrolimus for the treatment of skin disorders. Immunopharmacology 2000; 47: 203–13.

Jegasothy BV, Ackerman CD, Todo S, et al. Tacrolimus (FK 506) – a new therapeutic agent for severe recalcitrant psoriasis. Arch Dermatol 1992; 128: 781–5.

Remitz A, Reitamo S, Erkko P, et al. Tacrolimus ointment improves psoriasis in a microplaque assay. Br J Dermatol 1999; 141: 103–7.

Vente C, Reich K, Rupprecht R, Neumann C. Erosive mucosal lichen planus: response to topical treatment with tacrolimus. Br J Dermatol 1999; 140: 338–42.

Weichert G, Saucher DN. Efficacy of tacrolimus (FK 506) in idiopathic treatment-resistant pyoderma gangrenosum. J Am Acad Dermatol 1998; 39: 648–50.

Tacrolimus, Topical (Protopic)

Dose and Administration

Apply a thin layer of ointment twice daily. Treatment should be continued for 1 week after signs and symptoms have cleared. The 0.1% strength is for adults only; the 0.03% strength may be used in adults and children. Do not use with occlusive dressings.

Use

FDA-approved: Moderate-to-severe atopic dermatitis (short-term and intermittent long-term), in patients 2 years of age and older in whom the use of alternative, conventional therapies are inadvisable due to potential risks, inadequate response, or intolerance.

Other: Limited documentation for psoriasis, oral lichen planus, and seborrheic dermatitis. When combined with salicylic acid to increase penetration it is effective in treatment of plaque psoriasis.

Pharmacology

Immunomodulator that presumably inhibits T-cell activation by inhibiting calcineurin.

Adverse Effects/Precautions

No information with use in clinically infected atopic dermatitis; allow infections to clear. Predisposition to superficial skin infection such as varicella zoster virus, herpes simplex virus, or eczema herpeticum.

Evaluate etiology of any treatment-emergent lymphadenopathy.

Patients should minimize or avoid exposure to artificial or natural sunlight.

Local symptoms, such as burning or pruritus, may occur but usually resolve as lesions heal.

Pregnancy: FDA category C.

Drug Interactions

Unlikely, based on minimal absorption, but use caution with drugs that inhibit or induce the CYP3A hepatic microsomal enzyme system.

Preparation *Rx*

Ointment   0.1 & 0.03%   Protopic   30, 60 & 100 g

Selected References

Carroll CL, Clarke J, Camacho F, et al. Topical tacrolimus ointment combined with 6% salicylic acid gel for plaque psoriasis treatment. Arch Dermatol 2005; 141: 43–6

Carroll CL, Fleischer AB Jr. Tacrolimus ointment: the treatment of atopic dermatitis and other inflammatory cutaneous disease. Expert Opin Pharmacother 2004; 5: 2127-37.

Hodgson TA, Sahni N, Kaliakatsou F, et al. Long-term efficacy and safety of topical tacrolimus in the management of ulcerative/erosive oral lichen planus. Eur J Dermatol 2003; 13: 466-70.

Housman TS, Norton AB, Feldman ST, et al. Tacrolimus ointment: utilization patterns in children under age 2 years. Dermatol Online J 2004; 10: 2.

Remitz A, Reitamo S, Erkko P, et al. Tacrolimus ointment improves psoriasis in a microplaque assay. Br J Dermatol 1999; 141: 103-7.

Thalidomide (Thalomid)

WARNING: Thalidomide can cause severe birth defects even with a single dose. Women of childbearing age who receive thalidomide should use at least two forms of reliable contraception 1 month prior to the first dose, during treatment, and for 1 month after the last dose of thalidomide. In addition, these women should have regular pregnancy tests.

Dose and Administration

Erythema nodosum leprosum	100–400 mg/day
Severe, recurrent aphthous stomatitis	50–400 mg/day
Behçet's syndrome	200–400 mg/day
Prurigo nodularis	5–300 mg/day
Actinic prurigo	100–300 mg/day
Erythema multiforme	100–200 mg/day
Graft-versus-host disease	100–800 mg/day
Discoid lupus erythematosus	100–400 mg/day
Sarcoidosis	100–200 mg/day
Rheumatoid arthritis	300–600 mg/day
Pyoderma gangrenosum	100–400 mg/day
Jessner–Kanof disease	100 mg/day
Postherpetic neuralgia	100–300 mg/day
Uremic pruritus	100 mg/day
Palmoplantar pustulosis	100–200 mg/day
AIDS-associated proctitis	300 mg/day
Bullous pemphigoid	50–100 mg/day
Cicatricial pemphigoid	50–100 mg/day

Indications

FDA-approved: Acute treatment of the cutaneous manifestations of moderate to severe erythema nodosum leprosum. It is also used for the prevention of graft-versus-host disease, treatment and maintenance of reactional lepromatous leprosy, severe or recurrent aphthous stomatitis and ulcers, Kaposi's sarcoma, prurigo nodularis, actinic prurigo, lupus erythematosus (discoid and subacute cutaneous), Behçet's disease, palmoplantar pustulosis, sarcoidosis, rheumatoid arthritis, histiocytosis X, pyoderma gangrenosum, uremic pruritus, Jessner–Kanof disease, recurrent erythema multiforme, cold hemagglutination disease, Weber–Christian disease, ulcerative colitis, postherpetic neuralgia, AIDS proctitis, bullous pemphigoid, cicatricial pemphigoid, and actinic prurigo.

Monitoring

It is vital that women on thalidomide use at least two effective forms of contraception for one month prior to starting therapy, for the duration of therapy, and for at least one month after cessation of therapy. A pregnancy test should be administered 24 hours prior to initiating therapy and monthly during therapy. Electrophysiologic testing should be considered prior to beginning therapy and should be performed every 3 to 6 months to detect asymptomatic neuropathy. Withdrawal of drug at the earliest possible stage of neuropathy increases the chances of full recovery of sensation.

Pharmacology

Thalidomide, initially marketed as a sedative, is an immune modulator with anti-inflammatory properties. It is believed to act by selectively inhibiting TNF-α production, without affecting production of IL-1, IL-6, GM-CSF, or general proteins. Thalidomide also induces inhibition of IFN-γ production and enhances IL-4 and IL-5 production. The drug has also been reported to inhibit neutrophil

Thalidomide (Thalomid)

chemotaxis, to decrease monocyte phagocytosis without cytotoxicity, and to reduce the generation of superoxide and hydroxyl radicals. Healthy volunteers given thalidomide showed a decrease in their circulating T-helper to T-suppressor cell ratio secondary to a significant decrease in T-helper cells and an apparent increase in T-suppressor cells. Patients with erythema nodosum leprosum who are treated with thalidomide may show a decrease in IgM and reduced antibody production in response to antigenic stimuli. Thalidomide may have a role in suppressing activation of latent HIV-1. The teratogenic mechanism of thalidomide is not known.

Thalidomide has a half-life of 5 to 7 hours. Peak plasma concentrations occur 3 to 6 hours after oral doses. It is highly protein bound and largely nonrenally excreted; the main degradative pathway is most likely to be nonenzymatic hydrolytic cleavage. Hepatic metabolism of thalidomide probably involves the cytochrome P450 enzymes.

Adverse Effects/Precautions

Thalidomide is a highly potent teratogen and can cause devastating birth defects (phocomelia) with only one dose. Thalidomide should be used with extreme caution in women of childbearing age only after all risks have been discussed with the patient.

Pregnancy: FDA category X.

Thalidomide can also be present in the semen of male patients receiving thalidomide; they must always use a latex condom during any sexual contact with women of childbearing potential.

Thalidomide can also cause peripheral neuropathy, characterized by predominantly symmetric painful paresthesias of the hands and feet, and frequently accompanied by sensory loss, muscle cramps, and slight tremor. Symptoms usually reverse on discontinuation of therapy but may worsen or show no improvement.

Neutropenia (incidence < 1%) has been reported with thalidomide. Sedation, drowsiness, and somnolence are frequently observed, especially at higher doses (200 to 400 mg/day). Thalidomide may be administered at bedtime to minimize daytime drowsiness.

Nausea, vomiting, dry mouth, constipation, dizziness, red palms, brittle nails, increased appetite, menstrual abnormalities, and decreased libido, pruritus, rash, and hypersensitivity reactions may also occur.

Special Considerations

Patients must complete an informed consent form before thalidomide can be dispensed. Thalidomide can only be prescribed by physicians who are enrolled in the System for Thalidomide Education and Prescribing Safety (STEPS) program.

Preparation Rx

Capsules   50 mg   Thalomid

Selected References

Calabrese L, Fleischer AB. Thalidomide: current and potential clinical applications. Am J Med 2000; 108: 487–95.

Gaziev D, Galimberti M, Lucarelli G, Polchi P. Chronic graft-versus-host disease: is there an alternative to the conventional treatment? Bone Marrow Transplant 2000; 25: 689–96.

Marriott JB, Muller G, Dalgleish AG. Thalidomide as an emerging immunotherapeutic agent. Immunol Today 1999; 20: 538–40.

Ravot E, Lisziewicz J, Lori F. New uses for old drugs in HIV infection: the role of hydroxyurea, cyclosporin and thalidomide. Drugs 1999; 58: 953–63.

Sanchez MR. Miscellaneous treatments: thalidomide, potassium iodide, levamisole, clofazimine, colchicine, and D-penicillamine. Clin Dermatol 2000; 18: 131–45.

Thioguanine (Tabloid)

Dose and Administration

Pulse dosing of refractory psoriasis: Initially, 80 to 100 mg orally twice per week. Increase dose by 20 mg every 2 to 4 weeks to a maintenance dosage of 120 mg twice weekly, to 160 mg three times weekly.

Uses

Thioguanine is an antineoplastic agent used in treatment of refractory plaque-type psoriasis. Also used in acute nonlymphocytic leukemias and many other neoplasms.

Pharmacology

Thioguanine is a purine analogue, which acts as an antimetabolite in the S-phase of cell division. It is incorporated into the DNA and RNA of bone marrow cells and interferes with nucleic acid biosynthesis, leading to cell death.

Although thioguanine is administered primarily by the oral route, it is poorly absorbed following oral administration, and ingestion with food further decreases oral bioavailability. The drug distributes widely throughout the body tissues, concentrating in the bone marrow. Thioguanine is metabolized primarily in the liver, and both the unchanged drug and its metabolites are excreted in the urine.

Adverse Effects/Precautions

Absolute contraindications include bone marrow suppression, breastfeeding, current infection, neutropenia, and thrombocytopenia. Relative contraindications include pre-existing hepatic disease or biliary obstruction.

Liver function should be frequently monitored, and thioguanine should be discontinued in patients who develop decreased liver function, jaundice, hepatomegaly, or other signs of hepatotoxicity or biliary obstruction or stasis.

Lower dosages may be required in patients with hepatic and renal impairment. Tumor lysis syndrome may occur due to treatment with thioguanine, and appropriate measures must be taken to prevent hyperuricemia, including avoidance of uricosuric agents. Avoid vaccination and close contact with those receiving live vaccination.

Pregnancy: FDA category D.

Concomitant administration of thioguanine and busulfan has resulted in hepatotoxicity, esophageal varices, and portal hypertension in some patients, and caution should be used when administering these drugs concurrently.

Thioguanine can have a synergistic effect with carmustine, and concurrent use of thioguanine with other agents that cause bone marrow suppression may result in additive effects. Owing to the thrombocytopenic effects of thioguanine, an additive risk of bleeding may be seen in patients receiving anticoagulants, NSAIDs, aspirin, strontium-89 chloride, and thrombolytic agents. Sargramostim, GM-CSF, and filgrastim, G-CSF, are contraindicated for use in patients within 24 hours of treatment with antineoplastic agents.

Pancytopenia is the major and dose-limiting effect of thioguanine therapy. Adverse GI symptoms, more common at higher doses, include nausea, vomiting, anorexia, stomatitis, and diarrhea.

Preparation *Rx*

Tablets   40 mg   Tabloid

Selected Reference

Silvis NG, Levine N. Pulse dosing of thioguanine in recalcitrant psoriasis. Arch Dermatol 1999; 135: 433–7.

Antifungals

Fluconazole (Diflucan)

Uses, Dose and Administration

FDA-labeled

Vaginal candidiasis: 150 mg orally one time.

Oropharyngeal candidiasis: 200 mg day 1, then 100 mg daily for 2 weeks.

Esophageal candidiasis: 200 mg on day 1, followed by 100 mg once daily. Doses up to 400 mg/day may be used, based on the patient's response to therapy. Treat for at least 3 weeks (and at least 2 weeks following resolution of symptoms).

Cryptococcal meningitis: 400 mg orally on day 1, followed by 200 mg once daily for 10 to 12 weeks after the cerebrospinal fluid becomes culture negative. Doses up to 400 mg/day may be used, based on the patient's response to therapy. For suppression of relapse in HIV-infected patients, use 200 mg daily.

Also labeled for *Candida* systemic infections, urinary tract infections, peritonitis, and for prophylaxis of candidiasis in patients undergoing peripheral blood stem cell transplantation.

Other

Onychomycosis: 200 mg orally each week until the process has resolved.

Dosage

Adult Dose	Approximate Equivalent Pediatric Dose*
100 mg	3 mg/kg
200 mg	6 mg/kg
400 mg	12 mg/kg

*Do not exceed 600 mg/day

Renal dosage adjustment

Creatinine Clearance (ml/min)	% Recommended Dose
> 50	100%
≤ 50 (no dialysis)	50%
Routine dialysis	100% after each dialysis

Pharmacology

Fluconazole is a synthetic triazole antifungal agent. It is a highly selective inhibitor of fungal cytochrome P450 sterol C-14 α-demethylation. Oral bioavailability approaches 100%; therefore, oral and IV dosages are the same. Use of a loading dose twice the usual daily dose results in plasma concentrations close to steady state by the second day.

Adverse Effects/Precautions

Fluconazole is primarily excreted in the urine and requires dose adjustment in renal insufficiency.

The most common adverse reactions are mild-to-moderate headache, nausea and other gastrointestinal disturbances, and taste disturbance.

Hepatotoxicity may occur and is usually reversible. There is no obvious relationship to total daily dose or duration of therapy. Rare fatalities have been described. Fluconazole treatment should be discontinued in patients with signs or symptoms of liver disease.

Rare cases of anaphylaxis and exfoliative skin reactions have been reported.

Rare cases of QT prolongation and torsades de pointes, usually in significantly ill patients with co-morbidities such as structural heart disease, electrolyte abnormalities, or concomitant use of interacting medications.

Pregnancy: FDA category C.

Drug Interactions

Clinically or potentially significant drug interactions may occur between fluconazole and the following agents/classes:

- Oral hypoglycemics (increased plasma concentrations and effects of the hypoglycemic agent)
- Warfarin (increased prothrombin time)
- Phenytoin (increased phenytoin concentrations)
- Cyclosporine (increased cyclosporine concentrations)
- Rifampin (reduced fluconazole concentrations)
- Theophylline (increased serum theophylline levels)
- Tacrolimus (nephrotoxicity)

Preparation *Rx*

Tablets	50, 100, 150 & 200 mg
Oral suspension	350 mg/35 ml
Solution for injection	200 & 400 mg

Selected References

Elewski BE. Once-weekly fluconazole in the treatment of onychomycosis: introduction. J Am Acad Dermatol 1998; 38: S73–S76.

Gupta AK, Katz HI, Shear NH. Drug interactions with itraconazole, fluconazole, and terbinafine and their management. J Am Acad Dermatol 1999; 41: 237–49.

Schwarze R, Penk A, Pittrow L. Administration of fluconazole in children below 1 year of age. Mycoses 1999; 42: 3–16.

Griseofulvin (Fulvicin P/G, Grifulvin V, Gris-PEG)

Dose and Administration

Adult: 375 mg/day ultramicrosize or 500 mg/day microsize for tinea corporis. For tinea pedis, or tinea unguium, a divided dose of 750 mg of ultramicrosize or 1000 mg of microsize.

Children: Approximately 3.3 mg per *pound* per day of ultramicrosize or 5 mg per *pound* per day of microsize. For tinea capitis in children, doses of 15 to 20 mg per *pound* per day of microsize suspension are recommended.

Continue until the infecting organism is completely eradicated. Representative treatment periods are as follows: tinea capitis, 4 to 6 weeks; tinea corporis, 2 to 4 weeks; tinea pedis, 4 to 8 weeks; tinea unguium, fingernails, at least 4 months; toenails, at least 6 months.

Uses

Griseofulvin is indicated for 'ringworm' infections of the skin, hair, and nails; namely, tinea corporis, tinea pedis, tinea cruris, tinea barbae, tinea capitis, and tinea unguium when caused by *Trichophyton*, *Microsporum,* or *Epidermophyton* infection. The use of this drug is not justified in minor or trivial infections that will respond to topical antifungal agents alone. Griseofulvin is not effective in bacterial infections, candidiasis, histoplasmosis, actinomycosis, sporotrichosis, chromoblastomycosis, coccidioidomycosis, blastomycosis, cryptococcosis, tinea versicolor, and nocardiosis.

Monitoring

When patients are on long-term therapy, periodic monitoring of renal, hepatic, and hematologic systems has been recommended. Because long-term use of griseofulvin for the treatment of onychomycosis has been replaced by other medications, the necessity of any laboratory monitoring is not clear.

Pharmacology

Griseofulvin is fungistatic with *in vitro* activity against various species of *Microsporon, Epidermophyton,* and *Trichophyton.* It has no effect on bacteria or on other genera of fungi. It is deposited in keratin precursor cells with greater affinity for diseased tissue. The drug is tightly bound to new keratin, which becomes highly resistant to fungal invasion.

The gastrointestinal absorption of ultramicrocrystalline griseofulvin is approximately 1.5 times that of conventional microsized griseofulvin. Some individuals do not absorb microcrystalline griseofulvin as well, and better blood concentrations may be obtainable if the tablets are administered after a meal with a high fat content.

Adverse Effects/Precautions

The possibility of cross-sensitivity with penicillin has been suggested; however, penicillin-sensitive patients have been treated without difficulty.

Photosensitivity may occur, and patients should be warned to avoid exposure to intense natural or artificial sunlight.

Lupus erythematosus-like syndromes and exacerbations of existing lupus have been reported. Hypersensitivity may occur, including skin rashes, urticaria, and rarely angioedema and epidermal necrolysis, requiring withdrawal of therapy and appropriate countermeasures.

Griseofulvin (Fulvicin P/G, Grifulvin V, Gris-PEG)

Adverse effects reported occasionally are nausea, vomiting, epigastric distress, diarrhea, fatigue, dizziness, insomnia, and mental confusion. Headaches occur commonly but tend to dissipate with continued use of the drug.

Rare, serious effects are usually associated with high doses and long periods of therapy. Paresthesias of the hands and feet, proteinuria, nephrosis, leukopenia, hepatotoxicity, gastrointestinal bleeding, and menstrual irregularities have been reported rarely.

Griseofulvin is contraindicated in patients with porphyria, hepatocellular failure, or hypersensitivity to the drug.

The dosage in children aged 2 years and younger has not been established.

Griseofulvin should not be prescribed to pregnant patients or to patients intending to become pregnant within 1 month following cessation of therapy. Males should wait at least 6 months after completing griseofulvin therapy before fathering a child.

Drug Interactions

Griseofulvin reduces the effect of warfarin. The effects of alcohol may be increased. Griseofulvin may increase hepatic enzyme activity and thereby decrease the effects of oral contraceptive agents. Barbiturates usually depress griseofulvin activity.

Preparation *Rx*

Griseofulvin microsize

Tablets	250 & 500 mg	Fulvicin UF
Tablets	125, 250 & 500 mg	Grifulvin V
Suspension	125 mg/5 ml	

Griseofulvin ultramicrosize

| Tablets | 125 & 250 mg | Gris-PEG |

Selected References

Albengres E, Le Louet H, Tillement JP. Systemic antifungal agents. Drug interactions of clinical significance. Drug Saf 1998; 18: 83–97.

Chaumeil JC. Micronization: a method of improving the bioavailability of poorly soluble drugs. Methods Find Exp Clin Pharmacol 1998; 20: 211–15.

Friedlander SF. The evolving role of itraconazole, fluconazole and terbinafine in the treatment of tinea capitis. Pediatr Infect Dis J 1999; 18: 205–10.

Temple ME, Nahata MC, Koranyi KI. Pharmacotherapy of tinea capitis. J Am Board Fam Pract 1999; 12: 236–42.

Itraconazole (Sporanox)

Dose and Administration

Blastomycosis and histoplasmosis: 200 mg by mouth daily up to a maximum of 400 mg daily in divided doses.

Onychomycosis: 200 mg by mouth daily for 12 weeks. For fingernail onychomycosis, give two pulses of 200 mg twice daily for 1 week separated by a 3-week period.

> *Note:* Pulse therapy is FDA-approved for the treatment of fingernail onychomycosis, while only the continuous dosage regimen has been FDA approved for the treatment of toenail onychomycosis. Nevertheless, pulse dosing (three pulses) is widely used for onychomycosis.

Oropharyngeal candidiasis (liquid, 10 mg/ml): 200 mg daily for 1 to 2 weeks. (Swish and swallow 10 ml at a time.) 100 mg twice daily for fluconazole-refractory patients.

Esophageal candidiasis (liquid, 10 mg/ml): 100 mg daily for 1 to 2 weeks. (Swish and swallow 10 ml.)

Uses

Indicated for treatment of blastomycosis, histoplasmosis, and aspergillus in immuno-compromised and nonimmunocompromised patients and for onychomycosis of the toenail and fingernail in nonimmunocompromised patients. Oral solution indicated for treatment of oropharyngeal and esophageal candidiasis.

Pharmacology

Oral availability of itraconazole is approximately 50% and is maximal when the capsules are taken with a full meal. The presence of stomach acid improves absorption, and absorption is increased when the drug is taken with 8 oz of a cola beverage. Renal insufficiency does not affect plasma concentrations.

In vitro studies have demonstrated that itraconazole inhibits the cytochrome P450-dependent synthesis of ergosterol, which is a vital component of fungal cell membranes. The drug exhibits *in vitro* activity against *Blastomyces, Histoplasma, Aspergillus, Candida, Cryptococcus,* and *Trichophyton* species.

Contraindications

Do not treat onychomycosis with itraconazole in patients with evidence of left ventricular dysfunction (e.g. congestive heart failure).

Co-administration of itraconazole with certain drugs metabolized by the P450 3A enzyme system may result in increased plasma concentrations of those drugs, leading to potentially serious adverse events. Currently available medications that are contraindicated include the following: pimozide; quinidine; dofetilide; levomethadyl; triazolam; midazolam; HMG-CoA reductase inhibitors, such as lovastatin and simvastatin; and ergot alkaloids, such as dihydroergotamine, ergonovine, ergotamine, and methylergonovine.

Adverse Effects/Precautions

Liver function tests (see Monitoring). Patients should report any signs of liver dysfunction including unusual fatigue, anorexia, nausea, vomiting, jaundice, dark urine or pale stool. There have been rare cases of reversible idiosyncratic hepatitis reported. There are cases of serious hepatotoxicity, including fatalities; however, the causal association is uncertain.

Adverse events include nausea, vomiting, diarrhea, abdominal pain, anorexia, edema, fatigue, fever, malaise, rash, and pruritus.

Although the causal relationship to itraconazole is uncertain, rare cases of alopecia, hypertriglyceridemia, neutropenia, and neuropathy have also been reported.

Itraconazole (Sporanox)

Itraconazole absorption may be decreased by the presence of decreased gastric acidity. Absorption may also be decreased by concomitant administration of acids or acid secretion suppressors. Administration with 8 oz of a cola beverage results in increased absorption of itraconazole in patients with relative or absolute achlorhydria.

Drug Interactions

See also Contraindications.

Itraconazole may elevate serum concentrations of the following drugs: warfarin, protease inhibitors, vinca alkaloids, midazolam, triazolam, diazepam, calcium channel blockers, HMG CoA reductase inhibitors, cyclosporine, tacrolimus, oral hypoglycemics, methylprednisolone, digoxin, and quinidine.

Drugs that decrease itraconazole concentrations include phenytoin, phenobarbital, carbamazepine, isoniazid, rifampin, rifabutin, and gastric acid suppressants.

Monitoring

Liver function tests should be monitored in patients with pre-existing liver function abnormalities. Also monitor periodically in all patients receiving continuous treatment for more than 1 month or any time a patient develops signs or symptoms suggestive of liver dysfunction.

Special Considerations

The oral solution is a different preparation from the capsules, and drug exposure is greater with the oral solution.

Pregnancy: FDA category C. Should not be used to treat onychomycosis in pregnant patients or women contemplating pregnancy. Excreted in human milk. Has been administered to pediatric patients for 2 weeks with no serious unexpected adverse events.

Preparation *Rx*

Capsules	100 mg	Blister packs of 3 by 10 capsules
		Bottles of 30 capsules
		Pulse Pack containing seven blister packs with four capsules each
Solution	10 mg/ml, 150 ml bottle	

Selected References

Amichai B, Grunwald MH. Adverse drug reactions of the new oral antifungal agents – terbinafine, fluconazole, and itraconazole. Int J Dermatol 1998; 37: 410–15.

De Doncker P, Gupta AK, Cel Rosso JQ, et al. Safety of itraconazole pulse therapy for onychomycosis. An update. Postgrad Med 1999; Spec No: 17–25.

De Rosso JQ, Gupta AK. Oral itraconazole therapy for superficial, subcutaneous, and systemic infections. A panoramic view. Postgrad Med 1999; Spec No: 46–52.

Friedlander SF. The evolving role of itraconazole, fluconazole and terbinafine in the treatment of tinea capitis. Pediatr Infect Dis J 1999; 18: 205–10.

Gupta AK, Adam P, Soloman R, Aly R. Itraconazole oral solution for the treatment of tinea capitis using the pulse regimen. Cutis 1999; 64: 192–4.

Gupta AK, Katz HI, Shear NH. Drug interactions with itraconazole, fluconazole, and terbinafine and their management. J Am Acad Dermatol 1999; 41: 237–49.

Leyden J. Pharmacokinetics and pharmacology of terbinafine and itraconazole. J Am Acad Dermatol 1998; 38: S42–S47.

Ketoconazole (Nizoral)

Dose and Administration

Systemic fungal infections: 200 mg orally once daily. In very serious infections or if clinical response is insufficient, the dose may be increased to 400 mg by mouth daily. In children over 2 years of age, a dose of 3.3 to 6.6 mg/kg per day has been used.

Continue therapy until confirmation that active fungal infection has improved. The minimum duration for candidiasis is 1 to 2 weeks. Patients with chronic mucocutaneous candidiasis usually require maintenance therapy. The minimum duration for other labeled systemic infections is 6 months.

Tinea versicolor: 400 mg by mouth once daily for 3 days. The minimum duration for recalcitrant dermatophyte infections is 4 weeks in cases involving glabrous skin. Palmar and plantar infections may respond more slowly.

Uses

FDA-approved for systemic fungal infections (candidiasis, candiduria, chronic mucocutaneous candidiasis, oral thrush, coccidioidomycosis, blastomycosis, histoplasmosis, chromomycosis, and paracoccidioidomycosis). Also indicated for the treatment of severe recalcitrant cutaneous dermatophyte infections (e.g. tinea versicolor) that have not responded to topical therapy or oral griseofulvin.

Pharmacology

Ketoconazole is an imidazole antifungal agent that impairs the synthesis of fungal ergosterol. It is a weak basic agent and requires acidity for dissolution and absorption. It is excreted in sweat. Ketoconazole is a potent inhibitor of the hepatic cytochrome P450 3A4 enzyme.

Adverse Effects/Precautions

The most frequent adverse reactions are nausea or vomiting (3%), abdominal pain (1%), and pruritus (1%). Other adverse effects have been rarely reported, including alopecia, paresthesias, and increased cranial pressure. Hypertriglyceridemia has also been reported.

Hepatocellular hepatotoxicity (1 : 10 000 patients), including rare fatalities, has been reported. The average duration of therapy in which hepatotoxicity occurred was approximately 28 days, although the range was extensive (as early as 3 days). The injury is not always reversible. Patients should be instructed to report any signs or symptoms that may suggest liver dysfunction, including unusual fatigue, anorexia, nausea, vomiting, jaundice, dark urine, or pale stools.

Serum testosterone may be lowered, particularly with doses of 800 mg per day or higher.

Anaphylaxis has been reported rarely after the first dose.

Pregnancy: FDA category C.

Monitoring

Liver function tests should be measured before starting treatment and at frequent intervals during treatment.

Ketoconazole (Nizoral)

Drug Interactions

Ketoconazole is a potent inhibitor of the CYP 450 3A4 isoenzyme and has the potential to interact with numerous medications. Administration with terfenadine, astemizole, triazolam or cisapride is contraindicated, although only triazolam is widely available in the USA.

Ketoconazole may enhance the effects of the following: midazolam, triazolam, digoxin, warfarin, oral hypoglycemic agents, cyclosporine, tacrolimus, methyl-prednisolone.

Concomitant administration with phenytoin may alter the metabolism of one or both of the drugs; monitor both ketoconazole and phenytoin.

Concomitant rifampin reduces ketoconazole blood levels.

Isoniazid is also reported to affect ketoconazole concentrations adversely and should not be given concomitantly.

Preparation *Rx*

Tablets   200 mg

Selected Reference

Rheney CC, Saddler CM. Oral ketoconazole in cutaneous fungal infections. Ann Pharmacother 1998; 32: 709–11.

Terbinafine (Lamisil)

Uses, Dose and Administration

Fingernail onychomycosis: 250 mg orally once daily for 6 weeks.

Toenail onychomycosis: 250 mg orally once daily for 12 weeks.

Pharmacology

Synthetic allylamine derivative that inhibits squalene epoxidase, a key enzyme in sterol biosynthesis in fungi. Depending on drug concentration and fungal species, the drug may be fungicidal. Bioavailability is approximately 40%. In patients with renal impairment or hepatic cirrhosis, clearance is decreased by approximately 50%. Terbinafine is distributed to the sebum and skin with a terminal half-life of 200 to 400 hours, representing the slow elimination from tissues such as skin and fat.

Adverse Effects/Precautions

Rare cases of liver failure (some fatal) in patients with and without pre-existing liver disease. Most patients had serious co-morbidities. Discontinue if laboratory or clinical signs of liver injury present. Not recommended in patients with pre-existing liver or renal impairment.

Decreases in absolute lymphocyte counts and cases of severe neutropenia have been observed. Discontinue if neutrophil count is < 1000 cells/mm^3.

Rare reports of serious skin reactions (including Stevens–Johnson syndrome). Discontinue if a skin rash progresses.

Most frequent adverse events: headache, diarrhea, dyspepsia, rash, itching, and liver enzyme abnormalities. Taste disturbances (3%) usually abate within several weeks after discontinuation.

Pregnancy: FDA category B.

Monitoring

Liver function tests are recommended in patients taking the drug for more than 6 weeks or in those who develop unexplained nausea, anorexia or fatigue. Complete blood counts are recommended if patients develop signs or symptoms suggestive of secondary infection.

Drug Interactions

Potent inhibitor of CYP 2D6, therefore monitor carefully with concomitant tricyclic antidepressants, selective serotonin reuptake inhibitors, β-blockers, and monoamine oxidase inhibitors.

There have been occasional reports of an increase or decrease in prothrombin time in patients receiving warfarin. The causal relationship is unknown.

Terbinafine clearance is increased by rifampin (100%) and decreased by cimetidine (33%).

Preparation *Rx*

Tablets   250 mg

Selected References

Amichai B, Grunwald MH. Adverse drug reactions of the new oral antifungal agents – terbinafine, fluconazole, and itraconazole. Int J Dermatol 1998; 37: 410–15.

Gupta AK, Adam P. Terbinafine pulse therapy is effective in tinea capitis. Pediatr Dermatol 1998; 15: 56–8.

Gupta AK, Katz HI, Shear NH. Drug interactions with itraconazole, fluconazole, and terbinafine and their management. J Am Acad Dermatol 1999; 41: 237–49.

McClellan KJ, Wiseman LR, Markham A. Terbinafine. An update of its use in superficial mycoses. Drugs 1999; 58: 179–202.

Ciclopirox 8% Lacquer (Penlac)

Dose and Administration

Apply topical nail lacquer solution to all affected nails with applicator brush. Solution should be applied to the entire nail plate and 5 mm of surrounding skin once daily, preferably at bedtime. The solution should also be applied under the surface of the nail plate, when it is free of the nail bed. Allow to dry for 30 seconds. Wait 8 hours before bathing. Apply daily for 7 days, and then remove lacquer with alcohol. Repeat cycle. May be used for 48 weeks. Patient is to keep nails trimmed and may use an emery file board to loosen nail material. Abrasion of the nail surface may facilitate drug penetration. In clinical trials, monthly professional removal of the unattached, infected nail was performed.

May use with occlusive dressings.

Use

FDA-approved for mild to moderate onychomycosis of the fingernails and toenails without lunula involvement.

Pharmacology

Ciclopirox is a topical broad-spectrum fungicidal agent against dermatophytes, yeasts, actinomycetes, molds, and fungal saprophytes. Its mechanism of action is unknown but is thought to act by blocking transport across the fungal membrane causing intracellular depletion of nutrients.

The 8% solution dries to a concentration of over 30%. This provides a concentration gradient that serves to promote drug penetration into the diseased nail.

Adverse Effects/Precautions

The most common dermatologic side-effects are erythema, pruritus, rash, skin irritation, and nail discoloration.

Pregnancy: FDA category B.

Preparation *Rx*

Nail lacquer   8%   Penlac   3 ml

Clotrimazole

Dose and Administration

Topical oral:

Treatment of oropharyngeal candidiasis: Dissolve one troche slowly in the mouth five times daily for 14 days.

Prophylaxis of oropharyngeal candidiasis: Dissolve one troche slowly in the mouth three times daily for the duration of chemotherapy or until steroid therapy is at maintenance dosing.

Topical: Apply cream, lotion, or solution to affected and surrounding area(s) twice daily, morning and evening.

Vaginal: (Cream): Insert one applicatorful at bedtime for 7 to 14 days.

(Tablet): Insert 100 mg tablet daily for 7 days, or 200 mg for 3 days.

Uses

FDA-approved

Topical oral: Oropharyngeal candidiasis, treatment or prophylaxis in patients immunocompromised by chemotherapy, radiotherapy, or steroid therapy used in the treatment of leukemia, solid tumors, or renal transplantation.

Topical: Dermatomycoses, including cutaneous candidiasis, tinea cruris, tinea corporis, tinea pedis, pityriasis versicolor.

Vaginal: Vulvovaginal candidiasis.

Other: There are no data from well-controlled trials to indicate efficacy and safety of oral clotrimazole in the prophylaxis of oropharyngeal candidiasis in patients immunosuppressed due to causes other than those listed above.

Monitoring

Periodic liver function tests (with topical oral therapy only).

Pharmacology

Broad-spectrum imidazole antifungal agent. Impairs biosynthesis of ergosterol, prohibiting its incorporation into fungal cell membranes, leading to increased membrane permeability and functional loss of membrane-bound enzyme systems.

Adverse Effects

Topical oral: Elevated liver function tests, typically minimal, in approximately 15% of patients. Nausea, vomiting, unpleasant mouth sensations.

Topical: Erythema, stinging, burning, pruritus, urticaria, edema.

Vaginal: Lower abdominal cramping, dysuria, urinary frequency, burning, irritation.

Precautions

Clotrimazole is inappropriate therapy for systemic fungal infections.

Females self-medicating with OTC vaginal preparations should do so only if they have been previously diagnosed with vulvovaginal candidiasis and are having symptom recurrence. Medical attention should be sought for persistent symptoms or recurrence within 2 months.

Pregnancy: FDA category: oral: C; vaginal, topical: B

Drug Interactions

Oral clotrimazole may increase tacrolimus serum concentrations via inhibition of the cytochrome P450 3A4 metabolizing isoenzyme.

Clotrimazole

Oral clotrimazole may potentiate ergotamine derivatives (e.g. Cafergot), and is listed as a warning for ergotamine products.

Preparation

Oral

Tablet	500 mg	Mycelex troche *Rx*

Topical

Cream	1%	Various generics
		Lotrimin
		Mycelex *Rx/OTC* sizes range from 12 to 45 g
Solution	1%	Various generics
		Lotrimin
		Mycelex *Rx/OTC* 10 & 30 ml
Lotion	1%	Lotrimin *Rx* 30 ml

Vaginal

Tablet	100 mg (7s)	Generic
		Gyne-Lotrimin
		Mycelex-7 *OTC*
Tablet	200 mg (3s)	Generic
		Gyne-Lotrimin-3 *OTC*
Cream	2%	Generic
		Gyne-Lotrimin-3
		Trivagizole-3 *OTC*
Cream	1%	Generics
		Mycelex-7
		Gyne-Lotrimin-7 *OTC* 15, 30 & 45 g

Vaginal combination packs

Tablets	100 mg (7)	Mycelex-7 Pack *OTC*
Topical cream	1%	
Tablets	200 mg (3)	Gyne-Lotrimin-3 Pack *OTC*
Topical cream	1%	

References

Centers for Disease Control and Prevention. Sexually Transmitted Diseases Treatment Guidelines – 2002. Morbid Mortal Weekly Rep 2002; 51(No. RR-06): 1–80.

David LM, Veien NK, Schmidt JD, et al. Topical clotrimazole in dermatophytosis. Curr Ther Res 1973; 15: 133–7.

Lebherz T, Guess E, Wolfson N. Efficacy of single- versus multiple-dose clotrimazole therapy in the management of vulvovaginal candidiasis. Am J Obstet Gynecol 1985; 152: 965–8.

Owens NJ, Nightingale CH, Schweizer RT, et al. Prophylaxis of oral candidiasis with clotrimazole troches. Arch Intern Med 1984; 144: 290-3.

Sawyer PR, Brogden RN, Pinder RM, et al. Clotrimazole: a review of its antifungal activity and therapeutic efficacy. Drugs 1975; 9: 424–47.

Cream Antifungal Formulations for the Skin

Generic Name	Brand Name	Class	Sizes	Rx/OTC	Indications	Frequency	Duration
Butenafine 1%	Mentax cream (Rx), Lotrimin Ultra (OTC)	Benzylamine	15, 30 g	Rx and OTC	Tinea corporis, Tinea cruris, Tinea pedis *	QD	2 weeks, *BID – 7 days OR QD – 4 weeks
Ciclopirox 0.77%	Loprox cream	Pyridone/Non-imidazole	15, 30, 90 g	Rx	Tinea corporis, Tinea cruris, Tinea pedis, Tinea versicolor*, Cutaneous candidiasis	BID	4 weeks, *2 weeks
Clotrimazole 1%	Lotrimin/Lotrimin AF/Mycelex	Imidazole	12, 15, 24, 30, 45, 90 g	Rx and OTC	Tinea corporis, Tinea cruris*, Tinea pedis, Tinea versicolor (Rx only), Cutaneous candidiasis (Rx only)	BID	4 weeks, *2 weeks
Econazole 1%	Spectizole	Imidazole	15, 30, 85 g	Rx	Tinea corporis*, Tinea cruris *, Tinea pedis**, Tinea versicolor*, Cutaneous candidiasis***	QD–BID	*QD – 2 weeks, **QD – 1 month, ***BID – 2 weeks
Ketoconazole 2%	Nizoral	Imidazole	15, 30, 60 g	Rx	Tinea corporis, Tinea cruris, Tinea pedis*, Tinea versicolor, Cutaneous candidiasis, Seborrheic dermatitis**	QD–BID	2 weeks, *6 weeks, **BID – 4 weeks or clear

continued

126

Cream Antifungal Formulations for the Skin *continued*

Generic Name	Brand Name	Class	Sizes	Rx/OTC	Indications	Frequency	Duration
Miconazole 2%	Micatin (OTC) Monistat-Derm (Rx)	Imidazole	15, 30, 90 g 14 g	Rx and OTC	Tinea corporis Tinea cruris Tinea pedis* Tinea versicolor** (RX only) Cutaneous candidiasis (RX only)	BID	2 weeks *1 month **QD – 2 weeks
Naftifine 1%	Naftin	Allylamine	15, 30, 60 g	Rx	Tinea corporis Tinea cruris Tinea pedis	QD	4 weeks
Nystatin	Mycostatin, Nystex cream	Polyene	15, 30 g	Rx	Cutaneous candidiasis Mucocutaneous candidiasis	BID–TID	3 weeks or until clear
Oxiconazole 1%	Oxistat	Imidazole	15, 30, 60 g	Rx	Tinea corporis Tinea cruris Tinea pedis * Tinea versicolor**	QD–BID	2 weeks *QD/BID – 1 month **QD – 2 weeks
Sertaconazole 2%	Ertaczo	Imidazole	15, 30 g	Rx	Tinea pedis	BID	4 weeks
Sulconazole 1%	Exelderm	Imidazole	15, 30, 60 g	Rx	Tinea corporis Tinea cruris Tinea pedis* Tinea versicolor	QD–BID	3–4 weeks *BID – 4 weeks
Terbinafine 1%	Lamisil AT	Allylamine	15, 30 g	OTC	Tinea corporis* Tinea cruris* Tinea pedis	BID	1–4 weeks *QD – 1 week

Non-cream Antifungal Formulations for the Skin

Generic Name	Brand Name	Class	Sizes	Rx/OTC	Indications	Frequency	Duration
Amphotericin B 3%	Fungizone Lotion	Polyene	30 ml	Rx	Cutaneous candidiasis Mucocutaneous candidiasis	4–6x/day	Location/depen. 1–4 weeks
Ciclopirox 0.77%	Loprox Gel	Pyridone/ Non-imidazole	30, 45, 100 g	Rx	Tinea corporis Tinea pedis Seborrheic dermatitis	BID	4 weeks
Ciclopirox 0.77%	Loprox Suspension	Pyridone/ Non-imidazole	30, 60 ml	Rx	Tinea corporis Tinea cruris Tinea pedis Tinea versicolor* Cutaneous candidiasis	BID	4 weeks *2 weeks
Ciclopirox 1%	Loprox Shampoo	Pyridone/ Non-imidazole	120 ml	Rx	Seborrheic dermatitis	2x/week with at least 3 days between washes	Re-evaluate if no improvement after 4 weeks
Ciclopirox 8%	Penlac Nail Lacquer	Pyridone/ Non-imidazole	3.3, 6.6 ml	Rx	Onychomycosis (T. rubrum)	Apply QD x 7 days, then remove Repeat	Up to 48 weeks
Clotrimazole 1%	Lotrimin AF Lotion	Imidazole	20 ml	Rx and OTC	Tinea corporis Tinea cruris* Tinea pedis Tinea versicolor (RX only) Cutaneous candidiasis (RX only)	BID	4 weeks *2 weeks

continued

Non-cream Antifungal Formulations for the Skin *continued*

Generic Name	Brand Name	Class	Sizes	Rx/OTC	Indications	Frequency	Duration
Ketoconazole 2%	Nizoral shampoo	Imidazole	120 ml	Rx	Tinea (pityriasis) versicolor, Dandruff*	One application *2x/week with 3 days between washes	*4 weeks
Miconazole 2%	Lotrimin AF, Micatin spray powder	Imidazole	~100 g	OTC	Tinea corporis, Tinea cruris, Tinea pedis*	BID	2 weeks, *1 month
Naftifine 1%	Naftin gel	Allylamine	20, 40, 60 g	Rx	Tinea corporis, Tinea cruris, Tinea pedis	BID	4 weeks
Nystatin	Mycostatin, Nystex ointment	Polyene	15, 30 g	Rx	Cutaneous candidiasis, Mucocutaneous candidiasis	BID	3 weeks or until clear
Nystatin powder	Mycostatin, Nystop powder	Polyene	15 g	Rx	Cutaneous candidiasis, Mucocutaneous candidiasis	BID	3 weeks or until clear
Salicylic acid 3%/ Benzoic acid 6%	Whitfield's ointment		30 g	OTC		BID	
Oxiconazole 1%	Oxistat lotion	Imidazole	30 ml	Rx	Tinea corporis, Tinea cruris, Tinea pedis *	QD–BID	2 weeks, *QD/BID 1 month
Sulconazole 1%	Exelderm solution	Imidazole	30 ml	Rx	Tinea corporis, Tinea cruris, Tinea versicolor	QD–BID	3–4 weeks, *BID – 4 weeks
Terbinafine 1%	Lamisil AT spray	Allylamine	30 ml	Rx	Tinea corporis, Tinea cruris, Tinea pedis*	QD	1–4 weeks, *BID – 1–4 weeks

Generic Name	Brand Name	Formulation	Strength	Sizes	Rx/OTC	Regimen
Butoconazole	Gynazole-1	Vaginal Cream	2%	1 prefilled	Rx	1 applicatorful intravaginally once
	Femstat 3	Vaginal Cream	2%	20 g, or 3 prefilled	OTC	1 applicatorful intravaginally QHS for 3 days
	Mycelex-3	Vaginal Cream	2%	20 g, or 3 prefilled	OTC	1 applicatorful intravaginally QHS for 3 days
Clotrimazole	Gyne-Lotrimin	Suppositories	200 mg	# 3	OTC	Insert 1 intravaginally QHS for 3 days
	Gyne-Lotrimin 3	Vaginal Cream	2%	21 g	OTC	1 applicatorful intravaginally QHS for 3 days
	Mycelex-7	Vaginal Cream	1%	45 g	OTC	1 applicatorful intravaginally QHS for 7 days
	Gyne-Lotrimin 7	Vaginal Cream	1%	45 g	OTC	1 applicatorful intravaginally QHS for 7 days
	Gyne-Lotrimin 3 Combination Pack	Suppositories	200 mg	# 3	OTC	Insert 1 intravaginally QHS for 3 days
		Topical Cream	1%	7 g		Apply to affected areas morning and evening for 7 days or as needed
	Gyne-Lotrimin 7 Combination Pack	Suppositories	100 mg	# 7	OTC	Insert 1 intravaginally QHS for 7 days
		Topical Cream	1%	7 g		Apply to affected areas morning and evening for 7 days or as needed
Miconazole	Monistat-7	Suppositories	100 mg	# 7	OTC	Insert 1 intravaginally QHS for 7 days
	Monistat	Topical Cream	2%	9 g	OTC	Apply to affected areas morning and evening as needed
	Monistat 3	Vaginal Cream	2%	35 g, 45 g, or 7 prefilled	OTC	1 applicatorful intravaginally QHS for 7 days
	Monistat 7	Vaginal Cream	2%	3 prefilled	OTC	1 applicatorful intravaginally QHS for 3 days
	Monistat 3	Suppositories	200 mg	# 3	OTC	Insert 1 intravaginally QHS for 3 days
	Combination Pack	Topical Cream	2%		OTC	Apply to affected areas morning and evening for 7 days or as needed

continued

Vaginal Preparations for Vaginal Candidiasis

continued

Generic Name	Brand Name	Formulation	Strength	Sizes	Rx/OTC	Regimen
	Monistat 7	Suppositories	100 mg	#7	OTC	Insert 1 intravaginally QHS for 7 days
	Combination Pack	Topical Cream	2%			Apply to affected areas morning and evening for 7 days or as needed
	Monistat 1	Suppositories	1200 mg	#1	OTC	Insert 1 intravaginally once
	Combination Pack	Topical Cream	2%	9 g		Apply to affected areas morning and evening for 7 days or as needed
Nystatin	Mycostatin	Suppositories	100 000 units	#15, #30	Rx	Insert 1 intravaginally daily for 2 weeks
Terconazole	Terazol 3	Vaginal Cream	0.8%	20 g	Rx	1 applicatorful intravaginally QHS for 3 days
	Terazol 3	Suppositories	80 mg	#3	Rx	Insert 1 intravaginally QHS for 3 days
	Terazol 7	Vaginal Cream	0.4%	45 g	Rx	1 applicatorful intravaginally QHS for 7 days
Tioconazole	1-Day	Vaginal Ointment	6.5%	1 prefilled	OTC	1 applicatorful intravaginally once
	Vagistat-1	Vaginal Ointment	6.5%	1 prefilled	OTC	1 applicatorful intravaginally once

Antihistamines

Cetirizine (Zyrtec)

Dose and Administration

Adults and children 6 years of age and older: 5 or 10 mg once daily.

Elderly (> 76 years of age): 5 mg once daily.

Children 2 to 5 years of age: 2.5 mg once daily; may increase to 5 mg once daily or 2.5 mg twice daily if needed.

Children 6 months up to 2 years of age: 2.5 mg once daily. For children 12 to 23 months, may increase to 2.5 mg twice daily.

Dose adjustment for hepatic impairment or renal insufficiency ($CL_{cr} < 30$ ml/min):

Adults and children 6 years of age and older: 5 mg once daily.

Children < 6 years of age: Not recommended.

Uses

FDA-approved: Relief of symptoms associated with seasonal allergic rhinitis. Relief of symptoms associated with perennial allergic rhinitis. Treatment of uncomplicated skin manifestations associated with chronic idiopathic urticaria.

Other: Higher than recommended doses have been used for atopic dermatitis and allergen-induced asthma.

Pharmacology

Antihistamine with selective peripheral H_1-receptor antagonist properties. Chemically, the carboxylated metabolite of hydroxyzine and therefore less sedating.

Adverse Effects/Precautions

Most common include somnolence, fatigue, dry mouth. In addition, pediatric patients have also experienced headache, pharyngitis, abdominal pain.

Pregnancy: FDA category B.

Drug Interactions

No interactions were detected in pharmacokinetic studies with ketoconazole, erythromycin, or azithromycin.

One multiple dose study demonstrated a 16% reduction in clearance of cetirizine when administered concurrently with theophylline.

Preparation Rx

Tablets	5 & 10 mg
Chewable tablets	5 & 10 mg
Syrup	1 mg/ml, in 120 ml and 1 pint amber glass bottles

Selected References

Broide D. Clinical studies with cetirizine in allergic rhinitis and chronic urticaria. Allergy 1995; 50(Suppl 24): 31–5.

Gonzalez MA, Estes KS. Pharmacokinetic overview of oral second-generation H_1 antihistamines. Int J Clin Pharmacol Ther 1998; 36: 292–300.

Malick A, Grant JA. Antihistamines in the treatment of asthma. Allergy 1997; 52(Suppl 34): 55–66.

Spencer CM, Faulds D, Peters DH. Cetirizine. A reappraisal of its pharmacological properties and therapeutic use in selected allergic disorders. Drugs 1993; 46: 1055–80.

Chlorpheniramine (Various)

Dose and Administration

Adults and children 12 years of age and older

Oral: 4 mg every 4 to 6 hours; sustained release, 8 mg or 12 mg twice daily.

Parenteral (IM, IV, SC): 10 mg (range, 5–20 mg) per dose; maximum 40 mg per day.

Children 6 to 12 years of age

Oral: 2 mg every 4 to 6 hours.

Parenteral: 0.35 mg/kg per day in four divided doses.

Children 2 to 6 years of age

Oral: 1 mg every 4 to 6 hours.

Uses

FDA-labeled: Relief of symptoms associated with seasonal and perennial allergic rhinitis and vasomotor rhinitis.

Pharmacology

An alkylamine first generation H_1-receptor antihistamine. The alkylamines are the least sedating of the first-generation antihistamines.

Adverse Effects/Precautions

Sedation (although comparatively less sedating versus other first-generation antihistamines), blurred vision, dizziness, nervousness, changes in appetite, weight gain, nausea/vomiting, constipation or diarrhea. Acute overdose produces dry mouth, initial CNS excitation, followed by CNS depression, fixed pupils, urinary retention, and flushing.

Contraindicated in patients with narrow-angle glaucoma, prostatic hypertrophy, urinary retention, stenosing peptic ulcer.

Pregnancy: FDA category B. (*Note:* Many products containing chlorpheniramine also contain other agents which may define a different pregnancy category.)

Drug Interactions

Other CNS depressants, alcohol.

Preparation

Tablets	4 mg *OTC*
	8 mg, 12 mg extended release *OTC*
Syrup	2 mg/5 ml *OTC*
Injection	10 mg/ml *Rx*

Selected references

Schuller DE, Turkewitz D. Adverse effects of antihistamines. Postgrad Med 1986; 79: 75–86.

Simons FE, Simons KJ. H_1 receptor antagonists: clinical pharmacology and use in allergic disease. Pediatr Clin North Am 1983; 30: 899–914.

Simons FE, Simons KJ, Chung M, Yeh J. The comparative pharmacokinetics of H_1-receptor antagonists. Ann Allergy 1987; 59: 20–4.

Cromolyn (Gastrocrom) Oral Concentrate

Dose and Administration

Dose

Adults and children ≥ 13 years of age: 200 mg (two ampules) four times daily, $\frac{1}{2}$ hour prior to meals and at bedtime.

Children 2 to 12 years of age: 100 mg (one ampule) four times daily, $\frac{1}{2}$ hour prior to meals and at bedtime.

Children < 2 years of age: Not recommended.

Administration

Break ampule(s) open and squeeze liquid into glass of water. Stir and drink.

Uses

Management of symptoms in patients with mastocytosis. Improvement has been shown in the following symptoms: nausea, vomiting, diarrhea, abdominal pain, headaches, flushing, urticaria, itching. Beneficial effects appear within 2 to 6 weeks.

Pharmacology

Mast cell stabilizer.

Adverse Effects/Precautions

Consider dosage reduction in patients with renal or hepatic impairment.

Adverse effects are uncommon. Those reported in clinical trials may have been associated with the underlying disease: nausea, headache, diarrhea, pruritus, myalgia.

Pregnancy: FDA category B.

Preparation *Rx*

Oral Concentrate Solution   100 mg per 5-ml ampule; 8 ampules per foil pouch
NOT FOR INJECTION OR INHALATION

Selected References

Ferkovic TJ, Lanese TR, Long BD. Use of oral cromolyn sodium in systemic mastocytosis. Clin Pharm 1982; 1: 377–9.

Soter NA, Austen KF, Wasserman SI. Oral disodium cromoglycate in the treatment of systemic mastocytosis. N Engl J Med 1979; 301: 465–9.

Desloratadine (Clarinex)

Dose and Administration

Adults and children 12 years of age and older: 5 mg once daily.

Patients with liver failure or renal insufficiency (GFR < 30 ml/min): 5 mg every other day as starting dose.

Uses

FDA-approved: Treatment of chronic idiopathic urticaria. Relief of nasal and non-nasal symptoms of seasonal and perennial allergic rhinitis.

Pharmacology

Long-acting tricyclic antihistamine with selective peripheral H_1-receptor antagonism. A major active metabolite of loratadine.

Adverse Effects/Precautions

Pharyngitis, dry mouth, myalgia, fatigue, somnolence.

Pregnancy: FDA category C; manufacturer recommends to exercise caution.

Drug Interactions

Ketoconazole, erythromycin, cimetidine increase plasma concentrations of desloratadine, although no prolongation of QT_c interval has been demonstrated.

Preparation *Rx*

Tablets	5 mg
RediTabs (rapidly disintegrating tablets)	5 mg

(Use immediately after opening individual RediTab blister. Place one RediTab on the tongue and allow to slowly dissolve)

Selected References

Bonini S. Desloratadine: a new approach in the treatment of allergy as a systematic disease – pharmacology and clinical overview. Allergy 2001; 56(Suppl 65): 5–6.

Geha RS, Meltzer EO. Desloratadine: A new, nonsedating, oral antihistamine. J Allergy Clin Immunol 2001; 107: 751–62.

Limon L, Kockler DR. Desloratadine: a nonsedating antihistamine. Ann Pharmacother 2003; 37: 237–46.

Murdoch D, Goa KL, Keam SJ. Desloratadine: an update of its efficacy in the management of allergic disorders. Drugs 2003; 63: 2051–77.

See S. Desloratadine for allergic rhinitis. Am Fam Physician 2003; 68: 2015–16.

Diphenhydramine (Benadryl)

Dose and Administration

Adults and children 12 years of age and older
Oral: 25 to 50 mg every 4 to 6 hours.
Parenteral (IM, IV): 10 to 50 mg every 2 to 3 hours (maximum 400 mg/day).
Children 6 to 11 years of age
Oral: 12.5 mg every 4 to 6 hours (maximum 75 mg/day).
Parenteral (IM, IV): 1.25 mg/kg four times daily (maximum 300 mg/day).
Children 2 to 5 years of age
Oral: 6.25 mg every 4 to 6 hours (maximum 25 mg/day).

Uses

Used for a variety of hypersensitivity (type I) reactions, including relief of symptoms associated with seasonal and perennial allergic rhinitis, vasomotor rhinitis, allergic dermatosis, anaphylaxis. Also used as a night-time sedative, an antitussive (liquid), and to prevent motion sickness.

Pharmacology

An ethanolamine first-generation H_1-receptor antihistamine. It acts by competitively antagonizing histamine at the H_1 histamine receptor.

Adverse Effects/Precautions

Sedation, blurred vision, dizziness, nervousness, changes in appetite, weight gain, nausea/vomiting, constipation or diarrhea. Acute overdose produces dry mouth, initial CNS excitation, followed by CNS depression, fixed pupils, urinary retention, and flushing.

Contraindicated in patients with narrow-angle glaucoma, prostatic hypertrophy, urinary retention, stenosing peptic ulcer.

Pregnancy: FDA category B. (*Note:* Many products containing diphenhydramine also contain other agents which may define a different pregnancy category.)

Drug Interactions

Additive sedation in combination with other CNS depressants.

Preparation

Benadryl, generics		
Capsules	25 & 50 mg	OTC
Tablets	25 & 50 mg	OTC
Tablets, chewable	12.5 mg	OTC
Liquid, Solution, Elixir	12.5 mg/5 ml	OTC
Injection (50 mg/ml)	1 & 10 ml	Rx

Selected References

Schuller DE, Turkewitz D. Adverse effects of antihistamines. Postgrad Med 1986; 79: 75–86.

Simons FE, Simons KJ. H_1 receptor antagonists: clinical pharmacology and use in allergic disease. Pediatr Clin North Am 1983; 30: 899–914.

Simons FE, Simons KJ, Chung M, Yeh J. The comparative pharmacokinetics of H_1-receptor antagonists. Ann Allergy 1987; 59: 20–4.

Fexofenadine (Allegra)

Dose and Administration

Adults and children 12 years of age and older: 60 mg twice daily.

Children 6–11 years of age: 30 mg twice daily.

Patients with CL_{cr} < 80 ml/min or those receiving hemodialysis: one dose daily.

A dose of 180 mg daily may be given for allergic rhinitis. Higher doses have been used (180 to 240 mg daily) for treatment of chronic idiopathic urticaria.

Uses

FDA-approved: Relief of symptoms associated with seasonal allergic rhinitis.

Treatment of uncomplicated skin manifestations of chronic idiopathic urticaria (significantly reduces pruritus and the number of wheals).

Pharmacology

Antihistamine with selective peripheral H_1-receptor antagonist properties. Chemically, the carboxylated metabolite of terfenadine.

Adverse Effects/Precautions

Headache, viral infection, nausea, dysmenorrhea, drowsiness, fatigue, dyspepsia.

Pregnancy: FDA category C.

Drug Interactions

Plasma concentrations of fexofenadine were significantly elevated with co-administration of erythromycin or ketoconazole, although the levels were within the range observed in controlled trials of fexofenadine. No differences in QT_c interval or adverse events were detected with concomitant erythromycin or ketoconazole.

Preparation *Rx*

Tablets	30, 60 & 180 mg
Capsules	60 mg

Selected References

Bernstein DI, Schoenwetter WF, Nathan RA, et al. Efficacy and safety of fexofenadine hydrochloride for treatment of seasonal allergic rhinitis. Ann Allergy Asthma Immunol 1997; 79: 443–8.

Horak F, Stubner UP. Comparative tolerability of second generation antihistamines. Drug Saf 1999; 20: 385–401.

Markham A, Wagstaff AJ. Fexofenadine. Drugs 1998; 55: 269–74.

Mason J, Reynolds R, Rao N. The systemic safety of fexofenadine HCl. Clin Exp Allergy 1999; 29(Suppl 3): 163–70.

Pratt C, Brown AM, Rampe D, et al. Cardiovascular safety of fexofenadine. Clin Exp Allergy 1999; 29(Suppl 3): 212–16.

Hydroxyzine (Various)

Dose and Administration

Pruritus

Adults: 25 mg orally three or four times daily.

Children > 6 years: 50 mg to 100 mg orally per day, divided every 6 to 8 hours.

Children < 6 years: 50 mg orally per day, divided every 6 to 8 hours.

Anxiety

Adults: 50 mg to 100 mg orally four times daily.

Children > 6 years: 50 mg to 100 mg orally per day, divided every 6 hours.

Children < 6 years: 50 mg orally per day, divided every 6 hours.

Pre- or postoperative sedation or analgesia

Adults:	Oral: 50 mg to 100 mg.
	Intramuscular: 25 mg to 100 mg.
Children:	Oral: 0.6 mg/kg.
	Intramuscular: 1 mg/kg.

Uses

FDA-approved: Relief of pruritus. Relief of anxiety/tension associated with psychoneurosis. Adjunctive therapy for anxiety associated with organic disease states. Pre- and/or postoperative sedation and/or potentiation of analgesia. Parenteral administration has been employed in the management of symptoms associated with alcohol withdrawal (e.g. delirium tremens), as adjunctive therapy in various states of agitation, and as an antiemetic.

Pharmacology

H_1-receptor antagonist with central nervous system depressant, anticholinergic, antispasmodic, antiemetic, and local anesthetic effects, in addition to its antihistaminic activity. Chemically, a piperazine antihistamine.

Adverse Effects/Precautions

Sedation, dry mouth, possible nausea, constipation, abdominal pain, headache.

Necrosis and gangrene have occurred with inadvertent intra-arterial administration; parenteral administration should be limited to the intramuscular route.

Drug Interactions

Increase in adverse effects with concomitant central nervous system depressants or anticholinergics.

Preparation *Rx*

As hydrochloride

Tablet	10, 25, 50 & 100 mg	Atarax
		Generics
Syrup	10 mg/5 ml	Atarax
		Generics

Injection	25 & 50 mg/ml	Vistaril
(for IM use only)		Generics
As pamoate		
Capsule	25, 50 & 100 mg	Vistaril
		Generics
Oral Suspension	25 mg/5 ml	Vistaril
		Generics

Selected References

Breneman DL. Cetirizine versus hydroxyzine and placebo in chronic idiopathic urticaria. Ann Pharmacother 1996; 30: 1075–9.

Einarson A, Bailey B, Jung J, et al. Prospective controlled study of hydroxyzine and cetirizine in pregnancy. Ann Allergy Asthma Immunol 1997; 78: 183–6.

Loratadine (Claritin, Alavert)

Dose and Administration

Adults and children 6 years of age and older: 10 mg once daily.

Children 2–5 years of age: 5 mg once daily.

Patients with liver failure or GFR < 30 ml/min: dose every other day.

Uses

FDA-approved: Treatment of chronic idiopathic urticaria. Relief of nasal and non-nasal symptoms of seasonal allergic rhinitis.

Pharmacology

Long-acting tricyclic antihistamine with selective peripheral H_1-receptor antagonism.

Adverse Effects/Precautions

Headache, fatigue, somnolence, dry mouth, tachycardia/palpitation.

Pregnancy: FDA category B; manufacturer recommends to exercise caution.

Drug Interactions

None significant.

Preparation *OTC*

Tablets	10 mg
Orally disintegrating tablets	10 mg
Syrup	1 mg/ml 2-ounce & 4-ounce bottles

Selected References

Bradley CM, Nicholson AN. Studies on the central effects of the H_1-antagonist, loratadine. Eur J Clin Pharmacol 1987; 32: 419–21.

Gonzalez MA, Estes KS. Pharmacokinetic overview of oral second-generation H_1 antihistamines. Int J Clin Pharmacol Ther 1998; 36: 292–300.

Haria M, Fitton A, Peters DH. Loratadine: a reappraisal of its pharmacological properties and therapeutic use in allergic disorders. Drugs 1994; 48: 617–37.

Monroe EW. Loratadine in the treatment of urticaria. Clin Ther 1997; 19: 232–42.

Histamine-2 Receptor Antagonists

Generic	Brand	Availability[1]	Uses[2]	Adult Dose[3]	Adverse Effects
Cimetidine[4]	Tagamet	Tablets: 200 mg (OTC), 300 mg, 400 mg, 800 mg Liquid: 300 mg/5 ml Injection: 150 mg/ml; 300 mg/50 ml	Duodenal ulcer Gastric ulcer GI hypersecretory conditions Gastroesophageal reflux (GERD)	Acute: 800 mg HS Maintenance: 400 mg HS Acute: 800 mg HS or 300 mg ACHS 300 mg ACHS 800 mg BID or 400 mg QID	All agents well-tolerated. Rare: leukopenia, granulocytopenia, thrombocytopenia, agranulocytosis, aplastic anemia, pancytopenia.
Famotidine	Pepcid	Tablets: 10 mg (OTC), 20 mg, 40 mg Chewable tablets: 10 mg (OTC) Gelcaps: 10 mg (OTC) Powder for suspension: 40 mg/5 ml Injection: 10 mg/ml Premixed injection: 20 mg/50 ml in 0.9% sodium chloride	Duodenal ulcer Gastric ulcer Gastroesophageal reflux (GERD) GI hypersecretory conditions Erosive esophagitis	Acute: 40 mg HS or 20 mg BID Maintenance: 20 mg HS Acute: 40 mg HS 20 mg BID 20 mg QID Acute: 20–40 mg BID	Cimetidine has been uncommonly associated with reversible mental status changes and other CNS effects
Nizatidine	Axid	Tablets: 75 mg (OTC) Capsules: 150 mg, 300 mg Oral Solution: 15 mg/ml	Duodenal ulcer Gastric ulcer Gastroesophageal reflux (GERD) Erosive esophagitis	Acute: 300 mg HS or 150 mg BID Maintenance: 150 mg HS Acute: 150 mg BID or 300 mg HS 150 mg BID 150 mg BID	(e.g. agitation, psychosis, hallucinations), particularly in the elderly or severe illness.

Continued overleaf

continued

Generic	Brand	Availability[1]	Uses[2]	Adult Dose[3]	Adverse Effects
Ranitidine	Zantac	Tablets: 75 mg (OTC), 150 mg, 300 mg Capsules: 150 mg, 300 mg Tablets for solution: 25 mg, 150 mg (EFFERdose) Granules for solution: 150 mg packet (EFFERdose) Solution: 75 mg/5 ml Injection: 25 mg/ml Premixed injection: 50 mg/50 ml in 0.45% sodium chloride	Duodenal ulcer Gastric ulcer GI hypersecretory conditions Gastroesophageal reflux (GERD) Erosive esophagitis	Acute: 300 mg HS or 150 mg BID Maintenance: 150 mg HS Acute: 150 mg BID Maintenance: 150 mg HS 150 mg BID, maximum 6 g/day 150 mg BID Acute: 150 mg QID Maintenance: 150 mg BID	These agents inhibit the hepatic microsomal enzyme CYP450 3A4, although only cimetidine appears to do so to a clinically significant degree. Cimetidine is therefore associated with a number of drug interactions, including those with theophylline, phenytoin, warfarin, and quinidine, among others.

1. Rx status unless otherwise noted OTC strength indicated for heartburn.
2. Literature reports describe uses relating to dermatology which include the prevention and management of various allergic processes (e.g. acute urticaria), psoriasis, and porphyria cutanea tarda. Results have been mixed. In general, these agents potentiate histamine-induced bronchoconstriction and produce variable effects on cutaneous reactions.
3. Adjustment for renal impairment (CrCL <50 ml/min): extend the dosing interval.
4. Cimetidine has been used as a treatment for warts in doses of 20–40 mg/kg per day given in divided doses TID.

Anti-inflammatory Agents

Ibuprofen (Motrin, Advil)

Dose and Administration

Adults

Pain/fever/dysmenorrhea: 200 to 400 mg every 4 to 6 hours as needed.

Inflammatory disease: 1200 to 3200 mg/day, divided into three or four daily doses.

Children

Pain: 4–10 mg/kg per dose every 6 to 8 hours.

Fever: 5 mg/kg per dose (may give 10 mg/kg per dose if > 102.5°F (39°C)), may repeat every 6 to 8 hours. Maximum daily dose is 40 mg/kg.

Juvenile rheumatoid arthritis: 30–50 mg/kg per day, divided into four daily doses.

Uses

Nonsteroidal anti-inflammatory drugs (NSAIDs) have been used for their ability to treat pain and reduce fever. In addition, they are useful in the treatment (often adjunctive) of various inflammatory diseases, including rheumatoid arthritis, juvenile rheumatoid arthritis, osteoarthritis, UVB inflammation, vasculitis, and erythema nodosum. Also has been used in psoriasis.

Monitoring

Occult blood loss, complete blood count, renal function (serum creatinine, blood urea nitrogen (BUN), urine output), liver function tests, weight gain/edema, mental status changes, ophthalmologic examination if visual disturbances present.

Pharmacology

NSAID that possesses analgesic, anti-inflammatory, and antipyretic properties. Inhibits the formation of prostaglandins from arachidonic acid via the inhibition of the enzyme cyclo-oxygenase. The actions of prostaglandins are varied and include (1) mediation of pain sensations and inflammation; (2) maintenance of the protective mucous and bicarbonate barrier in the gut; and (3) maintenance of renal blood flow.

Precautions

Avoid in patients with demonstrated hypersensitivity/allergy (e.g. anaphylaxis, urticaria, angioedema, asthma) to aspirin or other NSAIDs. History of or active gastrointestinal ulceration, bleeding, or perforation. Coagulation disorders. Hypertension and congestive heart failure patients may experience worsening of disease (due to fluid retention and edema). Renal or hepatic dysfunction.

Has rarely been associated with the development of aseptic meningitis, particularly in patients with systemic lupus erythematosus. Presenting symptoms have included fever, chills, nausea/vomiting, nuchal rigidity, and mental status changes. Consider the possibility of NSAID involvement in these scenarios.

Adverse Effects

Gastrointestinal: Primarily upper gastrointestinal ulcerations, bleeding, perforations. Patients most prone include the elderly, those with a history of gastrointestinal bleeding, and those receiving concomitant corticosteroids, anticoagulants, or antiplatelet agents. Other gastrointestinal effects include nausea, vomiting, and indigestion.

Renal: Primarily acute renal failure. Highest risk in those with congestive heart failure, elderly, pre-existing renal impairment, and others dependent on prostaglandins for maintenance of renal blood flow.

Cardiovascular: Fluid retention and edema, which may exacerbate hypertension and congestive heart failure.

Hematologic: Inhibition of platelet aggregation with resultant prolongation of bleeding time. Other effects (uncommon) include anemia, aplastic anemia, hemolytic anemia, agranulocytosis, neutropenia, thrombocytopenia, agranulocytosis.

Hepatic: Mild elevation of liver function tests. Less than 1% have experienced clinically significant elevations in transaminases.

Central nervous system: Dizziness, somnolence, hallucinations (more common in elderly). Aseptic meningitis (see Precautions).

Dermatologic: Rash, pruritus (< 10%).

Other: Visual disturbances, tinnitus, hearing loss (uncommon).

Drug Interactions

NSAIDs may antagonize the natriuretic and/or antihypertensive effects of angiotensin converting enzyme (ACE) inhibitors, β-blockers, loop diuretics, and thiazide diuretics. May increase levels of phenytoin and lithium. Consider additive bleeding with concomitant anticoagulants (e.g. warfarin). Possible increased (temporary) risk of hypoglycemia with concomitant sulfonylureas.

Preparation

(Motrin, Nuprin, Advil, generics)

Tablets, Capsules, and/or Caplets	100 & 200 mg *OTC*
	300, 400, 600 & 800 mg *Rx*
Tablets, chewable	50 & 100 mg *OTC*
Suspension	100 mg/5 ml *Rx* and *OTC*
Drops	40 mg/ml *OTC*

Selected Reference

Lichtenstein J, Flowers F, Sherertz EF. Nonsteroidal anti-inflammatory drugs. Their use in dermatology. Int J Dermatol 1987; 26: 80–7.

Naproxen/Naproxen Sodium (Naprosyn, Anaprox, Naprelan, Aleve)

Dose and Administration

Adults

Pain/dysmenorrhea: 250 mg (275 mg naproxen sodium) every 6 to 8 hours; may give an initial dose of 500 mg (550 mg naproxen sodium).

Controlled release tablets: 1000 mg once daily.

Inflammatory disease: 250 to 500 mg twice daily (275 to 550 mg naproxen sodium).

Delayed release tablets: 375 to 500 mg twice daily.

Controlled release tablets: 750 to 1000 mg once daily.

Children

Pain: 5 to 7 mg/kg per dose every 8 to 12 hours.

Inflammatory disease: Usual dose 10 to 15 mg/kg per day, divided twice daily. Doses up to 20 mg/kg per day have been used.

Uses

Nonsteroidal anti-inflammatory drugs (NSAIDs) have been used for their ability to treat pain and reduce fever. In addition, they are useful in the treatment (often adjunctive) of various inflammatory diseases, including rheumatoid arthritis, juvenile rheumatoid arthritis, osteoarthritis, UVB inflammation, vasculitis, and erythema nodosum. Also has been used in psoriasis.

Monitoring

Occult blood loss, complete blood count, renal function (serum creatinine, BUN, urine output), liver function tests, weight gain/edema, mental status changes, ophthalmologic examination if visual disturbances are present.

Pharmacology

NSAID that possesses analgesic, anti-inflammatory, and antipyretic properties. Inhibits the formation of prostaglandins from arachidonic acid via the inhibition of the enzyme cyclo-oxygenase. The actions of prostaglandins are varied and include (1) mediation of pain sensations and inflammation; (2) maintenance of the protective mucous and bicarbonate barrier in the gut; and (3) maintenance of renal blood flow.

Precautions

Avoid in patients with demonstrated hypersensitivity/allergy (e.g. anaphylaxis, urticaria, angioedema, asthma) to aspirin or other NSAIDs. History of or active gastrointestinal ulceration, bleeding, or perforation. Coagulation disorders.

Hypertension and congestive heart failure patients may experience worsening of disease (due to fluid retention and edema). Renal or hepatic dysfunction.

Has rarely been associated with the development of aseptic meningitis, particularly in patients with systemic lupus erythematosus. Presenting symptoms have included fever, chills, nausea/vomiting, nuchal rigidity, and mental status changes. Consider the possibility of NSAID involvement in these scenarios.

Adverse Effects

Gastrointestinal: primarily upper gastrointestinal ulcerations, bleeding, perforations. Patients most prone include the elderly, those with a history of gastrointestinal bleeding, and those receiving concomitant corticosteroids, anticoagulants, or

Naproxen/Naproxen Sodium (Naprosyn, Anaprox, Naprelan, Aleve)

antiplatelet agents. Other gastrointestinal effects include nausea, vomiting, and indigestion.

Renal: primarily acute renal failure. Highest risk in those with congestive heart failure, the elderly, those with pre-existing renal impairment, and others dependent on prostaglandins for maintenance of renal blood flow.

Cardiovascular: fluid retention and edema, which may exacerbate hypertension and congestive heart failure.

Hematologic: inhibition of platelet aggregation with resultant prolongation of bleeding time. Other effects (uncommon) include anemia, aplastic anemia, hemolytic anemia, agranulocytosis, neutropenia, thrombocytopenia, and agranulocytosis.

Hepatic: mild elevation of liver function tests. Less than 1% have experienced clinically significant elevations in transaminases.

Central nervous system: dizziness, somnolence, hallucinations (more common in the elderly). Aseptic meningitis (see Precautions).

Dermatologic: rash, pruritus (< 10%).

Other: visual disturbances, tinnitus, hearing loss (uncommon).

Drug Interactions

NSAIDs may antagonize the natriuretic and/or antihypertensive effects of angiotensin converting enzyme (ACE) inhibitors, β-blockers, loop diuretics, and thiazide diuretics. May increase levels of phenytoin and lithium. Consider additive bleeding with concomitant anticoagulants (e.g. warfarin). Possible increased (temporary) risk of hypoglycemia with concomitant sulfonylureas.

Preparation

Naproxen

Tablets	250, 375 & 500 mg	*Rx* Naprosyn / Generic
Tablets, delayed-release	375 & 500 mg	*Rx* Naprosyn EC / Generic
Suspension	125 mg/5 ml	*Rx* Naprosyn / Generic

Naproxen sodium

Tablets	220 mg (200 mg naproxen)	*OTC* Aleve / Generic
	275 mg (250 mg naproxen)	*Rx* Anaprox / Generic
	550 mg (500 mg naproxen)	*Rx* Anaprox DS / Generic

Tablets controlled release

	375 mg naproxen (412.5 mg naproxen sodium)	*Rx* Naprelan
	500 mg naproxen (550 mg naproxen sodium)	*Rx* Naprelan

Selected Reference

Lichtenstein J, Flowers F, Sherertz EF. Nonsteroidal anti-inflammatory drugs. Their use in dermatology. Int J Dermatol 1987; 26: 80–7.

Prednisone (Deltasone, Orasone)

Dose and Administration

Usual oral dose: Depends on disease state, acute treatment versus maintenance therapy, and response. Give 1 to 2 mg/kg orally per day, divided two to four times daily, in acute exacerbations and titrate to response. Titration time frame can vary from 1 week to 1 month with a slow taper, decreasing by a consistent dosage. Maintenance therapy for chronic disease can range from 5 to 30 mg/day orally, or as needed for suppression of symptoms.

Uses

Treatment of angioedema, ankylosing spondylitis, asthma, atopic dermatitis, dermatitis, gout, graft-versus-host disease, idiopathic thrombocytopenia, juvenile rheumatoid arthritis, kidney transplant rejection prophylaxis, mycosis fungoides, pemphigus vulgaris, bullous pemphigoid, polymyositis, psoriasis, rheumatoid arthritis, sarcoidosis, Stevens–Johnson syndrome, systemic lupus erythematosus, thyroiditis, ulcerative colitis, urticaria, Wegener's granulomatosis.

Pharmacology

Glucocorticoids are naturally synthesized steroid hormones that regulate protein transcription at the genomic level. They curtail the inflammatory response by decreasing transcription of inflammatory proteins, interfering with the function of inflammatory mediators, and inhibiting leukocyte migration to the site of inflammation. Prednisone is a glucocorticoid that is metabolized by the liver to its active form, prednisolone, a naturally produced steroid hormone. It is approximately four times as potent as hydrocortisone. It is extremely bioavailable through the gastrointestinal tract and is widely systemically available.

Contraindications

Hypersensitivity, systemic fungal infections.

Adverse Effects/Precautions

Increase dosage in times of physical and emotional stress (before, during, and after the event).

Corticosteroids may mask symptoms of infection and should be avoided in situations where the bacterial or viral infection is not well controlled by antibiotic agents.

Decreased wound healing.

Corticosteroids have been shown to cause posterior subcapsular cataracts and may exacerbate glaucoma symptoms. Those on chronic steroid therapy should be routinely assessed for cataract formation.

Patients on immunosuppressive doses (2 mg/kg per day or 20 mg/day) should not be administered live-virus vaccines. If vaccination is desired, it should be completed no less than 2 weeks prior to the course of immunosuppressive therapy.

Use with caution in patients with Cushing's syndrome.

Avoid prolonged use in children because of the possibility of retarded bone growth.

Prednisone (Deltasone, Orasone)

Abrupt discontinuation of corticosteroids is discouraged, owing to the possibility of acute adrenal insufficiency as a result of prolonged hypothalamic–pituitary–adrenal axis suppression. Tapering is usually only necessary after regimens of at least 10 mg prednisone (or equivalent) for 2 weeks.

Side-effects include decreased lymphocyte or monocyte count, blue toe syndrome, leukemoid reactions, hypertension, mood instability, Cushing's syndrome, diabetes mellitus, osteoporosis, acne, and other cardiovascular and neurologic abnormalities.

Pregnancy: FDA category B.

Drug Interactions

Rifabutin and rifampin increase the hepatic metabolism of prednisone and prednisolone via hepatic enzyme induction; increased dosages may be needed. The use of NSAIDs or aspirin with prednisone increases the risk of gastrointestinal ulceration. Hypokalemia may result from the potassium-wasting effect of prednisone with a potassium-depleting diuretic.

Preparation *Rx*

Syrup	5 mg/ml	Prednisone Intensol
	1 mg/ml & 0.1 mg/ml	Prednisone liquid
Tablets	1, 2.5 & 5 mg	Deltasone
	10, 20 & 50 mg	Orasone
		Generics

Selected Reference

Frey B, Frey FJ. Clinical pharmacokinetics of prednisone and prednisolone. Clin Pharmacokinet 1990; 19: 126–46.

Nonsteroidal Anti-inflammatory Drugs (NSAIDs)

Generic	Brand	Availability	Daily Dosage[1]	Maximum Daily Dosage
Salicylates				
Aspirin	Ecotrin, Bayer, various	Tablets: 81 mg, 165 mg, 325 mg, 500 mg, 650 mg, 975 mg; Tablets, extended release: 650 mg; Tablets, controlled release: 800 mg; Suppositories: 120 mg, 200 mg, 300 mg, 600 mg	325–650 mg q4 h prn; 3200–6000 mg divided TID or QID	6000 mg
Salsalate	Salflex, Amigesic, generics	Tablets: 500 mg, 750 mg	3000 mg divided BID or TID	3000 mg
Choline magnesium salicylate	Trilisate, generic	Tablets: 500 mg, 750 mg, 1000 mg; Liquid: 500 mg/5 ml	1000–4500 mg divided BID or TID	4500 mg
Non-salicylate NSAIDs				
Diclofenac potassium	Cataflam, generic	Tablets: 50 mg	100–200 mg divided BID, TID, or QID	200 mg
Diclofenac sodium	Voltaren, generic	Tablets: 25 mg, 50 mg, 75 mg	100–200 mg divided BID, TID, or QID	200 mg
	Voltaren XR, generic	Tablets, extended release: 50 mg, 75 mg, 100 mg	100 mg (may increase to BID)	
Etodolac	Lodine, generic	Capsules: 200 mg, 300 mg; Tablets: 400 mg, 500 mg	200–400 mg q6–8 h prn or 600–1000 mg divided BID, TID, or QID	1200 mg
	Lodine XL	Tablets, extended release: 400 mg, 500 mg, 600 mg	800–1200 mg QD	
Fenoprofen	Nalfon, generic	Capsules: 200 mg, 300 mg; Tablets: 600 mg	900–2400 mg divided TID or QID	3200 mg
Flurbiprofen	Ansaid, generic	Tablets: 50 mg, 100 mg	200–300 mg divided BID, TID, or QID	300 mg

continued

Generic	Brand	Availability	Daily Dosage[1]	Maximum Daily Dosage
Ibuprofen[2]	Advil, Motrin, generic	Tablets, Caplets, and/or Capsules: 100 mg, 200 mg, 300 mg, 400 mg, 600 mg, 800 mg Tablets, chewable: 50 mg, 100 mg Suspension: 100 mg/5 ml Drops: 40 mg/ml	1200–3200 mg divided TID or QID	3200 mg
Indomethacin	Indocin, generic	Capsules: 25 mg, 50 mg Suspension: 25 mg/5 ml Suppositories: 50 mg	50–150 mg divided BID, TID, or QID	200 mg
	Indocin SR, generic	Capsules, sustained release: 75 mg	75–150 mg divided QD or BID	150 mg
Ketoprofen	Orudis KT, generic	Tablets: 12.5 mg	12.5 mg q4–6h prn	75 mg
	Orudis, generic	Capsules: 25 mg, 50 mg, 75 mg	150–200 mg divided TID or QID	300 mg
	Oruvail, generic	Capsules, extended release: 100 mg, 150 mg, 200 mg	100–200 mg QD 200 mg	200 mg
Ketorolac tromethamine	Toradol, generic	Tablets: 10 mg	10 mg q4–6h prn (for short-term use only)	40 mg
Meclofenamate sodium	Meclomen, generic	Capsules: 50 mg, 100 mg	50–100 mg q4–6h prn 200–400 mg divided TID or QID	400 mg
Mefenamic acid	Ponstel	Capsules: 250 mg	1000 mg divided QID	1000 mg
Meloxiam	Mobic	Tablets: 7.5 mg	7.5 mg QD	15 mg
Nabumetone	Relafen	Tablets: 500 mg, 750 mg	1000–2000 mg divided BID or QD	2000 mg
Naproxen[2]	Naprosyn, generic	Tablets: 250 mg, 375 mg, 500 mg Suspension: 125 mg/5 ml	500–1000 mg divided BID	1500 mg
	EC-Naprosyn	Tablets, delayed release: 375 mg, 500 mg	750–1000 mg divided BID	

continued overleaf

continued

Generic	Brand	Availability	Daily Dosage[1]	Maximum Daily Dosage
Naproxen sodium[2]	Aleve, generic	Tablets: 220 mg	220 mg q8–12 h prn	660 mg
	Anaprox, generic	Tablets: 275 mg	550–1100 mg divided BID	1500 mg
	Anaprox DS, generic	Tablets: 550 mg		
	Naprelan	Tablets, controlled release: 375 mg, 500 mg as naproxen	750–1000 mg QD	
Oxaprozin	Daypro	Tablets: 600 mg	600–1200 mg QD	1800 mg
Piroxicam	Feldene, generic	Capsules: 10 mg, 20 mg	20 mg QD (or 10 mg BID)	20 mg
Sulindac	Clinoril, generic	Tablets: 150 mg, 200 mg	300–400 mg divided BID	400 mg
Tolmetin sodium	Tolectin, generic	Tablets: 200 mg, 600 mg	600–1800 mg divided TID	1800 mg
	Tolectin DS, generic	Capsules: 400 mg		
Cyclo-oxygenase-2 (COX-2) inhibitor NSAID				
Celecoxib	Celebrex	Capsules: 100 mg, 200 mg	200–400 mg divided BID	400 mg

[1] Adult dosage. Consult product labeling for dosage adjustment(s) in renal and/or hepatic failure.
[2] See complete monograph elsewhere in text.

Topical Corticosteroids

Topical corticosteroids are available in different potencies. They are classified into seven potency classes, with class 1 representing the most potent. The most potent topicals are used for thick, chronic processes (such as neurodermatitis), while the least potent preparations are generally used on the face and intertriginous areas, and in infants and young children.

Except for vehicle effects, there is probably little to no difference between the safety and efficacy of steroids from the same class. Vehicle effects may be important, however. Creams, gels, lotions, and foam-based products are more cosmetically pleasing than ointment vehicles. Ointments may provide greater moisturizing for dry skin processes (such as psoriasis and atopic dermatitis) and often contain fewer potential irritants.

The risks of topical corticosteroid use include atrophy, striae (stretch marks), telangiectasias, and potential systemic effects of adrenal suppression and growth retardation. Glaucoma and cataracts are other potential risks, especially with application near the eyes. Local side-effects are more likely to occur with prolonged use of the more potent preparations, especially when used in sensitive skin areas (face and intertriginous areas).

Vehicle: Topical Creams

Prescription required; generally applied twice daily. Elocon is approved for once daily application.

Class	Brand	Generic	%
1	Temovate	Clobetasol propionate	0.05
1	Temovate-E	Clobetasol propionate	0.05
1	Ultravate	Halobetasol propionate	0.05
2	Dermacin	Fluocinonide	0.05
2	Diprolene AF	Augmented betamethasone dipropionate	0.05
2	Halog	Halcinonide	0.1
2	Halog-E	Halcinonide	0.1
2	Lidex	Fluocinonide	0.05
2	Maxivate	Betamethasone dipropionate	0.05
2	Psorcon	Diflorasone diacetate	0.05
2	Topicort	Desoximetasone	0.25
3	Alphatrex	Betamethasone dipropionate	0.05
3	Aristocort	Triamcinolone acetonide	0.5
3	Aristocort A	Triamcinolone acetonide	0.5
3	Cyclocort	Amcinonide	0.1
3	Diprosone	Betamethasone dipropionate	0.05
3	Florone	Diflorasone diacetate	0.05
3	Florone E	Diflorasone diacetate	0.05
3	Kenalog	Triamcinolone acetonide	0.5
3	Lidex-E	Fluocinonide	0.05

continued overleaf

Topical Corticosteroids

continued

Class	Brand	Generic	%
3	Maxiflor	Diflorasone diacetate	0.05
3	Telador	Betamethasone dipropionate	0.05
4	Aristocort	Triamcinolone acetonide	0.1
4	Delta-Tritex	Triamcinolone acetonide	0.1
4	Elocon	Mometasone furoate	0.1
4	Kenalog	Triamcinolone acetonide	0.1
4	Topicort-LP	Desoximetasone	0.05
4	Triderm	Triamcinolone acetonide	0.1
5	Betatrex	Betamethasone valerate	0.1
5	Cloderm	Clocortolone pivalate	0.1
5	Cordran SP	Flurandrenolide	0.05
5	Cutivate	Fluticasone propionate	0.05
5	Dermatop	Prednicarbate	0.1
5	Locoid	Hydrocortisone butyrate	0.1
5	Synalar	Fluocinolone acetonide	0.025
5	Westcort	Hydrocortisone valerate	0.2
6	Aclovate	Alclometasone dipropionate	0.05
6	Aristocort	Triamcinolone acetonide	0.025
6	Aristocort A	Triamcinolone acetonide	0.1
6	Aristocort A	Triamcinolone acetonide	0.025
6	Cordran SP	Flurandrenolide	0.025
6	DesOwen	Desonide	0.05
6	Kenalog	Triamcinolone acetonide	0.025
6	Synalar	Fluocinolone acetonide	0.025
6	Tridesilon	Desonide	0.05

Vehicle: Topical Ointments

Prescription required; generally applied twice to three times daily. Elocon is approved for once daily application.

Class	Brand	Generic	%
1	Diprolene	Augmented betamethasone dipropionate	0.05
1	Psorcon	Augmented diflorasone diacetate	0.05
1	Temovate	Clobetasol propionate	0.05
1	Ultravate	Halobetasol propionate	0.05
2	Alphatrex	Betamethasone dipropionate	0.05
2	Aristocort	Triamcinolone acetonide	0.5
2	Cyclocort	Amcinonide	0.1
2	Diprosone	Betamethasone dipropionate	0.05
2	Florone	Diflorasone diacetate	0.05
2	Lidex	Fluocinonide	0.05
2	Maxiflor	Diflorasone diacetate	0.05

continued overleaf

Topical Corticosteroids

continued

Class	Brand	Generic	%
2	Maxivate	Betamethasone dipropionate	0.05
2	Topicort	Desoximetasone	0.25
3	Aristocort A	Triamcinolone acetonide	0.1
3	Betatrex	Betamethasone valerate	0.1
3	Cutivate	Fluticasone propionate	0.005
3	Delta-Tritex	Triamcinolone acetonide	0.1
3	Halog	Halcinonide	0.1
4	Aristocort	Triamcinolone acetonide	0.1
4	Cordran	Flurandrenolide	0.05
4	Elocon	Mometasone furoate	0.1
4	Kenalog	Triamcinolone acetonide	0.1
4	Synalar	Fluocinolone acetonide	0.025
4	Westcort	Hydrocortisone valerate	0.2
5	Locoid	Hydrocortisone butyrate	0.1
6	Aclovate	Alclometasone dipropionate	0.05
6	DesOwen	Desonide	0.05
6	Tridesilon	Desonide	0.05

Vehicle: Gels

Prescription required. Apply twice daily.

Class	Brand	Generic	%
1	Clobevate	Clobetasol propionate	0.05
1	Diprolene	Augmented betamethasone dipropionate	0.05
1	Temovate	Clobetasol propionate	0.05
2	Lidex	Fluocinonide	0.05
2	Topicort	Desoximetasone	0.05

Vehicle: Lotions

Prescription required. Apply twice daily.

Class	Brand	Generic	%
1	Clobex	Clobetasol propionate	0.05
3	Cyclocort	Amcinonide	0.1
5	Cordran	Flurandrenolide (with menthol)	0.05
5	Kenalog	Triamcinolone acetonide	0.1
5	Locoid Emulsion	Hydrocortisone butyrate	0.1
6	DesOwen	Desonide	0.05
6	Kenalog	Triamcinolone acetonide	0.025

Topical Corticosteroids

Vehicle: Solutions

Prescription required. Usually applied twice daily. Most useful for scalp conditions.

Class	Brand	Generic	%
1	Cormax scalp application	Clobetasol propionate	0.05
1	Diprolene lotion	Augmented betamethasone dipropionate	0.05
1	Temovate scalp application	Clobetasol propionate	0.05
2	Lidex	Fluocinonide	0.05
3	Halog	Halcinonide	0.1
3	Maxivate lotion	Betamethasone dipropionate	0.05
4	Elocon lotion	Mometasone furoate	0.1
5	Alphatrex lotion	Betamethasone dipropionate	0.05
5	Betatrex lotion	Betamethasone valerate	0.1
5	Diprosone lotion	Betamethasone dipropionate	0.05
5	Locoid	Hydrocortisone butyrate	0.1
6	Fluonid	Fluocinolone acetonide	0.01
6	Synalar	Fluocinolone acetonide	0.01

Vehicle: Other

Prescription required.

Tape vehicles (Cordran) are most useful for prurigo lesions and other heavily rubbed lesions as seen in neurodermatitis, lichen simplex chronicus, and some lesions of psoriasis. Foam preparations (Olux, Luxiq) are designed to deliver topical corticosteroids to hair-bearing areas; these preparations contain alcohol and may cause a transient burning sensation on sensitive skin. Derma-Smoothe/FS oil is also used for scalp application, particularly for thick, hyperkeratotic scalp processes such as severe scalp psoriasis or tinea amiantacea. It may also be useful for atopic dermatitis. Commonly used overnight on the scalp, it may be best removed in the morning with dishwashing detergent followed by use of a medicated shampoo.

Class	Brand	Generic	Preparation
1	Cordran tape	Flurandrenolide	$4\,\mu g/cm^2$
1	Olux	Clobetasol propionate	0.05%; 50 g, 100 g foam, for scalp application
3	Luxiq	Betamethasone valerate	0.12%; 50 g, 100 g foam, for scalp application
5	Derma-Smoothe/FS	Fluocinolone acetonide oil	0.01% in mineral/peanut oil vehicle

continued overleaf

Topical Corticosteroids

continued

Class	Brand	Generic	Preparation
—	Kenalog aerosol	Triamcinolone acetonide	0.147 mg/g
—	Beconase AQ nasal spray	Beclomethasone dipropionate	42 µg/spray
—	Flonase nasal spray	Fluticasone propionate	50 µg/spray
—	FS Shampoo	Fluocinolone acetonide	0.01%
—	Kenalog in Orabase paste	Triamcinolone acetonide	0.1%
—	Nasacort AQ nasal spray	Triamcinolone acetonide	55 µg/spray
—	Nasalide nasal spray	Flunisolide	25 µg/spray
—	Nasarel nasal spray	Flunisolide	25 µg/spray
—	Nasonex nasal spray	Mometasone fumarate	50 µg/spray
—	Rhinocort Aqua nasal spray	Budesonide	32 µg/spray
—	Vancenase AQ nasal spray	Beclomethasone dipropionate	42 µg & 84 µg/spray

Triamcinolone Acetonide Injection (Kenalog)

Uses, Dose and Administration

FDA-approved

Intradermal (10 mg/ml): 1 mg per injection site, with injection sites separated by at least 1 cm, weekly for the treatment of: discoid lupus, alopecia areata, psoriasis, keloids, necrobiosis, lipoidica diabeticorum, lichen planus lesions.

Intramuscular (40 mg/ml): 40–80 mg once weekly for the treatment of: bullous dermatitis herpetiformis, exfoliative dermatitis, pemphigus vulgaris, Stevens–Johnson syndrome, psoriasis, seborrheic dermatitis, systemic lupus erythematosus, contact dermatitis, atopic dermatitis.

Intra-articular (10 mg/ml or 40 mg/ml): 2.5–40 mg once weekly for the treatment of: osteoarthritis, rheumatoid arthritis, bursitis, gouty arthritis, epicondylitis, tenosynovitis.

Pharmacology

Triamcinolone is a synthetic glucocorticoid used for its anti-inflammatory and immunosuppressive properties. In pharmacologic doses, triamcinolone inhibits the release of inflammatory mediators, inhibits diapedesis of leukocytes and macrophages, and reduces capillary permeability and edema.

Immunosuppressive properties include reducing the concentration of immunoglobulin and complement as well as immune complex transfer across the capillary membrane.

Adverse Effects/Precautions

Adverse dermatologic effects related to intralesional/intramuscular injection include the following: acne vulgaris, skin atrophy, bruising, dermatitis, erythema, exfoliative dermatitis, ecchymoses, hirsutism, impaired wound healing, folliculitis, injection site reaction, striae, telangiectasia, skin hyper/hypopigmentation, urticaria, sterile abscesses, lupus erythematosus-like lesions, and suppressed reactions to skin tests.

Pregnancy: FDA category C.

Preparation *Rx*

40 mg/ml suspension for intramuscular and intra-articular use

10 mg/ml suspension for intradermal and intra-articular use

Antiparasitics

Ivermectin (Stromectol)

Uses, Dose and Administration

FDA-approved

Strongyloidiasis: single oral dose of 200 micrograms per kg body weight.

Onchocerciasis: single oral dose of 150 micrograms per kg body weight.

Other

Scabies: single oral dose of 200 to 250 micrograms per kg body weight.

Pharmacology

Semi-synthetic anthelmintic drug derived from the avermectin class of antiparasitic drugs. Binds to glutamate-gated chloride channels on membranes of invertebrate nerve and muscle cells, ultimately causing paralysis and death of the parasite. Poor penetration across the blood–brain barrier.

Adverse Effects/Precautions

Generally has low side-effect profile as established by decades of use in the treatment of various nematode infections. Severe adverse reactions include the Mazzotti-type reaction in the treatment of filiariasis, thought to be an allergic response to the actual dying filia. Reported minor adverse effects include the following, although not specifically reported during the treatment of scabies: fatigue, abdominal pain, anorexia, constipation, diarrhea, nausea, vomiting, dizziness, pruritus, urticaria, abnormal sensation of eyes, eyelid edema, and conjunctivitis.

Pregnancy: FDA category C; has been shown to be excreted in human milk, and should be avoided in nursing mothers.

Safety and efficacy have not been established in infants weighing less than 15 kg.

In immunocompromised hosts with intestinal strongyloidiasis, further treatment is usually required.

Monitoring

Strongyloidiasis: Repeat stool examination to document clearance of organism.

Onchocerciasis: Further treatment usually required.

Scabies: No laboratory monitoring recommended.

Drug Interactions

No known drug interactions.

Preparation *Rx*

Tablets   3 & 6 mg

References

Abramowicz M. Drugs for head lice. Med Lett Drugs Ther 1997; 39: 6–7.

Chouela EN, Abeldano AM, Pellerano G, et al. Equivalent therapeutic efficacy and safety of ivermectin and lindane in the treatment of human scabies. Arch Dermatol 1999; 135: 651–5.

Meinking TL, Taplin D, Hermida JL, et al. The treatment of scabies with ivermectin. N Engl J Med 1995; 333; 26–30.

Usha V, Nair TV. A comparative study of oral ivermectin and topical permethrin cream in the treatment of scabies. J Am Acad Dermatol 2000; 42: 236–40.

Lindane (Kwell)

Use, Dose and Administration

Available in a lotion and shampoo. The lotion is indicated for treatment of ectoparasitic infestations, such as *Sarcoptes scabiei* (scabies). Lindane shampoo is indicated for treatment of pediculosis capitis, pediculosis pubis and their ova.

In both conditions, lindane is second-line treatment and is indicated when the patient cannot tolerate or has had failed other agents.

Lindane Lotion: S. scabiei

ONE application of a thin film to entire body (neck down). Leave for 8 to 12 hours, and then remove by bathing. All potentially exposed garments and bed sheets, pillow cases and towels should be either dry-cleaned or washed in hot water.

Lindane Shampoo: pediculosis capitis, pediculosis pubis

Wash hair with regular shampoo, then completely dry hair. Massage lindane into dry hair, leave for 4 to 5 minutes. After several minutes, add a small quantity of water, until hair lathers. Rinse hair, and proceed to remove nits with nit comb.

Hair Length	Dosage
Short	30 ml
Medium	45 ml
Long	60 ml

Post-treatment pruritus is expected with both lindane lotion and shampoo but does not warrant further treatment. Retreatment is not recommended. Person applying the lotion or shampoo should wear rubber gloves or wash hands immediately afterward.

Pharmacology

Lindane is a chlorocyclohexane compound with ectoparasiticidal and ovicidal properties. It is directly absorbed by the parasites and ova. It permeates the dermis and accumulates in lipid tissues, such as the white matter of the brain.

Contraindications

Premature neonates, patients with a history of seizure disorder, and those with a known sensitivity to the product or its constituents.

Adverse Effects/Precautions

Permeates the skin and is associated with possibility of CNS toxicity. Neurotoxicity manifested as generalized seizures and bone marrow suppression has been reported, most commonly following exposure to high doses due to misuse, overuse or ingestion. Irritant dermatitis (1/100) has also been reported.

Pregnancy: FDA category B/C. Lindane can be potentially excreted in human milk, and it should be avoided in nursing mothers.

Lindane (Kwell)

Avoid use in infants and young children, because of the high incidence of adverse reactions.

Drug Interactions

Avoid concomitant use of oils, lotions or creams, as these may promote transdermal absorption of lindane. Use caution with concomitant drugs that lower the seizure threshold.

Preparation *Rx*

Lindane Lotion or Shampoo USP	1%	60 ml or pint containers

References

Finkelstein LE, Mendelson MH. Stopping the spread of scabies. Am J Nurs 1997; 10: 68–9.

Fischer TF. Lindane toxicity in a 24-year-old woman. Ann Emerg Med 1994; 24: 972–4.

Franz TJ, Lehman PA, Franz SF, Guin JD. Comparative percutaneous absorption of lindane and permethrin. Arch Dermatol 1996; 132: 901–5.

Malathion (Ovide)

Use, Dose and Administration

Fast-acting pediculocide with a high degree of ovicidal activity. Indicated for treatment of *Pediculus humanus capitis* and their ova.

Apply Malathion to dry hair, and leave for 8 to 12 hours. Follow with shampooing of hair and use nit comb to remove lice and ova. If lice present 7 to 9 days after initial treatment, may repeat application.

Pharmacology

An organophosphate that is an irreversible inhibitor of cholinesterase. Malathion is hydrolyzed and detoxified by plasma carboxylesterases much more rapidly in mammals than in insects.

Contraindication

Neonates and infants (scalp more permeable, possibility of increased absorption).

Adverse Effects/Precautions

Transdermal absorption has not been extensively studied at this time. No systemic adverse effects have yet been reported. Malathion 0.5% is carried in 78% isopropanol, which may cause irritation at the application site. Avoid contact with eyes, as this may result in mild conjunctivitis.

Malathion poisoning is possible and manifests as cholinergic hyperactivity causing abdominal cramps, diarrhea, vomiting, excessive salivation, sweating, lacrimation, miosis, respiratory distress, seizures and skeletal muscle weakness. Patient will be bradycardic, but may present with initial tachycardia. If overdose is suspected, the airway should be maintained and gastric lavage undertaken; administer activated charcoal. Atropine may be needed to overcome cholinergic overactivity.

Safety and efficacy have not been studied in children under 6 years old.

Pregnancy: FDA category B; not to be used by nursing mothers, as potential for excretion in human milk does exist.

Drug Interactions

No known drug interactions.

Preparation *Rx*

Lotion   0.5%   60 ml

References

Abramowicz M. Malathion for treatment of head lice. Med Lett Drugs Ther 1999; 41: 73–4.

Chosidow O. Scabies and pediculosis. Lancet 2000; 355: 819–26.

Eichenfield LF, Colon-Fontanez F. Treatment of head lice. Pediatr Infect Dis J 1998; 17: 419–20.

Permethrin (Nix, Elimite, Acticin)

Use, Dose and Administration

Permethrin is available in a 1% cream (Nix) for the treatment of pediculosis capitis and approved for prophylactic therapy during outbreaks. Permethrin is also approved for the treatment of *Sarcoptes scabiei* (scabies) infestation, available in 5% creams (Elimite, Acticin).

Nix for pediculosis capitis: wash hair with regular shampoo, rinse and dry then massage Nix cream into hair and scalp. Leave for 10 minutes then rinse with water. Remove nits with nit comb. One application is generally sufficient, but may re-treat if lice present 7 days after initial treatment. For prophylactic use, a second application is warranted 2 weeks after the initial treatment.

Elimite or Acticin for *S. scabiei*: apply cream to entire body from head (excluding scalp) to soles of feet. Leave for 8–14 hours then remove by bathing. One application is generally sufficient, but if live mites present at 2 weeks, re-treatment is indicated. Post-treatment pruritus is expected and may persist, but this is not an indication for re-treatment.

Pharmacology

Synthetic compound based on the insecticidal components of natural pyrethrins, which are extracts from chrysanthemum flowers. Essentially disrupts sodium channels in the nerve cell membrane, resulting in paralysis of the pest. It is absorbed poorly from the skin and is 20 times less permeable through human skin as compared with lindane. It is rapidly metabolized to inactive compounds and excreted in urine.

Adverse Effects/Precautions

Generally a very safe drug, with low side-effect profile, primarily attributed to its minimal transdermal absorption. Avoid contact with mucous membranes and eyes, as this may cause irritation.

Local erythema, pruritus and swelling may occur. May precipitate asthmatic attack in susceptible individuals.

Not for use in children under 2 months old.

Pregnancy: FDA category B. Avoid in nursing mothers because of potential excretion in human milk.

Monitoring

Pediculosis capitis: lack of living lice on scalp. Scabies: lack of live mites. Pruritus may persist for up to 2 weeks post-treatment, but if no living mites are present, re-treatment is not warranted.

Drug Interactions

No known drug interactions.

Preparation

Rx

Cream	5%	Elimite	60 g tube
Cream	5%	Acticin	60 g tube

OTC

Cream	1%	Nix	60 ml bottle

References

Abramowicz M. Drugs for head lice. Med Lett Drug Ther 1997; 39: 6–7.

Franz TJ, Lehman PA, Franz SF, Guin DJ. Comparative percutaneous absorption of lindane and permethrin. Arch Dermatol 1996; 132: 901–5.

Meinking TL, Taplin D. Safety of permethrin vs lindane for the treatment of scabies. Arch Dermatol 1996; 132: 959–62.

Antipruritics and Topical Anesthetics

Capsaicin (Zostrix)

Dose and Administration

Adults: Apply to affected area(s) three to four times daily. Wash hands thoroughly after application (unless treating hands).

Children: Limited experience, although similar dosing has been utilized in children 2 years of age and older.

Use

Pain relief associated with postherpetic neuralgia, pruritus, arthritis, backache, strains, and sprains.

Pharmacology

Depletion and inhibition of synthesis of substance P in peripheral sensory neurons. Substance P is a neurotransmitter, responsible for pain and itch transmission and sensation.

Adverse Effects/Precautions

Burning sensation with application, usually resolves with routine use. Heat may worsen the burning sensation. Do not wrap the area after application. Do not apply to broken/damaged skin. Avoid mucous membranes.

Preparation *OTC*

Cream	0.025%	Zostrix	2 oz
	0.075%	Zostrix-HP	2 oz

Lotion and gel also available

References

Bernstein JE, Korman NJ, Bickers DR, et al. Topical capsaicin treatment of chronic postherpetic neuralgia. J Am Acad Dermatol 1989; 21: 265–70.

Dubinsky RM, Kabbani H, El-Chami Z, et al. Quality Standards Subcommittee of the American Academy of Neurology. Practice parameter: treatment of postherpetic neuralgia: an evidence-based report of the Quality Standards Subcommittee of the American Academy of Neurology. Neurology 2004; 63: 959–65.

Plaghki L, Adriaensen H, Morlion B, et al. Systematic overview of the pharmacological management of postherpetic neuralgia. Dermatology 2004; 208: 206–16.

Diphenhydramine (Benadryl) Topical

Use

Temporary relief of itching due to minor skin disorders, such as those associated with insect bites, stings, sunburn, and poison ivy, oak, or sumac.

Administration

Apply up to 3 to 4 times daily.

2% preparations are intended for adults and children 12 years of age and older.

1% preparations are appropriate for adults and children 2 years of age and older.

Pharmacology

Antihistamine with some local anesthetic properties when applied topically.

Precautions

Do not apply to blistered skin, oozing skin, or around the eyes or mucous membranes. Do not use on chicken pox or measles.

Selected Preparations *OTC*

Cream	2%	Benadryl Maximum Strength	15 & 30 g
	2% with 0.1% zinc acetate	Benadryl Itch Stopping Cream Extra Strength	14 g
	1% with 0.1% zinc acetate	Benadryl Itch Stopping Cream Original Strength	14 g
Gel	1%	Benadryl Itch Stopping Gel Original	4 oz
	1% with 1% zinc acetate	Benadryl Itch Stopping Gel Children's	4 oz
	2%	Benadryl Itch Stopping Gel Extra Strength	4 oz
	2% with 1% zinc acetate	Benadryl Itch Stopping Gel Maximum Strength	4 oz
Spray	1% with zinc acetate 0.1%	Benadryl Itch Stopping Spray Original	2 oz
	2%	Benadryl Maximum Strength	60 ml
	2% with zinc acetate 0.1%	Benadryl Itch Stopping Spray Extra Strength	2 oz
Stick	2% with zinc acetate 0.1%	Benadryl Itch Relief Stick Extra Strength	14 ml

Doxepin, Topical (Zonalon)

Use, Dose and Administration

Short-term management (up to 8 days) of moderate pruritus associated with the following forms of eczematous dermatitis: atopic dermatitis, lichen simplex chronicus. Apply a thin film four times daily with at least 3 to 4 hours between applications. Occlusive dressings should not be utilized with doxepin cream.

Pharmacology

A dibenzoxepin tricyclic compound with antipruritic properties. Precise mechanism is unknown; believed to be due to potent histamine-1 and histamine-2 receptor antagonism. In patients with pruritic atopic dermatitis, addition of doxepin cream to corticosteroid (e.g. hydrocortisone, triamcinolone) monotherapy has resulted in improved symptom resolution.

Adverse Effects/Precautions

Drowsiness (> 20%), particularly when applied to > 10% of body surface area. Burning or stinging at application site (20% of patients; 25% of these considered severe). Exacerbation of pruritus or eczema, dryness/tightness of skin, paresthesias, edema (1 to 10%). Irritation, tingling, scaling, cracking (< 1%). Other anticholinergic effects may be observed (e.g. dry mouth, 10%; dry eyes).

Contraindicated in patients with untreated narrow-angle glaucoma and predisposition to urinary retention.

Pregnancy: FDA category B.

Use in pediatric patients is not recommended.

Drug Interactions

Caution with concurrent CNS depressants, as drowsiness may be enhanced.

Since the potential exists for absorption sufficient to produce doxepin serum concentrations similar to those seen with oral therapy, the potential for drug interactions with the following medications cannot be ruled out: monoamine oxidase inhibitors, cimetidine, alcohol. Doxepin is metabolized by CYP 2D6, therefore co-administration with inducers (e.g. carbamazepine, rifampin, phenytoin) or inhibitors (e.g. cimetidine, type 1C antiarrhythmics, certain selective serotonin reuptake inhibitors (SSRIs)) of this enzyme should be with caution.

Preparation Rx

Cream   5%   30 & 45 g

References

Berberian BJ, Breneman DL, Drake LA, et al. The addition of topical doxepin to corticosteroid therapy: an improved treatment regimen for atopic dermatitis. Int J Dermatol 1999; 38: 145–8.

Drake LA, Fallon JD, Sober A. Relief of pruritus in patients with atopic dermatitis after treatment with topical doxepin cream. J Am Acad Dermatol 1994; 31: 613–16.

Drake LA, Millikan LE. The antipruritic effect of 5% doxepin cream in patients with eczematous dermatitis. Arch Dermatol 1995; 131: 1403–8.

Lidocaine Patch (Lidoderm)

Dose and Administration

Remove release liner from patch and apply to *intact* skin, covering the most painful area(s). A maximum of three patches for up to 12 hours per 24-hour period may be used. Patches may be cut prior to removing the release liner. Patches should be removed if irritation or burning occurs and not reapplied until these symptoms resolve.

Use

Relief of pain associated with postherpetic neuralgia.

Pharmacology

A local anesthetic (amide-type) that stabilizes neuronal membranes by inhibiting sodium ion influx necessary for impulse generation and conduction. May require several hours to observe onset of clinical effect.

Precautions

Contraindicated in patients sensitive to amide anesthetics. Discarded patches contain significant amounts of lidocaine and should be out of reach of children. Dosing in amounts and durations in excess of those recommended may result in increased lidocaine absorption and predisposition to adversities/toxicity. Patients with hepatic disease will metabolize absorbed lidocaine less efficiently. Safety and efficacy in pediatric patients have not been established.

Pregnancy: FDA category B.

Adverse Effects

Redness, swelling, abnormal sensation at the application site; typically resolve within minutes to hours. Allergic reactions, generally rare, may occur. Systemic adversities unlikely (due to limited absorption); if occur, include CNS excitation and/or depression, cardiovascular depression.

Drug Interactions

Additive effects with other local anesthetics, systemic class I antiarrhythmic agents.

Preparation *Rx*

Patch   5%   Lidoderm

Each patch is packaged in a child-resistant envelope. Cartons of 30. Each patch is 10 x 14 cm

References

Galer BS, Rowbotham MC, Perander J, et al. Topical lidocaine patch relieves postherpetic neuralgia more effectively than a vehicle topical patch: results of an enriched enrollment study. Pain 1999; 80: 533–8.

Rowbotham MC, Davies PS, Verkempinck C, et al. Lidocaine patch: double-blind controlled study of a new treatment method for post-herpetic neuralgia. Pain 1996; 65: 39–44.

Lidocaine/Prilocaine Cream (EMLA)

Dose and Administration

Adults

Minor dermal procedures (e.g. venipuncture): Apply 2.5 g of EMLA Cream over 20 to 25 cm^2 of skin surface (and cover with occlusive dressing); OR 1 EMLA Anesthetic Disc (1 g over 10 cm^2) for at least 1 hour.

Major dermal procedures (e.g. split thickness skin graft harvesting): Apply 2 g of EMLA Cream per 10 cm^2 of skin and allow to remain in contact with the skin for at least 2 hours (covered with occlusive dressing).

Adult male genital skin (adjunct prior to local anesthetic infiltration): Apply a thick layer of EMLA Cream (1 g/10 cm^2) to the skin surface for 15 minutes. Local anesthetic infiltration should be performed immediately after removal of EMLA Cream.

Post-herpetic neuralgia: Doses of 5 to 10 g, occluded for 24 hours, have been used.

Children

Controlled studies of EMLA Cream in children < 7 years of age have shown less overall benefit than in older children or adults.

Dosage for Infants and Children

Age and weight guidelines	Maximum total EMLA dose	Maximum application area	Maximum application time
0–3 months or < 5 kg	1 g	10 cm^2	1 hour
3–12 months and > 5 kg	2 g	20 cm^2	4 hours
1–6 years and > 10 kg	10 g	100 cm^2	4 hours
7–12 years and > 20 kg	20 g	200 cm^2	4 hours

Uses

Topical anesthesia for use on normal intact skin for local analgesia. Local anesthetic/analgesic uses have included minimizing pain associated with venous/arterial cannulation, refractory postherpetic neuralgia, circumcision, and various dermatologic procedures (e.g. split skin graft harvesting, laser ablation of white-heads, laser treatment of port-wine stains).

Pharmacology

Amide-type local anesthetics that stabilize neuronal membranes (inhibition of sodium ion influx necessary for impulse generation and conduction). Clinical effect is dependent on dose and duration of application. Dermal analgesia can be expected to increase for up to 3 hours under occlusive dressing and persist for 1 to 2 hours after removal of the cream.

Precautions

Contraindicated in patients sensitive to amide anesthetics. Not recommended for use on mucous membranes (other than genital) due to increased absorption. Not recommended for use when there is the possibility of drug diffusion past the tympanic membrane. Should not be used in patients with congenital or idiopathic methemoglobinemia and in infants receiving treatment with methemoglobin-inducing agents. Excess dosage or duration may result in increased lidocaine absorption and predisposition to adversities/toxicity. Patients with hepatic disease will metabolize absorbed lidocaine less efficiently.

Pregnancy: FDA category B.

Adverse Effects

Methemoglobinemia has been reported in infants and children (20–30%) when EMLA has been used in excessive doses, durations, surface area, concomitant administration of methemoglobin-inducing agents, or infants less than 3 months of age with immature metabolism capabilities. Most patients have recovered spontaneously after removal of the cream. Treatment with IV methylene blue may be effective if required.

Redness, swelling, abnormal sensation at the application site (typically resolves within minutes to hours). Allergic reactions, generally rare, may occur. Systemic adversities unlikely (due to limited absorption); if occur, include CNS excitation and/or depression, cardiovascular depression.

Drug Interactions

Use caution with concomitant class I antiarrhythmic drugs (additive adversities). Prilocaine may contribute to methemoglobin formation in patients treated with other methemoglobinemia-inducing agents.

Availability *Rx*

Each gram of EMLA contains lidocaine 25 mg and prilocaine 25 mg as active ingredients.

Cream

5 g tube, box of one, contains two Tegaderm dressings (6 x 7 cm)

5 g tube, box of five, contains 12 Tegaderm dressings (6 x 7 cm)

30 g tube, box of one

EMLA Anesthetic Disc

1 g; box of two, box of 10

The Anesthetic Disc is a single-dose unit contained within an occlusive dressing. It is composed of a laminate backing, an absorbent cellulose disc, and an adhesive tape ring. The active contact surface is approximately 10 cm^2. The surface area of the entire anesthetic disc is approximately 40 cm^2.

References

Ashinoff R, Geronemus RG. Effect of topical anesthetic EMLA on the efficacy of pulsed dye laser treatment of port-wine stains. J Dermatol Surg Oncol 1990; 16: 1008–11.

Goodacre RE, Sanders R, Watts DA, et al. Split skin grafting using topical local anaesthesia (EMLA): a comparison with infiltrated anaesthesia. Br J Plastic Surg 1988; 41: 533–8.

Litman SJ, Vitkun SA, Poppers PJ. Use of EMLA cream in the treatment of post-herpetic neuralgia. J Clin Anesth 1996; 8: 54–7.

Manner T, Kanto J, Iisalo E, et al. Reduction of pain at venous cannulation in children with a eutectic mixture of lidocaine and prilocaine (EMLA cream): comparison with placebo cream and no local premedication. Acta Anaesthesiol Scand 1987; 31: 735–9.

Pepall LM, Cosgrove MP, Cunliffe WJ. Ablation of whiteheads by cautery under topical anesthesia. Br J Dermatol 1991; 125: 256–9.

Smith M, Gray M, Ingram S, Jewkes DA. Double-blind comparison of topical lignocaine–prilocaine cream (EMLA) and lignocaine infiltration for arterial cannulation in adults. Br J Anaesth 1990; 65: 240–2.

Stow PJ, Glynn CJ, Minor B. EMLA cream in the treatment of post-herpetic neuralgia. Pain 1989; 39: 301–5.

Taddio A, Stevens B, Craig K, et al. Efficacy and safety of lidocaine–prilocaine cream for pain during circumcision. N Engl J Med 1997; 336: 1197–1201.

Selected Topical Anesthetics

Rx/OTC	Generic	Brand	Availability	Other ingredients	Comments
Amides					
OTC	Dibucaine	Nupercainal, generics	Ointment, 1%; 30 g	In Nupercainal: acetone, sodium bisulfite, lanolin, mineral oil, white petrolatum	
OTC	Lidocaine	Nupercainal	Cream, 0.5%; 42.5 g	Acetone, sodium bisulfite, glycerin	
OTC		Solarcaine Aloe Extra Burn Relief	Cream, 0.5%; 120 g	Aloe, lanolin oil, lanolin, camphor, propylparaben, eucalyptus oil, EDTA, menthol, tartrazine	
OTC		Solarcaine Aloe Extra Burn Relief	Gel, 2.5%; 120 g, 240 g	Aloe vera gel, glycerin, EDTA, isopropyl alcohol, menthol, diazolidinyl urea, tartrazine	
OTC		DermaFlex	Gel, 2.5%; 15 g	Alcohol, 79%	
OTC		Solarcaine Aloe Extra Burn Relief	Spray, 0.5%; 120 ml	Aloe vera gel, glycerin, EDTA, diazolidinyl urea, vitamin E, parabens	
Rx		Xylocaine	Spray, 10%; 1 ml disposable, 30 ml	Saccharin, cetylpyridinium, alcohol (flavored)	For oral anesthesia
OTC		Xylocaine	Ointment, 2.5%; 37.5 g	Water-soluble carbowaxes	
Rx		Xylocaine	Ointment, 5%; 3.5 g, 35 g	Saccharin (in flavored product); also unflavored	Suitable for oropharynx, minor burns, insect bites
Rx		Xylocaine, generics	Solution, 4%; 50 ml		Suitable for oral and nasal membranes, proximal digestive tract
Rx		Xylocaine Viscous, generics	Solution, 2%; 20 ml UD, 50 ml, 100 ml, 450 ml	In Xylocaine: sodium carboxymethylcellulose, parabens, saccharin	Suitable for mouth and pharynx

Continued overleaf

Selected Topical Anesthetics

Rx/OTC	Generic	Brand	Availability	Other ingredients	Comments
Rx		Xylocaine	Jelly, 2%; 30 ml	Hydroxypropylmethylcellulose base, parabens	For urethral areas, endotracheal intubation
OTC	Benzocaine	Americaine Anesthetic	Spray, 20%; 60 ml		
OTC		Dermoplast	Spray, 20%; 82.5 ml	Menthol 0.5%, methylparaben, aloe, lanolin	
OTC		Lanacane	Spray, 20%; 113 ml	Benzethonium chloride 0.1%, ethanol 36%, aloe extract	
OTC		Solarcaine Medicated First Aid	Spray, 20%; 90 ml	Triclosan 0.13%, alcohol	
OTC		Solarcaine	Aerosol, 20%; 90 ml, 120 ml	Triclosan 0.13%, SD alcohol 40 35%, tocopheryl acetate	
OTC		Dermoplast	Lotion, 8%; 90 ml	Menthol 0.5%, aloe, glycerin, parabens, lanolin	
OTC		Solarcaine	Lotion; 120 ml	Triclosan, mineral oil, alcohol, aloe extract, tocopheryl acetate, menthol, camphor, parabens, EDTA	
OTC		Lanacane	Cream, 6%; 28 g, 56 g	Benzethonium chloride 0.1%, aloe, parabens, castor oil, glycerin, isopropyl alcohol	
OTC		Anbesol	Liquid, 6.3%; 9.3, 22.2 ml	0.5% phenol, povidone-iodine, 70% alcohol, camphor, menthol	For oral use
OTC		Maximum Strength Anbesol	Gel, 6.3%; 7.5 g; Liquid, 20%; 9 ml	0.5% phenol, 70% alcohol; Alcohol 50%, saccharin	
OTC		Orajel Mouth-Aid	Liquid, 20%; 13.5 ml	Cetylpyridinium chloride 0.1%, ethyl alcohol 70%, tartrazine, saccharin	

Continued overleaf

continued

Rx/OTC	Generic	Brand	Availability	Other ingredients	Comments
OTC			Gel, 20%; 5.6 g, 10 g	Benzalkonium chloride 0.02%, zinc 0.1%, EDTA, saccharin	
OTC		Zilactin-B	Gel, 10%; 0.25 oz	Boric acid, hydroxypropylcellulose, propylene glycol, salicylic acid; alcohol, tannic acid	
Esters					
OTC	Tetracaine	Pontocaine	Ointment, 1%; 28.35 g	Glycerin, light mineral oil, methylparaben, sodium metabisulfite	
OTC			Cream, 1%; 28.35 g	Light mineral oil, methylparaben, sodium metabisulfite	
OTC	Pramoxine	Itch-X	Spray, 1%; 60 ml	Benzyl alcohol 10%, aloe vera gel, SD alcohol 40	
OTC			Gel, 1%; 35.4 g	Benzyl alcohol 10%, aloe vera gel, diazolidinyl urea, SD alcohol 40, parabens	
OTC		ProctoFoam NS	Aerosol (foam suspension), 1%; 15 g	Parabens (does not contain a steroid)	
Combination products					
OTC	Lidocaine 2.5%, benzalkonium chloride 0.13%	Bactine Antiseptic	Spray: 60 ml, 120 ml, 480 ml; Liquid; 473 ml; Aerosol; 90 g	EDTA, alcohol 13.7%	

Continued overleaf

continued

Rx/OTC	Generic	Brand	Availability	Other ingredients	Comments
OTC	Pramoxine 1%, zinc acetate 0.1%	Caladryl Clear	Lotion: 180 ml	Alcohol, camphor, diazolidinyl urea, glycerin, parabens, propylene glycol	
OTC	Calamine, 6.971%, zinc oxide, 6.971%	Calamine Lotion	Lotion: 240 ml	Bentonite, calcium hydroxide, glycerin	
OTC	Benzocaine 14%, tetracaine 2%, butamben 2%	Cetacaine	Aerosol; 56 g Liquid; 56 ml Ointment; 37 g Gel; 29 g	Benzalkonium chloride 0.5%, cetyl dimethyl ethyl ammonium bromide 0.005% in a water-soluble base	
OTC	Calamine 14%, diphenhydramine 2%	Ivarest Maximum Strength Cream	Cream; 56 g	Lanolin oil, petrolatum, propylene glycol	
OTC	Zinc acetate 2%, benzyl alcohol 10%	Ivy-Dry Super Lotion Extra Strength	Spray; 180 ml	Alcohol, camphor, menthol, acetic acid, parabens	
OTC	Lidocaine 2%, benzalkonium chloride 0.13%	Medi-Quik	Spray; 85 ml Aerosol; 90 ml	Camphor, benzyl alcohol	
OTC	Benzocaine, resorcine	Vagisil	Cream; 30 g, 60 g	Lanolin alcohol, parabens, trisodium EDTA, mineral oil, sodium sulfite	

Antiviral and Wart Treatments

Acyclovir (Zovirax) Oral and Injection

Uses, Dose and Administration

Note: See **Special Precautions** for dosage adjustment with renal dysfunction.

Herpes zoster (shingles), acute treatment

Oral: Adult: 800 mg every 4 hours, five times daily for 7 to 10 days.

Injection (immunocompromised patients):

≥ 12 years of age: 10 mg/kg every 8 hours for 7 days.

< 12 years of age: 20 mg/kg every 8 hours for 7 days.

Genital herpes (HSV), initial episode

Oral: Adult: 200 mg every 4 hours, five times daily for 7 to 10 days; OR 400 mg three times daily for 7 to 10 days.

Injection (severe episodes, ≥ 12 years of age): 5 mg/kg every 8 hours for 5 days.

Genital herpes (HSV), intermittent therapy of recurrent episodes

Oral: Adult: 200 mg every 4 hours, five times daily for 5 days; OR 400 mg three times daily for 5 days.

Genital herpes (HSV), chronic suppression for recurrent episodes

Oral: Adult: 400 mg twice daily. Alternatives include 200 mg three to five times daily. Re-evaluate after 1 year of therapy.

Chickenpox (varicella), treatment

Oral:

Adult (and child > 40 kg): 800 mg four times daily for 5 days.

Child (< 2 years of age): 20 mg/kg per dose (maximum 800 mg per dose) four times daily for 5 days.

Mucocutaneous herpes simplex in immunocompromised patients

Injection (initial or recurrent):

≥ 12 years of age: 5 mg/kg every 8 hours for 7 days.

< 12 years of age: 10 mg/kg every 8 hours for 7 days.

Herpes simplex encephalitis

Injection:

≥ 12 years of age: 10 mg/kg every 8 hours for 10 days.

3 months to 12 years: 20 mg/kg every 8 hours for 10 days.

Neonatal herpes infections

Injection: Birth to 3 months: 10 mg/kg every 8 hours for 10 days.

Doses of 15 mg/kg or 20 mg/kg have been used; safety and efficacy of these doses are not known.

Acyclovir (Zovirax) Oral and Injection

Pharmacology

Inhibitory activity against herpes simplex (HSV-1 and HSV-2) and varicella-zoster (VZV) viruses. Guanosine analogue with preferential affinity (versus normal cells) for viral thymidine kinase, the enzyme responsible for acyclovir monophosphorylation. Acyclovir triphosphate is produced via further phosphorylation and is incorporated into viral DNA in place of guanosine. Viral DNA polymerase is also inactivated, preventing elongation of the viral DNA chain.

Adverse Effects

Generally well-tolerated, however, nausea, vomiting, diarrhea, headache, or rash may occur.

Transient renal impairment ($\leq 10\%$) due to crystal nephropathy is most closely associated with rapid intravenous administration but has also occurred with oral use. Risk factors for development of renal dysfunction include dehydration, concomitant nephrotoxic agents, and underlying renal disease. Phlebitis with intravenous administration may also occur (associated with high pH). Adequate hydration and infusion over 1 hour is recommended to minimize these adversities.

Neurotoxicity ($\leq 1\%$) is more likely in patients receiving high doses, intravenous therapy, and concurrent neurotoxic drugs, and in those with renal impairment.

Special Precautions

Weight-based dosing should be based on lean body weight.

Intravenous administration: Infuse each dose over 1 hour. Ensure adequate hydration.

Dosage reduction for pre-existing renal impairment:

Dosage Adjustment for Renal Impairment, Intravenous Administration

Creatinine Clearance (ml/min per 1.73 m^2)	Percent of Recommended Dose	Dosing Interval (hours)
> 50	100	8
25–50	100	12
10–25	100	24
0–10	50	24

Dosage Adjustment for Renal Impairment, Oral Administration

Normal Dosage Regimen (5 times daily)	Creatinine Clearance (ml/min per 1.73 m^2)	Dosage	Adjusted Dosage Regimen Adjusted Interval
200 mg every 4 hours	> 10	200 mg	Every 4 hours, 5 times daily
	0–10	200 mg	Every 12 hours
400 mg every 12 hours	> 10	400 mg	Every 12 hours
	0–10	200 mg	Every 12 hours
800 mg every 4 hours	> 25	800 mg	Every 4 hours, 5 times daily
	10–25	800 mg	Every 8 hours
	0–10	800 mg	Every 12 hours

For hemodialysis patients, adjust the regimen so that a dose will be given just after dialysis

Acyclovir (Zovirax) Oral and Injection

Drug Interactions

Concomitant nephrotoxic agents.

Preparation *Rx*

Oral

Tablets	400 & 800 mg
Capsules	200 mg
Suspension	200 mg/5 ml

Injection

Solution	50 mg/ml (as sodium)
Powder for injection	500 & 1000 mg vials (as sodium)

References

Becker BN, Fall P, Hall C, et al. Rapidly progressive acute renal failure due to acyclovir: case report and review of the literature. Am J Kidney Dis 1993; 22: 611–15.

Centers for Disease Control and Prevention. Sexually Transmitted Diseases Treatment Guidelines – 2002. Morbid Mortal Weekly Rep 2002; 51(No. RR-06): 1–80.

de Ruiter A, Thin RN. Genital herpes: a guide to pharmacological therapy. Drugs 1994: 47: 297–304.

Wagstaff AJ, Faulds D, Goa KL. Acyclovir: a reappraisal of its antiviral activity, pharmacokinetic properties and therapeutic efficacy. Drugs 1994; 47: 153–205.

Acyclovir (Zovirax) Topical

Uses, Dose and Administration

Herpes labialis (cold sores), treatment of recurrent episodes

Cream: ≥ 12 years of age: Apply five times per day for 4 days. Initiate during prodrome or when lesions appear. Apply only to external lips and face and not inside the mouth or nose.

Note: Topical therapy may reduce the duration of viral shedding and pain in immunocompromised patients; no benefit is seen in immunocompetent patients.

Genital herpes (HSV), initial episode

Ointment: $^1/_2$-inch ribbon per 4-inch^2 surface area every 3 hours, six per day for 7 days.

Note: Topical is less effective than systemic therapy and therefore generally discouraged.

Mucocutaneous herpes simplex in immunocompromised patients

Ointment (initial non-life-threatening episode only): $^1/_2$-inch ribbon per 4-inch^2 surface area every 3 hours, six per day for 7 days.

Note: Topical is less effective than systemic therapy and therefore generally discouraged.

Pharmacology

Inhibitory activity against herpes simplex (HSV-1 and HSV-2) and varicella-zoster (VZV) viruses. Guanosine analogue.

Adverse Effects

Cream: Dry lips, desquamation, dryness of skin, cracked lips, burning skin, pruritus, flakiness of skin, stinging on skin (all < 1%).

Ointment: Mild pain, including transient burning/stinging, 30%; local pruritus < 5%.

Special Precautions

Wear protective glove(s) during ointment application for genital herpes to prevent spread of virus to non-infected areas.

Preparation *Rx*

Ointment	5%	3 & 15 g tubes
Cream	5%	2 g tubes

References

Centers for Disease Control and Prevention. Sexually Transmitted Diseases Treatment Guidelines – 2002. Morbid Mortal Weekly Rep 2002; 51(No. RR-06): 1–80.

de Ruiter A, Thin RN. Genital herpes: a guide to pharmacological therapy. Drugs 1994; 47: 297–304.

Wagstaff AJ, Faulds D, Goa KL. Acyclovir: a reappraisal of its antiviral activity, pharmacokinetic properties and therapeutic efficacy. Drugs 1994; 47: 153–205.

Bleomycin (Blenoxane)

Dose and Administration

Dosing formerly in mg, replaced by units: 1 mg = 1 unit.

Warts: Intralesional injection of 0.1% (1 unit/ml) aqueous solution. Use a bifurcated vaccination needle to inject at multiple sites within the lesion.

Cutaneous malignancies: Electrochemotherapy (intralesional therapy combined with electric pulses) may be successful for local treatment for cutaneous malignancies, including basal cell carcinoma, advanced metastatic melanoma, squamous cell carcinoma, and Kaposi's sarcoma.

Bleomycin Intralesional Dosage Based on Lesion Size

up to 100 mm^3	0.5 units
100 to 150 mm^3	0.75 units
150 to 500 mm^3	1.0 unit
500 to 1000 mm^3	1.5 units
1000 to 2000 mm^3	2 units
2000 to 3000 mm^3	2.5 units
3000 to 4000 mm^3	3 units
4000 to 5000 mm^3	3.5 units

Following bleomycin, inject 1% lidocaine with epinephrine solution at the site, followed by 6 to 8, 99-microsecond pulses of electricity at an amplitude of 1.3 kV/cm

In pediatric patients, the efficacy and safety of bleomycin is uncertain but it may be used for intralesional injection of hemangiomas and lymphangiomas.

Uses

FDA-approved: Squamous cell carcinoma of cervix, head and neck, and nasopharynx; Hodgkin's and non-Hodgkin's lymphoma; malignant pleural effusion; testicular carcinoma.

Other uses: Intralesional therapy of warts, head and neck lymphangioma, keratoacanthoma centrifugum marginatum, and hemangiomas. Topical therapy for dysplastic oral leukoplakia. Injection therapy for childhood germ cell tumors, esophageal carcinoma, histiocytic lymphoma, hypercalcemia of malignancy, Kaposi's sarcoma, non-small-cell lung carcinoma, metastatic melanoma, osteosarcoma, ovarian carcinoma, pelvic lymphoceles, penile carcinoma, and verrucous carcinoma.

Pharmacology

Water-soluble antibiotic from bacterial cultures. Cytotoxicity is secondary to excision of free bases after binding to DNA, thus leading to single strand breaks. 60–70% renal excretion.

Adverse Effects/Precautions

Most common reactions, especially with systemic therapy: pulmonary fibrosis and interstitial pneumonitis (10% incidence with up to 60% mortality; increased age and total dose, lung radiation, concurrent chemotherapy, and poor pulmonary reserve are predisposing factors for pulmonary toxicity); thrombocytopenia; severe coronary artery disease; drug-induced hyperpyrexia (25–50% of patients on intramuscular/intravenous treatment but preventable with acetaminophen (paraceta-

Bleomycin (Blenoxane)

mol) and antihistamine pretreatment); mucositis/stomatitis (30% of patients); taste impairment (10% of patients).

Dermatologic effects include hyperpigmentation, hyperkeratosis of hands and nails, and edema and erythema of the hands and feet in about 50% of patients. Increased dermal toxicity at high doses of 200 to 300 units where erythema followed by painful white vesicles on hands and feet is noted. 8% of patients develop a bleomycin-induced rash on pressure areas and creases within days and up to 2 to 3 weeks after bleomycin therapy. Dermal toxicity is reversible. Other skin reactions include reports of diffuse scleroderma, alopecia, flagellate dermatitis, flagellate erythema, and onycholysis.

Extensive necrosis and a severe Raynaud's syndrome-like phenomenon may occur with intralesional injection on acral sites.

Rare effects include transient decreases in GFR, hepatic injury, and visual changes.

Drug Interactions

Cisplatin and Bleomycin: delayed bleomycin elimination.

Digoxin and Bleomycin: decreased bioavailability of digoxin.

Phenytoin and Bleomycin: decreased phenytoin concentration.

Monitoring

Associated pulmonary toxicity, therefore monitor chest X-rays. Also, carefully monitor patients after the first and second doses of bleomycin for possible idiosyncratic reaction.

Special Considerations

Increased incidence of dose-related pulmonary fibrosis if cumulative lifetime dose of bleomycin exceeds 400 units. Consider a lower lifetime limit for the elderly.

In moderate renal failure (GFR 10–50 ml/min) give 75% of normal dose, and in severe renal failure (GFR < 10 ml/min) give 50% of dose.

Pregnancy: FDA category D.

Do not give live vaccines to patients on immunosuppressive therapy.

Body waste disposal precautions include using gloves and disposable linens or plastic bags when handling the urine, feces, or vomitus of patients.

Preparation *Rx*

15 units/vial or 30 units/vial for intravenous, intramuscular or subcutaneous use.

Selected References

Chan S, Middleton RK. Bleomycin treatment of warts. DICP Ann Pharmacother 1990; 24: 952–3.

de la Torre C, Losada A, Cruces MJ. Keratocanthoma centrifugum marginatum: treatment with intralesional bleomycin. J Am Acad Dermatol 1997; 37: 1010–11.

Evans WE, Yee GC, Crom WR, et al. Clinical pharmacology of bleomycin and cisplatin. Head Neck Surg 1981; 4: 98–110.

Heller R, Jaroszeki MJ, Reintgen DS, et al. Treatment of cutaneous and subcutaneous tumors with electrochemotherapy using intralesional bleomycin. Cancer 1998; 83: 148–9.

Shelley WB, Shelley ED. Intralesional bleomycin sulfate therapy for warts: a novel bifurcated needle puncture technique. Arch Dermatol 1991; 127: 234–6.

Docosanol (Abreva)

Dose and Administration

Adults and children 12 years or over: Apply to affected area on face or lips at the first sign of lesion. Apply five times daily until healed.

Use

Treats cold sores/fever blisters on the face or lips. Reduces time to healing by 1 day.

Pharmacology

Antiviral agent. Inhibits lipid-enveloped viruses that enter cells by fusion with the plasma membrane of the cell. Forces the virus to remain on the cell surface. No direct viricidal activity.

Adverse Effects/Precautions

Do not use near eyes or on genitalia. Not appropriate for genital herpes. No significant adversities. Low frequency (3%) of dermatologic effects, such as application site reactions, rash, pruritus, or dry skin.

Preparation *OTC*

Cream   10%   Abreva 2 g

Selected Reference

Alrabiah FA, Sacks SL. New antiherpesvirus agents: their targets and therapeutic potential. Drugs 1996; 52: 17–32.

Famciclovir (Famvir)

Uses, Dose and Administration

Herpes zoster (shingles), treatment: 500 mg every 8 hours for 7 days.

Genital herpes (HSV), initial episode: 250 three times daily for 7 to 10 days.

Genital herpes (HSV), recurrent episode:

Immunocompetent patients: 125 mg twice daily for 5 days.

HIV-infected patients: 500 mg twice daily for 7 days.

Note: Efficacy of famciclovir has not been established when treatment is initiated more than 6 hours after onset of symptoms or lesions.

Genital herpes (HSV), chronic suppression: 250 mg twice daily for up to 1 year.

Orolabial herpes simplex, recurrent episodes in HIV-infected patients: 500 mg twice daily for 7 days.

Dosage Adjustment for Renal Impairment

| | Creatinine Clearance (ml/min) | | | |
Indication	≥ 60	40–59	20–39	< 20
Herpes zoster	500 mg every 8 h	500 mg every 12 h	500 mg every 24 h	500 mg every 24 h
Genital herpes, recurrent	125 mg every 12 h	125 mg every 12 h	125 mg every 24 h	125 mg every 24 h
Genital herpes, suppression	250 mg every 12 h	250 mg every 12 h	125 mg every 12 h	125 mg every 24 h
Recurrent genital or orolabilal herpes, HIV-infected patient	500 mg every 12 h	500 mg every 12 h	500 mg every 24 h	250 mg every 24 h

For hemodialysis patients, adjust the regimen so that a dose will be given just after dialysis

Pharmacology

Famciclovir undergoes rapid biotransformation to the active antiviral compound penciclovir, which exhibits inhibitory activity against herpes simplex (HSV-1 and HSV-2) and varicella-zoster (VZV) viruses. Within these viruses, thymidine kinase initiates penciclovir phosphorylation. Penciclovir triphosphate competes with deoxyguanosine triphosphate, inhibits DNA polymerase, and subsequently prevents viral DNA synthesis and replication.

Adverse Effects/Precautions

Patients may experience headache, dizziness, nausea, or diarrhea. Acute renal failure has occurred in patients with underlying renal disease administered doses in excess of those appropriate for their level of renal function. Adjust dosage for renal impairment (see above).

Pregnancy: FDA category B.

Safety and efficacy have not been established in children < 18 years of age.

Famciclovir (Famvir)

Drug Interactions

Concurrent probenecid use may increase penciclovir concentrations. No clinically significant drug interactions have been demonstrated with cimetidine, digoxin, or theophylline.

Preparation *Rx*

Tablets   125, 250 & 500 mg

References

Centers for Disease Control and Prevention. Sexually Transmitted Diseases Treatment Guidelines – 2002. Morbid Mortal Weekly Rep 2002; 51(No. RR-06): 1–80.

Diaz-Mitoma F, Sibbald RG, Shafran SD, et al. Oral famciclovir for the suppression of recurrent genital herpes: a randomized controlled trial. JAMA 1998; 280: 887–92.

Perry CM, Wagstaff AJ. Famciclovir: a review of its pharmacological properties and therapeutic efficacy in herpesvirus infections. Drugs 1995; 50: 396–415.

Schacker T, Hu HL, Koelle DM, et al. Famciclovir for the suppression of symptomatic and asymptomatic herpes simplex virus reactivation in HIV-infected persons. Ann Intern Med 1998; 128: 21–8.

Tyring SK. Advances in the treatment of herpesvirus infection: the role of famciclovir. Clin Ther 1998; 20: 661–70.

Imiquimod (Aldara)

Dose and Administration

Note: Handwashing is recommended before and after application.

External genital warts: Apply a thin layer of cream to external genital/perianal warts three times weekly, just prior to normal sleeping hours. Cream should be left on for 6 to 10 hours then removed with mild soap and water. Continue treatment until complete clearance of warts or a maximum of 16 weeks.

Actinic keratosis (AK): Apply twice weekly for 16 weeks to a defined treatment area on the face or scalp (but not both concurrently). The treatment area should be a single contiguous area (approximately 25 cm^2). Wash the area, apply the cream prior to normal sleeping hours, leave on skin for 8 hours, then wash with mild soap and water. Safety of additional treatment courses (i.e. after completing 16 weeks) has not been established.

Superficial basal cell carcinoma (sBCC): Apply five times weekly for 6 weeks. Application should cover a 1 cm margin of skin around the tumor. Wash the area, apply the cream prior to normal sleeping hours, leave on skin for 8 hours, then wash with mild soap and water.

sBCC Tumor Diameter	Cream Droplet Diameter	Amount of Cream
0.5 to < 1.0 cm	4 mm	10 mg
≥ 1.0 to < 1.5 cm	5 mm	25 mg
≥ 1.5 to 2.0 cm	7 mm	40 mg

Uses

FDA-approved:

Treatment of external genital and perianal warts/condyloma acuminata (≥ 12 years of age).

Actinic keratoses (clinically typical, nonhyperkeratotic, nonhypertrophic) on the face and scalp in immunocompetent adults.

Biopsy-confirmed, superficial basal cell carcinoma in immunocompetent adults (maximum tumor diameter of 2 cm), located on trunk, neck, or extremities (excluding hands and feet), and only when surgical methods are medically less appropriate and patient follow-up can be reasonably assured. (Use not established for face, head, or anogenital area.)

Pharmacology

The mechanism of imiquimod in the treatment of genital/perianal warts is unknown. Animal models suggest immune response modification via cytokine induction, particularly interferon-α, as an immunomodulating action that mimics an antiviral response. Other cytokines induced include tumor necrosis factor-α and interleukins 1, 6, and 8. Imiquimod possesses no direct antiviral activity *in vitro*.

Adverse Effects/Precautions

Local skin reactions are common and include erythema, erosion, excoriation/flaking, or edema; therapy may be interrupted until these subside. Some reports of localized

Imiquimod (Aldara)

hypo- and hyperpigmentation (may be permanent). May exacerbate inflammatory skin conditions.

Heightened sunburn susceptibility. Minimize exposure to natural or artificial sunlight. Use sunscreen.

Use only after skin has completely healed from other drug or surgical treatment.

Pregnancy: FDA category B. The CDC states, however, that podofilox, podophyllin, and imiquimod should be avoided during pregnancy. Many specialists advocate removal of genital warts during pregnancy.

Special Considerations

Discard partially used packets. Avoid contact with eyes, lips, or nostrils. May use nonocclusive dressings to cover the affected area; avoid occlusive dressings. Applications should not be on successive days. Sexual contact should be avoided while cream is on the genital/perianal area.

Preparation *Rx*

Available as 5% cream in single-use packets of 250 mg each, 12 packets per box. Each packet contains an amount of cream sufficient to cover an area of 20 cm^2. For AK and sBCC, patients should be prescribed no more than three boxes (36 packets) for the 16-week treatment period.

Selected References

Centers for Disease Control and Prevention. Sexually Transmitted Diseases Treatment Guidelines – 2002. Morbid Mortal Weekly Rep 2002; 51(No. RR-06): 1–80.

Geisse J, Caro I, Lindholm J, et al. Imiquimod 5% cream for the treatment of superficial basal cell carcinoma: results from two phase III, randomized, vehicle-controlled studies. J Am Acad Dermatol 2004; 50: 722–33.

Lebwohl M, Dinehart S, Whiting D, et al. Imiquimod 5% cream for the treatment of actinic keratosis: results from two phase III, randomized, double-blind, parallel group, vehicle-controlled trials. J Am Acad Dermatol 2004; 50: 714–21.

Penciclovir (Denavir)

Use, Dose and Administration

Treatment of recurrent herpes labialis: Apply to lesion(s) every 2 hours while awake for 4 days. Initiate treatment as soon as possible (during prodrome or at first sign of lesions).

Pharmacology

Exhibits inhibitory activity against herpes simplex (HSV-1 and HSV-2) and varicella-zoster (VZV) viruses. Within these viruses, thymidine kinase initiates penciclovir phosphorylation. Penciclovir triphosphate competes with deoxyguanosine triphosphate, inhibits DNA polymerase, and subsequently prevents viral DNA synthesis and replication.

Adverse Effects

Headache and application site reactions have been reported, but at lower incidences than placebo.

Precautions

Use only on the lips and/or face.

Efficacy/safety have not been established in immunocompromised individuals, or in pediatrics.

Special Considerations

Controlled clinical trials show statistically significant efficacy compared with placebo, however, the degree of difference between the two groups was small. Time to healing improved from 5 days in the placebo group to 4.5 days in the active drug group.

Preparation *Rx*

Cream   1% (10 mg/g)   1.5 g tube

Reference

Spruance SL, Rea TL, Thoming C, et al. Penciclovir cream for the treatment of herpes simplex labialis. JAMA 1997; 277: 1374–9.

Podofilox (Condylox)

Dose and Administration

Patients should wash hands prior to and after application. Prescriber should demonstrate appropriate application site(s) and technique.

Adults

Solution: Using cotton-tipped applicator supplied with product, apply twice daily for 3 consecutive days, followed by 4 consecutive days with no application. Repeat cycle until no warts are visible to a maximum of four cycles. Limit treatment area to ≤ 10 cm². No more than 0.5 ml per day should be used. Allow solution to dry after each application before allowing opposing skin surfaces to return to normal position. Dispose of applicator after single use.

Gel: Using applicator tip or finger, apply twice daily for 3 consecutive days, followed by 4 consecutive days with no application. Repeat cycle until no warts are visible to a maximum of four cycles. Limit treatment area to ≤ 10 cm². No more than 0.5 g per day should be used. Allow gel to dry after each application before allowing opposing skin surfaces to return to normal position.

Uses

FDA-labeled

Solution: Topical treatment of external genital warts (condylomata acuminata). Not indicated for perianal or mucous membrane warts (e.g. urethra, rectum, vagina).

Gel: Topical treatment of anogenital warts. Not indicated for mucous membrane warts (e.g. urethra, rectum, vagina).

Pharmacology

Also known as podophyllotoxin. Chemically synthesized or purified from the plant families Coniferae and Berberidaceae. An antimitotic agent; inhibits tubulin and associated microtubular function. Is also the primary active component of podophyllin (podophyllum resin), which contains 4–20 times higher concentrations of podofilox in addition to caustic components.

Adverse Effects/Precautions

Local inflammation, burning, itching, pain, erosion (solution, 50–80%; gel, 20–30%).

Pregnancy: FDA category C. The CDC states, however, that podofilox, podophyllin, and imiquimod should be avoided during pregnancy. Many specialists advocate removal of genital warts during pregnancy.

Special Considerations

Therapy is not a cure, nor does it prevent transmission of human papilloma virus (HPV). Fewer than 50% of patients using podofilox or podophyllin (podophyllum resin) become wart-free. Approximately one-third of patients using podofilox will have wart recurrence. Benefits of podofilox versus podophyllin include 1) a standardized formulation/concentration of active substances, and 2) a reduced extent

Podofilox (Condylox)

of systemic absorption. The CDC recommends that practitioners should be familiar with both patient- and practitioner-applied genital wart regimens.

Preparation Rx

Solution	0.5%	3.5 ml bottles with child-resistant screw caps
Gel	0.5%	3.5 g tubes with applicator tips

Selected References

Beutner KR, Ferenczy A. Therapeutic approaches to genital warts. Am J Med 1997; 102: 28–37.

Centers for Disease Control and Prevention. Sexually Transmitted Diseases Treatment Guidelines – 2002. Morbid Mortal Weekly Rep 2002; 51(No. RR-06): 1–80.

Tyring S, Edwards L, Cherry LK, et al. Safety and efficacy of 0.5% podofilox gel in the treatment of anogenital warts. Arch Dermatol 1998; 134: 33–8.

Podophyllin (Podocon-25)

Dose and Administration

Podophyllin should only be administered by the health-care provider. This product is not for patient self-application.

Apply sparingly to intact lesions, avoiding contact with healthy surfaces. Allow to dry. Contact time for the first administration should be approximately 30 minutes to determine patient tolerability. Subsequent contact times may be 1 to 4 hours, depending on condition of the lesion and patient. After elapsed contact time, thoroughly remove product with alcohol or soap and water. Consider limiting application volume to no more than 0.5 ml or application surface area to less than $10\,cm^2$ per visit.

Uses

FDA-labeled: Topical treatment of external genital warts (condylomata acuminata).

Pharmacology

Also known as podophyllum resin. Is a mixture of resins obtained from the May apple or Mandrake (*Podophyllum peltatum* Linne) plant of the northern and middle United States. This mixture differs from that of India. Primary active component is podofilox. Other nonstandard quantities of caustic and cytotoxic components are present as well. An antimitotic agent; inhibits tubulin and associated microtubular function.

Adverse Effects/Precautions

Paresthesia, polyneuritis, paralytic ileus, pyrexia, leukopenia, thrombocytopenia, coma, death. Severe systemic reactions typically associated with widespread use on multiple lesions. Onset of symptoms may occur within hours and last for up to several years.

Not for use in diabetics, patients on concomitant corticosteroids, or those with poor circulation. Do not apply to bleeding warts or those with hair growing from them, birthmarks, or moles.

Pregnancy: not recommended.

Special Considerations

Therapy is not a cure, nor does it prevent transmission of human papilloma virus (HPV). Fewer than 50% of patients using podofilox or podophyllin (podophyllum resin) become wart-free. Approximately 40% of patients using podophyllin will have wart recurrence. Benefits of podofilox versus podophyllin include 1) a standardized formulation/concentration of active substances, and 2) a reduced extent of systemic absorption. The CDC recommends that practitioners should be familiar with both patient- and practitioner-applied genital wart regimens.

Preparation *Rx*

Liquid   25% in benzoin tincture   15 ml with applicator tip

Selected References

Beutner KR, Ferenczy A. Therapeutic approaches to genital warts. Am J Med 1997; 102: 28–37.

Centers for Disease Control and Prevention. Sexually Transmitted Diseases Treatment Guidelines – 2002. Morbid Mortal Weekly Rep 2002; 51(No. RR-06): 1–80.

Topical Salicylic Acid Preparations

WARNING: Salicylic acid should not be used in patients with known sensitivity to aspirin or salicylic acid. Heavy use of medications containing salicylic acid may cause salicylism, marked by tinnitus, nausea and vomiting. Patients with hepatic and renal dysfunction are at an increased risk of salicylism. Other common adverse effects are stinging, burning, and dryness of the skin. Surrounding tissues may be irritated with prolonged use.

Keratolytics should be used with caution in patients with diabetes. Diabetic patients with poor peripheral circulation may not be able to properly heal areas of tissue exposed to keratolytics.

SAC, Salicylic Acid

Keratolytics

Brand Name	Composition	Size
Keralyt Gel	6% SAC	28.4 g
Hydrisalic Gel	5% SAC	28.3 g
Calicylic Crème	5% SAC/10% urea	60 g
MG 217 Sal-Acid ointment	3% SAC	60 g
MG 217 Sal-Acid solution	3% SAC	60 ml
Whitfield's ointment	3% SAC/6% benzoic acid	30 g
Panscol lotion	3% SAC/2% phenol	120 ml
Panscol solution	3% SAC/1% phenol	90 g

Wart/Callous Medications

Brand Name	Composition	Size
Compound W One Step Wart Remover Pads	40% SAC	14/pack
Dr. Scholl's One-Step Callous Removers	40% SAC in rubber-based vehicle	4, 6/pack
Dr. Scholl's Clear Away Wart Remover Pads	40% SAC in rubber-based vehicle	14, 18, 24/pack
Dr. Scholl's Corn Removers	40% SAC in rubber-based vehicle	6, 9/pack
Duofilm patch	40% SAC in rubber-based vehicle	18/box
Mediplast plasters	40% SAC plaster	25/box
Sal-Acid plasters	40% SAC plaster in collodion-like vehicle	14/box
Compound W gel	17% SAC with collodion	0.25 oz
Dr. Scholl's Clear Away Wart Remover Gel	17% SAC with collodion	0.5 oz
Duofilm Liquid	17% SAC with collodion	10 ml
Duoplant Gel	17% SAC with collodion	15 g

Continued overleaf

Topical Salicylic Acid Preparations

continued

Brand Name	Composition	Size
Occlusal HP solution	17% SAC in polyacrylic solution	10 ml
Salactic Film	17% SAC in collodion-like vehicle + lactic acid	15 ml
Tinamed	17% SAC with collodion	14.8 ml
Wart-Off Maximum Strength Solution	17% SAC with collodion	13.5 ml
Trans-Ver-Sal Wart Remover	15% SAC in karaya gum	20 mm (15/box) 12 mm (10, 25/box) 6 mm (12, 40/box)
Compound W Liquid	17% SAC with collodion	9.3 ml

Trichloroacetic Acid (TCAA) Topical Solution

Dose and Administration

Prescriber-applied treatment: Apply small amount of an 80–90% solution to warts, taking care not to apply to surrounding area(s). Allow to dry (a white 'frosting' will develop) and powder with talc or baking soda to remove unreacted acid/excess solution. Repeat at 1–2-week intervals.

Uses

Alternative to cryotherapy with liquid nitrogen for genital warts and anal warts. Especially appropriate alternative for pregnant patients requiring therapy, as alternatives such as podophyllin and podofilox should not be used during pregnancy.

Pharmacology

Exfoliative agent that works by destroying the epidermis and the upper dermis.

Minimally absorbed, therefore appropriate choice for pregnant patients.

Adverse Effects/Precautions

If penetration to the dermis occurs, may prolong healing time, promote scar formation, and lead to patient discomfort. May neutralize with topical sodium bicarbonate administration to alleviate patient discomfort.

Special Considerations/Preparations

Not commercially available as a solution. Trichloroacetic acid, USP (crystals) may be added to distilled water. 100 g added to 100 ml produces a 100% solution, which can then be diluted to the desired concentration. Store in brown glass bottles.

Selected References

Centers for Disease Control and Prevention. Sexually Transmitted Diseases Treatment Guidelines – 2002. Morbid Mortal Weekly Rep 2002; 51(No. RR-06): 1–80.

Gabriel F, Thin RN. Treatment of anogenital warts. Comparison of trichloroacetic acid and podophyllin versus podophyllin alone. Br J Vener Dis 1983; 59: 124–6.

Godley MJ, Bradbeer CS, Gellan M, et al. Cryotherapy compared with trichloroacetic acid in treating genital warts. Genitourin Med 1987; 63: 390–2.

Schwartz DB, Greenberg MD, Daoud Y, et al. Genital condylomas in pregnancy: use of trichloroacetic acid and laser therapy. Am J Obstet Gynecol 1988; 158: 1407–16.

Valacyclovir (Valtrex)

Uses, Dose and Administration

Indication	Days of Therapy	≥ 50	30–49	10–29	< 10 *
Herpes zoster (shingles) ¶	7	1 g every 8 hours	1 g every 12 hours	1 g every 24 hours	500 mg every 24 hours
Genital herpes, initial episode¶	10	1 g every 12 hours	No adjustment necessary	1 g every 24 hours	500 mg every 24 hours
Genital herpes, recurrent episode¶	3	500 mg every 12 hours		500 mg every 24 hours	500 mg every 24 hours
Genital herpes, suppressive therapy 2 options	—	1 g every 24 hours		500 mg every 24 hours	500 mg every 24 hours
	—	500 mg every 24 hours#		500 mg every 48 hours	500 mg every 48 hours
Genital herpes, reduction of transmission (source partner)	—	500 mg every 24 hours#		500 mg every 48 hours	500 mg every 48 hours
Genital herpes, suppressive therapy, HIV-infected patients	‡	500 mg every 12 hours		500 mg every 24 hours	500 mg every 24 hours
Herpes labialis¶	1	two 2-g doses, approx. 12 hours apart	two 1-g doses, approx. 12 hours apart	two 500-mg doses, approx. 12 hours apart	500 mg one-time dose

*For hemodialysis patients, adjust the regimen so that a dose will be given just after dialysis.
¶Initiate therapy as soon as symptoms appear.
#This regimen is an alternative in patients with < 10 recurrences per year.
‡Safety/efficacy beyond 6 months in HIV-infected patients is not established.

Pharmacology

Valacyclovir is orally well absorbed, and subsequent serum acyclovir concentrations approximate those with intravenous acyclovir administration.

Exhibits inhibitory activity against herpes simplex (HSV-1 and HSV-2) and varicella-zoster (VZV) viruses. Valacyclovir is the L-valyl ester of acyclovir and is rapidly and extensively converted to the active compound. Acyclovir is a guanosine analogue with a preferential affinity (versus normal cells) for viral thymidine kinase, the enzyme responsible for acyclovir monophosphorylation. Acyclovir triphosphate is produced via further phosphorylation and is incorporated into viral DNA in place of guanosine. Viral DNA polymerase is also inactivated, preventing elongation of the viral DNA chain.

Adverse Effects/Precautions

Some patients may experience headache, nausea, vomiting, or diarrhea.

Valacyclovir (Valtrex)

Acute renal failure and central nervous system symptoms have occurred in patients with underlying renal disease administered doses in excess of those appropriate for their level of renal function.

Thrombotic thrombocytopenic purpura/hemolytic uremic syndrome has occurred in patients with advanced HIV disease and in bone marrow and renal transplant recipients at doses of 8 g of valacyclovir per day.

Pregnancy: FDA category B.

Safety and effectiveness in pre-pubertal pediatric patients have not been established.

Preparation *Rx*

Caplets   500 mg & 1 g

References

Beutner KR, Friedman DJ, Forszpaniak C, et al. Valaciclovir compared with acyclovir for improved therapy for herpes zoster in immunocompetent adults. Antimicrob Agents Chemother 1995; 39: 1546–53.

Centers for Disease Control and Prevention. Sexually Transmitted Diseases Treatment Guidelines – 2002. Morbid Mortal Weekly Rep 2002; 51(No. RR-06): 1–80.

Fife KH, Barbarash RA, Rudolph T, et al. Valacyclovir versus acyclovir in the treatment of first-episode genital herpes infection. Sex Transm Dis 1997; 24: 481–6.

Perry CM, Faulds D. Valaciclovir: a review of its antiviral activity, pharmacokinetic properties and therapeutic efficacy in herpesvirus infections. Drugs 1996; 52: 754–72.

Tyring SK, Douglas JM, Corey L, et al. A randomized, placebo-controlled comparison of oral valacyclovir and acyclovir in immunocompetent patients with recurrent genital herpes infections. Arch Dermatol 1998; 134: 185–9.

Hair Growth and Reduction Medications

Eflornithine Cream (Vaniqa)

Dose and Administration

Apply a thin layer twice daily, at least 8 hours apart, to affected areas of the face and under the chin. Rub in thoroughly and do not wash the area for 4 hours. Cosmetics and sunscreens may be applied after the treated area has dried. Hair removal techniques should be continued during eflornithine treatment until desired results have been achieved.

Uses

FDA-approved: The reduction of unwanted facial hair in women.

Pharmacology

Eflornithine inhibits ornithine decarboxylase, an enzyme used in the synthesis of polyamines, inhibiting hair follicle cell growth. Less than 1% of the applied dose is absorbed.

In clinical trials, women were treated twice daily for up to 24 weeks. Marked or better improvement (protocol definition of success) was seen in 32% of patients and occurred after 24 weeks of treatment. Nearly 60% of patients demonstrated improvement at 24 weeks. Improvement in hair growth may be seen as early as 8 weeks. Hair growth approaches pretreatment levels within 8 weeks of treatment withdrawal. If no benefit is observed after 4 months of therapy, eflornithine should be discontinued.

Adverse Effects/Precautions

Local adverse effects of acne, pseudofolliculitis barbae, and local irritation (including stinging or burning on application) may occur.

Pregnancy: FDA category C.

Preparation *Rx*

Cream   13.9%   Vaniqa   30 g

Selected References

Azziz R. The evaluation and management of hirsutism. Obstet Gynecol 2003; 101: 995–1007.

Balfour JA, McClellan K. Topical eflornithine. Am J Clin Dermatol 2001; 2: 197–201; discussion 202.

Malhotra B, Noveck R, Behr D, Palmisano M. Percutaneous absorption and pharmacokinetics of eflornithine HCl 13.9% cream in women with unwanted facial hair. J Clin Pharmacol 2001; 9: 972–8.

Finasteride (Propecia)

WARNING: Finasteride is not indicated for use in women. Administration to a woman who is or may become pregnant can interfere with the genitalia development of a male fetus.

Dose and Administration

Androgenetic alopecia: Take 1 mg by mouth once daily.

Hirsutism: Take 5 mg by mouth once daily.

Uses

FDA-approved: Treatment of androgenetic alopecia in men with mild to moderate hair loss of the vertex and anterior middle scalp area. It has also been used in women for hirsutism.

Pharmacology

Finasteride is a competitive inhibitor of type II 5(α)-reductase, which normally catalyzes the conversion of testosterone to 5(α)-dihydrotestosterone. Elevated concentrations of dihydrotestosterone are associated with the manifestations of androgenetic alopecia (e.g. miniaturization of hair follicles, shortened anagen (growth) phase of hair cycle, decrease in the diameter and length of hair shaft). Finasteride administration results in reduced concentrations of dihydrotestosterone in the serum and scalp with a noted improvement in hair counts and increased scalp coverage as compared with baseline. Effects are most notable at the vertex and anterior middle scalp area. Increased 5(α)-reductase activity is also present in hirsutism, thus making finasteride a potential treatment option. Finasteride is extensively metabolized in the liver and should be used cautiously in patients with hepatic insufficiency.

Adverse Effects/Precautions

The most common adverse effects include decreased libido, erectile dysfunction, and ejaculatory disorder (primarily decreased ejaculate volume). Women who are or may become pregnant should not handle crushed finasteride tablets and should avoid exposure to semen of men taking finasteride because of the risk of teratogenicity to a male fetus. Pregnancy: FDA category X. Use in women can result in feminization of a male fetus.

Special Considerations

The beneficial effects of finasteride generally appear within 3 months of initiating therapy. These effects continue with prolonged therapy but reverse on discontinuation of therapy within 12 months. Men more than 60 years of age may not respond to finasteride because type II 5(α)-reductase activity is generally decreased in older men.

Preparation *Rx*

Tablets	1 mg	Propecia
Tablets	5 mg	Proscar

Selected References

Leyden J, Dunlap F, Miller B, et al. Finasteride in the treatment of men with frontal male pattern hair loss. J Am Acad Dermatol 1999; 40: 930–7.

Moghetti P, Tosi F, Tosti A, et al. Comparison of spironolactone, flutamide, and finasteride efficacy in the treatment of hirsutism: a randomized, double blind, placebo-controlled trial. J Clin Endocrinol Metab 2000; 85: 89–94.

Price VH. Drug therapy: treatment of hair loss. N Engl J Med 1999; 964–73.

Saraswat A, Kumar B. Minoxidil vs. finasteride in the treatment of men with androgenetic alopecia. Arch Dermatol 2003; 139: 1219–21.

Minoxidil Topical Solution (Rogaine)

Dose and Administration

Apply 1 ml of solution to the dry affected scalp area twice daily. Allow 15 minutes to elapse prior to using any other hair product.

Uses

FDA-approved: Indicated for hair regrowth in men and women with androgenetic alopecia. It has also been used to treat alopecia areata.

Pharmacology

The mechanism of action in hair growth is not fully understood. It appears to act at the level of the hair follicle, perhaps as a potassium-channel agonist or a direct stimulant. It reverses hair follicle miniaturization seen in androgenetic alopecia by normalizing the hair follicle cycle and increasing the length of the anagen (growth) period. Its beneficial effects on hair regrowth are thought to be unrelated to its vasodilatory actions, as increased scalp blood flow has not been demonstrated consistently. Percutaneous absorption from intact scalp is minimal.

Adverse Effects/Precautions

Local irritation is the most frequent adverse effect. Common adverse effects include pruritus, dryness, and scaling/flaky scalp. Hypertrichosis may be noted in women and typically occurs above the eyebrows, on the cheeks, upper lip, and chin.

Pregnancy: FDA category C.

Special Considerations

Minoxidil should not be applied to irritated scalp areas because increased absorption and systemic adverse effects may occur. Minoxidil is primarily effective in promoting hair regrowth on the vertex scalp and has no proven clinically significant effect on temporal recession. At least 4 months of therapy are required for a positive response, but up to 1 year of therapy may be necessary in some patients. Following therapy discontinuation, new hair is generally lost within 3 to 4 months; therefore, continuous therapy is required to maintain beneficial effects.

Preparation *OTC*

Solution	2%	Rogaine for Women	60 ml
	2%	Rogaine for Men	60 ml
	5%	Rogaine for Men Extra Strength	60 ml

Selected References

Fiedler-Weiss VC. Topical minoxidil solution (1% and 5%) in the treatment of alopecia areata. J Am Acad Dermatol 1987; 16: 745–8.

Price VH. Treatment of hair loss. N Engl J Med 1999; 341: 964–73.

Saraswat A, Kumar B. Minoxidil vs. finasteride in the treatment of men with androgenetic alopecia. Arch Dermatol 2003; 139: 1219–21.

Spironolactone (Aldactone)

Dose and Administration

Acne vulgaris: Take 150–200 mg by mouth once a day.

Androgenetic alopecia: Take 100 mg by mouth twice a day.

Hirsutism: Take 25–100 mg by mouth twice a day. Daily doses of 400 mg have been utilized. Cyclic therapy for 21 days has been recommended as an alternative to continuous therapy.

Uses

FDA-approved: Treatment of primary hyperaldosteronism, congestive heart failure, cirrhosis of the liver, nephrotic syndrome, essential hypertension, and hypokalemia. Other uses include acne vulgaris unresponsive to other therapies, androgenetic alopecia, and hirsutism.

Monitoring

Periodic monitoring of electrolytes may be appropriate if imbalance is suspected (e.g. hypomagnesemia, hyponatremia, hypochloremic alkalosis, hyperkalemia).

Pharmacology

Spironolactone is a potassium-sparing diuretic that competitively inhibits the actions of aldosterone on the distal renal tubules. It also displays several antiandrogenic effects. Specifically, spironolactone decreases testosterone synthesis by inhibiting 17α-hydroxylase, a key enzyme in the formation of testosterone. Binding of dihydrotestosterone to its receptors is also inhibited with a decrease in activity at target sites (e.g. hair follicles). Additionally, spironolactone decreases sebaceous gland activity via its antiandrogenic activity and decreases sebum excretion rates.

Adverse Effects/Precautions

Nausea, vomiting, diarrhea, and gastrointestinal ulceration have been reported.

Hypotension and polyuria may occur secondarily to its diuretic effects.

Gynecomastia, decreased libido, and impotence have occurred in males. In females, menstrual irregularities and breast tenderness have been reported.

Hyperkalemia can occur and is most common in patients receiving concomitant medications that increase serum potassium (e.g. potassium supplements, angiotensin converting enzyme inhibitors) and in those with renal insufficiency.

Hyponatremia may occur and is most common in patients receiving concomitant therapy with other diuretics.

Spironolactone is contraindicated in patients with severe renal insufficiency and hyperkalemia.

Pregnancy: FDA category D. Do not use in pregnancy unless benefit outweighs risk to fetus. Spironolactone administration to rats resulted in feminization in male offspring and enlarged uteri and ovaries in the female.

Spironolactone (Aldactone)

Drug Interactions

Spironolactone should not be used concurrently with other potassium-sparing diuretics (e.g. amiloride, triamterene). Concomitant therapy with angiotensin converting enzyme (ACE) inhibitors, potassium supplements, and nonsteroidal anti-inflammatory drugs (e.g. indomethacin) should be approached cautiously because of the risk of hyperkalemia. Spironolactone may increase serum concentrations of digoxin.

Preparation *Rx*

Tablets	25, 50 & 100 mg	Aldactone
		Various generics

Selected References

Adamopoulos DA, Karamertzanis M, Nicopoulou S, Gregoriou A. Beneficial effect of spironolactone on androgenic alopecia [letter]. Clin Endocrinol 1997; 47: 759–60.

Azziz R. The evaluation and management of hirsutism. Obstet Gynecol 2003; 101: 995–1007.

Goodfellow A, Alaghband-Zadeh J, Carter G, et al. Oral spironolactone improves acne vulgaris and reduces sebum excretion rates. Br J Dermatol 1988; 209–14.

Price VH. Treatment of hair loss. N Engl J Med 1999; 341: 964–73.

Rittmaster RS. Antiandrogen treatment of polycystic ovary syndrome. Endocrinol Metab Clin North Am 1999; 28: 409–21.

Ophthalmic and Otic Preparations

Ciprofloxacin (Ciloxan)
Ophthalmic Solution and Ointment

Uses, Dose and Administration

Conjunctivitis due to the following bacteria: *Haemophilus influenzae, Staphylococcus aureus, Staphylococcus epidermidis, Streptococcus pneumoniae, Streptococcus* (Viridans group).

Solution: Adults and children ≥1 year of age: Instill one or two drops into the conjunctival sac every 2 hours while awake for 2 days, then every 4 hours while awake for 5 additional days (total duration, 7 days).

Ointment: Adults and children ≥2 years of age: Apply a half-inch ribbon into the conjunctival sac three times daily for 2 days, then twice daily for 5 additional days (total duration, 7 days).

Corneal ulcers due to the following bacteria: *Pseudomonas aeruginosa, Serratia marcescens, S. aureus, S. epidermidis, S. pneumoniae, Streptococcus* (Viridans group).

Solution: Adults and children ≥1 year of age: Instill two drops into the affected eye(s) every 15 minutes for the first 6 hours, then two drops every 30 minutes for the remainder of the first day. On day 2, instill two drops into the affected eye(s) every hour. From days 3–14, instill two drops into the affected eye(s) every 4 hours (total duration, 14 days). Treatment may be continued if re-epithelialization does not occur after 14 days.

Pharmacology

Fluoroquinolone antibiotic (bactericidal) with a broad *in vitro* spectrum of activity. Inhibits bacterial DNA gyrase and therefore interferes with effective DNA coiling.

Adverse Effects/Precautions

Local burning/discomfort. White crystalline precipitates have been observed in corneal ulcer patients; these typically resolve and do not preclude continued treatment with this agent. Other ocular irritations (e.g. foreign body sensation, photophobia, blurred vision) have occurred in < 10% of patients.

Pregnancy: FDA category C.

Low systemic absorption poses negligible risk for arthropathy in pediatric patients. Experience is not available with the solution in children <1 year of age, and experience with the ointment is not available in children <2 years of age.

Preparation Rx

Ophthalmic solution	0.3%	Ciloxan	2.5, 5 & 10 ml dropper bottles
Ophthalmic ointment	0.3%	Ciloxan	3.5 g tubes

Selected References

Hu FR, Luh KT. Topical ciprofloxacin for treating nontuberculous mycobacterial keratitis. Ophthalmology 1998; 105: 269–72.

Leibowitz HM. Antibacterial effectiveness of ciprofloxacin 0.3% ophthalmic solution in the treatment of bacterial conjunctivitis. Am J Ophthalmol 1991; 112: 29S–33S.

Erythromycin (Ilotycin) Ophthalmic Ointment

Uses, Dose and Administration

FDA-approved

Treatment of superficial ocular infections of the conjunctiva and/or cornea caused by organisms susceptible to the drug (see **Pharmacology**): Apply 1 cm of ointment directly to the infected eye(s) up to six times daily, depending on the infection severity.

Prophylaxis of ophthalmia neonatorum caused by *Neisseria gonorrhoeae* or *Chlamydia trachomatis*: Apply 1 cm of ointment into each lower conjunctival sac immediately, or at least within 1 hour, after delivery. Use a new tube for each infant.

Note: Infants born to mothers with clinically apparent gonorrhea require systemic anti-infective therapy in addition to ophthalmic therapy. Neonates with gonococcal ophthalmia should receive systemic therapy; in these cases, ophthalmic therapy is not necessary.

Other

Adjunct to systemic therapy for trachoma and inclusion conjunctivitis: Apply to each eye twice daily (1) for 2 months, OR (2) for the first 5 days of each month for 6 months.

Pharmacology

Macrolide antibiotic that binds to the 50S subunit of the microbial ribosome. May be bacteriostatic or bactericidal. Erythromycin is most active against gram-positive bacteria (cocci and bacilli). Erythromycin also has a broad range of activity against gram-positive anaerobic organisms. Also active against many atypical bacteria, such as *C. trachomatis, Mycoplasma pneumoniae*, and *Legionella*. Some gram-negative cocci (e.g. *Neisseria* species) and bacilli (e.g. *Haemophilus influenzae*) are typically sensitive; however, this may be more variable.

Adverse Effects/Precautions

Ocular irritation, redness, hypersensitivity.

Pregnancy: FDA category B.

Preparation *Rx*

Ophthalmic ointment	0.5%	Ilotycin	3.5, 3.75 & 1 g tubes

Selected References

Centers for Disease Control. 1998 guidelines for treatment of sexually transmitted diseases. Morbid Mortal Weekly Rep 1998; 47(RR-1): 1–111.

Chen JY. Prophylaxis of ophthalmia neonatorum: comparison of silver nitrate, tetracycline, erythromycin and no prophylaxis. Pediatr Infect Dis J 1992; 11: 1026–30.

Zola EM. Evaluation of drugs used in the prophylaxis of neonatal conjunctivitis. Drug Intell Clin Pharm 1984; 18: 692–6.

Neomycin/Polymyxin B/Bacitracin/Hydrocortisone (Cortisporin) Ophthalmic Ointment

Uses, Dose and Administration

Steroid-responsive inflammatory ocular conditions in which a corticosteroid is indicated* and a bacterial infection exists or is suspected. The combination product is typically active against the following bacterial strains: *Staphylococcus aureus*, streptococci, *Escherichia coli*, *Haemophilus influenzae*, *Klebsiella/Enterobacter* species, *Neisseria* species, and *Pseudomonas aeruginosa*.

*Inflammatory conditions of the palpebral and bulbar conjunctiva, cornea, and anterior segment of the globe; chronic anterior uveitis; corneal injury from burns (chemical, radiation, thermal); penetration of foreign bodies.

Adults: Apply in affected eye(s) every 3 or 4 hours, depending on severity of condition. No more than 8 g should be used prior to re-evaluation (see **Precautions**).

Pharmacology

Neomycin: An aminoglycoside antibiotic (bactericidal). Binds to the 30S subunit of the microbial ribosome, altering mRNA function. Primarily active against gram-negative organisms (except *P. aeruginosa*), but does have some activity against gram-positive bacteria (*S. aureus*). All streptococci, gram-positive bacilli, and anaerobes are resistant.

Polymyxin B: Bactericidal antibiotic that is a cationic surface-active agent (detergent). Interferes with phospholipids of the bacterial plasma membrane. Spectrum of activity limited to gram-negative organisms and primarily includes *P. aeruginosa*, *E. coli*, *Klebsiella* species, and *Enterobacter*.

Bacitracin: A mixture of polypeptides derived from *Bacillus subtilis*. Prevents formation of peptidoglycan chains needed for cell wall synthesis and alters membrane permeability. Spectrum of activity includes gram-positive cocci, anaerobic cocci, most gonococci, meningococci, *Neisseria* species, and *H. influenzae*. Most gram-negative bacteria are resistant.

Hydrocortisone: Possesses anti-inflammatory, immunosuppressive, and antiproliferative properties.

Adverse Effects/Precautions

Prolonged use of ocular corticosteroids predisposes to ocular hypertension/glaucoma, secondary infection/impaired healing. Use beyond 8 g should occur only after examination with the aid of magnification (e.g. slit lamp biomicroscopy) and, if appropriate, fluorescein staining. Monitor intraocular pressure if treatment exceeds 10 days.

Hypersensitivity/allergic-type reactions may occur with the use of ocular antibiotics.

Pregnancy: FDA category C.

Preparation *Rx*

Cortisporin ophthalmic ointment: Ingredients per g, in 3.5 g tubes: Neomycin 3.5 g (as sulfate), polymyxin B 10 000 units (as sulfate), bacitracin 400 units (as zinc), hydrocortisone 10 mg (1%).

Neomycin/Polymyxin B/Hydrocortisone (Cortisporin) Ophthalmic Suspension

Uses, Dose and Administration

Steroid-responsive inflammatory ocular conditions in which a corticosteroid is indicated* and a bacterial infection exists or is suspected. The combination product is typically active against the following bacterial strains: *Staphylococcus aureus*, *Escherichia coli*, *Haemophilus influenzae*, *Klebsiella/Enterobacter* species, *Neisseria* species, and *Pseudomonas aeruginosa*. NOT active against streptococci.

> *Inflammatory conditions of the palpebral and bulbar conjunctiva, cornea, and anterior segment of the globe; chronic anterior uveitis; corneal injury from burns (chemical, radiation, thermal); penetration of foreign bodies.

Adults: Instill one or two drops in the affected eye(s) every 3 or 4 hours, depending on severity of condition. May use more frequently if necessary. No more than 20 ml should be used prior to re-evaluation (see **Precautions**).

Pharmacology

Neomycin: An aminoglycoside antibiotic (bactericidal). Binds to the 30S subunit of the microbial ribosome, altering mRNA function. Primarily active against gram-negative organisms (except *P. aeruginosa*), but does have some activity against gram-positive bacteria (*S. aureus*). All streptococci, gram-positive bacilli, and anaerobes are resistant.

Polymyxin B: Bactericidal antibiotic that is a cationic surface-active agent (detergent). Interferes with phospholipids of the bacterial plasma membrane. Spectrum of activity limited to gram-negative organisms and primarily includes *P. aeruginosa*, *E. coli*, *Klebsiella* species, and *Enterobacter*.

Hydrocortisone: Possesses anti-inflammatory, immunosuppressive, and antiproliferative properties.

Adverse Effects/Precautions

Prolonged use of ocular corticosteroids predisposes to ocular hypertension/glaucoma, secondary infection/impaired healing. Use beyond 20 ml should occur only after examination with the aid of magnification (e.g. slit lamp biomicroscopy) and, if appropriate, fluorescein staining. Monitor intraocular pressure if treatment exceeds 10 days.

Hypersensitivity/allergic-type reactions may occur with the use of ocular antibiotics.

Pregnancy: FDA category C.

Preparation *Rx*

Cortisporin ophthalmic suspension (shake well prior to each instillation).

Ingredients per g, in 7.5 ml dropper bottles: Neomycin 3.5 g (as sulfate), polymyxin B 10 000 units (as sulfate), hydrocortisone 10 mg (1%).

Sulfacetamide Sodium (Bleph-10) Ophthalmic Solution and Ointment

Uses, Dose and Administration

Treatment of conjunctivitis and other superficial ocular infections due to susceptible organisms (see **Pharmacology**):

Solution: Instill one or two drops into the conjunctival sac of the affected eye(s) every 1 to 4 hours. As improvement is observed, the dosage may be tapered by extending the dosing interval. Usual treatment duration is 7 to 10 days.

Ointment: Apply half-inch ribbon into the lower conjunctival sac of the affected eye(s) three to four times daily and at bedtime. As improvement is observed, the dosage may be tapered by extending the dosing interval. Usual treatment duration is 7 to 10 days.

Trachoma, adjunct to systemic sulfonamide treatment:

Solution: Instill two drops into the conjunctival sac of the affected eye(s) every 2 hours.

Pharmacology

Sulfonamide that inhibits the formation of dihydropteroic acid from *para*-aminobenzoic acid and pteridine. Dihydropteroic acid is the precursor to dihydrofolic acid. Inhibition of this pathway prevents formation of tetrahydrofolic acid and subsequent bacterial DNA synthesis. Organisms generally susceptible include *Escherichia coli*, *Streptococcus pneumoniae, Streptococcus* (Viridans group), *Haemophilus influenzae*, *Klebsiella* species, *Enterobacter* species. Although indicated for *Staphylococcus aureus*, many staphylococcal isolates are resistant.

Adverse Effects/Precautions

Local irritation, stinging, burning. Rarely, Stevens–Johnson syndrome.

Pregnancy: FDA category C.

Preparation *Rx*

Ophthalmic solution	10%	Bleph-10	5 & 15 ml dropper bottles
Ophthalmic ointment	10%	Bleph-10	3.5 g tubes

Selected Reference

Lohr JA, Austin RD, Grossman M, et al. Comparison of three topical antimicrobials for acute bacterial conjunctivitis. Pediatr Infect Dis J 1988; 7: 626–9.

Trifluridine (Viroptic)

Dose and Administration

Adults and children 6 years of age and older: Instill one drop into affected eye(s) every 2 hours while awake (maximum nine drops daily per eye). After complete re-epithelialization occurs, reduce administration frequency to every 4 hours while awake (minimum five drops daily per eye) and continue treatment for an additional 7 days. Consider other therapeutic intervention(s) if improvement is not observed after an initial 7 days or if complete re-epithelialization does not occur after 14 days of administration. Avoid use longer than 21 days.

Uses

FDA-labeled: Primary keratoconjunctivitis and recurrent epithelial keratitis caused by herpes simplex virus types 1 and 2. Has been effective in certain cases unresponsive to vidarabine.

Pharmacology

Fluorinated pyrimidine nucleoside, structurally resembling thymidine. Precise mechanism of antiviral action unknown; believed to inhibit thymidine synthetase, an enzyme required for DNA synthesis. *In vitro* and *in vivo* antiviral activity includes herpes simplex types 1 and 2.

Adverse Effects/Precautions

Transient burning/stinging (5%); other various ocular irritations (< 5%).

Preparation *Rx*

Ophthalmic solution   1%   7.5 ml dropper bottles

Selected References

Anon. Trifluridine (Viroptic) for herpetic keratitis. Med Lett Drug Ther 1980; 22: 46–8.

Carmine AA, Brogden RN, Heel RC, et al. Trifluridine: a review of its antiviral activity and therapeutic use in the topical treatment of viral eye infections. Drugs 1982; 23: 329–53.

Sugar J, Stark W, Binder PS, et al. Trifluorothymidine treatment of herpes simplex epithelial keratitis and comparison with idoxuridine. Ann Ophthalmol 1980; 12: 611–15.

Selected Ophthalmic Antibiotics, Corticosteroids, and Combinations

Generic	Brand	Availability	Dose	Adverse Effects
Antibiotics				
Ciprofloxacin[1]	Ciloxan	Solution, 0.3%; 2.5 ml, 5 ml, 10 ml Ointment, 0.3%; 3.5 g	Bacterial conjunctivitis: *Solution:* Adults and children ≥1 year: 1 or 2 drops into conjunctival sac q2h while awake for 2 days, then q4h while awake for 5 additional days (total, 7 days) *Ointment:* Adults and children ≥2 years: Apply half-inch ribbon into conjunctival sac 3 times daily for 2 days, then twice daily for 5 additional days (total, 7 days) Corneal ulcers: Adults and children ≥1year: 2 drops into affected eye(s) q15min for the first 6 h, then q30min for the rest of the 1st day. On day 2, 2 drops q1h. Days 3–14, 2 drops every 4 h	3
Erythromycin[1,2]	(generic)	Ointment, 0.5%; 3.5 g, 1 g	Superficial infections of conjunctiva and/or cornea: 1 cm of ointment directly to the infected eye(s) up to 6 times daily Adjunct to systemic therapy for trachoma and inclusion conjunctivitis: Apply to each eye twice daily (1) for 2 months; OR (2) for the first 5 days of each month for 6 months	3
Gentamicin	Garamycin, Gentacidin, Genoptic	Solution, 0.3%; 5 ml, 15 ml Ointment, 0.3%; 3.5 g	Instill 1 or 2 drops into affected eye(s) q4h. For severe infections, may administer up to 2 drops q1h Apply half-inch ribbon to affected eye(s) 2 to 3 times daily	3

Selected Ophthalmic Antibiotics, Corticosteroids, and Combinations

Generic	Brand	Availability	Dose	Adverse Effects
Levofloxacin	Quixin	Solution, 0.5%; 2.5 ml, 5 ml	Days 1 & 2: Instill 1–2 drops into the affected eye(s) q2h while awake up to 8 times daily Days 3–7: Instill 1–2 drops into the affected eye(s) q4h while awake up to 4 times daily	3
	Iquix	Solution, 1.5%; 5 ml	Days 1–3: Instill 1–2 drops into the affected eye(s) every 30 min–2 h while awake and approximately 4 & 6 hours after retiring Days 4 through treatment completion: Instill 1–2 drops into the affected eye(s) every 1–4 h while awake	3
Moxifloxacin	Vigamox	Solution, 0.5%; 3 ml	Bacterial conjunctivitis: Adults and children > 1 year old: Instill 1 drop into the affected eye(s) 3 times daily for 7 days	3
Ofloxacin	Ocuflox	Solution, 0.3%; 1 ml, 5 ml, 10 ml	Bacterial conjunctivitis: Days 1 & 2: 1–2 drops q2–4 h Days 3–7: 1–2 drops 4 times daily Corneal ulcers: Days 1 & 2: 1–2 drops q30min while awake. Awaken at 4 & 6 h after falling asleep and instill 1–2 drops Days 3–7 or 9: 1–2 drops q1h while awake Days 7 or 9 to completion: 1–2 drops 4 times daily	3
Sulfacetamide[1]	Bleph-10	Solution, 10%; 5 ml, 15 ml Ointment, 10%; 3.5 g	Bacterial conjunctivitis: Solution: 1 or 2 drops into conjunctival sac q1–4h. Taper by increasing dosing interval. Total duration, 7–10 days Ointment: half-inch ribbon into conjunctival sac 3–4 times daily & at bedtime. Taper by increasing dosing interval. Total duration, 7–10 days	3

Continued overleaf

Selected Ophthalmic Antibiotics, Corticosteroids, and Combinations

Generic	Brand	Availability	Dose	Adverse Effects
			Trachoma: *Solution:* 2 drops into conjunctival sac q2h. Must use adjunctive oral therapy	
Tobramycin	Tobrex	Solution, 0.3%; 5 ml	Instill 1 or 2 drops into affected eye(s) q4h. For severe infections, may administer up to 2 drops q1h	3
		Ointment, 0.3%; 3.5 g	Apply half-inch ribbon to affected eye(s) 2 to 3 times daily. For severe infections, may administer q3–4h	
Antibiotic Combinations				
Bacitracin/Polymyxin B	Polysporin	Ointment; 3.5 g	Apply q3–4h for 7–10 days	3
Neomycin/Polymyxin B/ Bacitracin	Neosporin, AK-Spore	Ointment; 3.5 g	Apply q3–4h for 7–10 days	3
Polymyxin B/ Neomycin/Gramicidin	Neosporin, AK-Spore	Solution; 10 ml	Instill 1 or 2 drops q4h for 7–10 days. For severe infections, may administer up to 2 drops q1h	3
Oxytetracycline/ Polymyxin B	Terak	Ointment; 3.5 g	Apply half-inch ribbon onto lower lid 2–4 times daily	3
Trimethoprim/ Polymyxin B	Polytrim	Solution; 10 ml	Instill 1 drop into affected eye(s) q3h (maximum 6 doses daily) for 7–10 days	3
Corticosteroids				
Dexamethasone	Decadron	Solution, 0.1%; 5 ml	1 or 2 drops q1h during the day and q2h during the night. Taper to q4h, then 3–4 times daily	4
		Ointment, 0.05%; 3.5 g	Apply 3–4 times daily. Taper to twice, then once daily	
Prednisolone	Pred-Forte	Suspension, 1%; 1 ml, 5 ml, 10 ml, 15 ml	1 to 2 drops 2–4 times daily. May administer more frequently for the first 24–48 h	4
	Pred-Mild	Suspension, 0.12%; 5 ml, 10 ml	1 to 2 drops 2–4 times daily. May administer more frequently for the first 24–48 h	

Selected Ophthalmic Antibiotics, Corticosteroids, and Combinations

Generic	Brand	Availability	Dose	Adverse Effects
Antibiotic/Corticosteroid Combinations				
Neomycin/ Dexamethasone	NeoDecadron	Solution; 5 ml	1 or 2 drops q1h during the day and q2h during the night. Taper to q4h, then 3–4 times daily	3,4
Neomycin/Polymyxin B/ Hydrocortisone[1]	Cortisporin	Suspension; 7.5 ml	1 or 2 drops in affected eye(s) q3–4h	
Neomycin/Polymyxin B/ Bacitracin/ Hydrocortisone[1]	Cortisporin	Ointment; 3.5 g	Apply to affected eye(s) q3–4h	
Prednisolone/ Neomycin/Polymyxin B	Poly-Pred	Suspension; 5 ml, 10 ml	1 or 2 drops q3–4h. Acute infections may require q30min frequency initially	
Prednisolone/ Gentamicin	Pred-G	Suspension, 1%/0.3%; 2 ml, 5 ml, 10 ml	1 drop 2–4 times daily. May administer q1h for first 24–48 h if needed	
	Pred-G	Ointment, 0.6%/0.3%; 3.5 g	Apply half-inch ribbon into conjunctival sac 1–3 times daily	
Tobramycin/ Dexamethasone	TobraDex	Suspension, 0.3%/0.1%; 2.5 ml, 5 ml, 10 ml	1 or 2 drops into conjunctival sac q4–6h. May administer q2h for first 24–48 h if needed	
		Ointment, 0.3%/0.1%; 3.5 g	Apply half-inch ribbon into conjunctival sac 3–4 times daily	
Sulfacetamide/ Prednisolone	Blephamide	Suspension, 10%/0.2%; 5 ml, 10 ml	Instill 1 drop 2–4 times daily	
		Ointment, 10%/0.2%; 3.5 g	Apply half-inch ribbon 3–4 times daily and once or twice at night	

1. See complete monograph elsewhere in text.
2. For ophthalmia neonatorum, see complete monograph.
3. Hypersensitivity/allergic-type reactions may occur with use of ocular antibiotics.
4. With prolonged corticosteroid use, increased intraocular pressure and secondary ocular infection may develop.

Ophthalmic Decongestants

Rx/OTC	Generic Name	Brand Name	Availability	Pharmacology	Dose/Age Group	Adverse Effects	Comments
Agents for allergic conjunctivitis							
Rx	Azelastine	Optivar	Solution, 0.05%; 6 ml	Histamine-1 antagonist	1 drop in affected eye(s) twice daily (≥3 years of age)	Ocular burning/stinging (30%), headache (15%), bitter taste (10%)	1
Rx	Emedastine	Emadine	Solution, 0.05%; 5 ml	Histamine-1 antagonist	1 drop in affected eye(s) up to four times daily (≥3 years of age)	Headache (11%), ocular burning/stinging (<5%)	1
Rx	Epinastine	Elestat	Solution, 0.05%; 5 ml, 10 ml	Histamine-1 antagonist; mast cell stabilizer	1 drop in affected eye(s) twice daily (≥3 years of age)	Ocular burning/stinging and other various ocular irritations (1–10%), headache, rhinitis (1–3%)	1
Rx	Ketorolac	Acular	Solution, 0.5%; 3 ml, 5 ml, 10 ml	Nonsteroidal anti-inflammatory drug (NSAID), inhibits prostaglandin synthesis	1 drop in affected eye(s) four times daily (≥12 years of age)	Ocular burning/stinging (up to 40%), other various ocular irritations (<5%)	Caution in aspirin- or NSAID-sensitive patients
Rx	Ketotifen	Zaditor	Solution, 0.025%; 5 ml, 7.5 ml	Histamine-1 antagonist; mast cell stabilizer	1 drop in affected eye(s) every 8 to 12 hours (≥3 years of age)	Headache, rhinitis (10–25%); other various ocular irritations (<5%)	1

Ophthalmic Decongestants

Rx/OTC	Generic Name	Brand Name	Availability	Pharmacology	Dose/Age Group	Adverse Effects	Comments
Rx	Levocabastine	Livostin	Suspension, 0.05%; 2.5 ml, 5 ml, 10 ml	Histamine-1 antagonist	1 drop in affected eye(s) four times daily (≥ 12 years of age)	Mild ocular stinging/burning (30%), headache (5%), other various ocular irritations (< 5%)	Shake well before each use
Rx	Olopatadine	Patanol	Solution, 0.1%; 5 ml	Histamine-1 antagonist; mast cell stabilizer	1 drop in affected eye(s) twice daily, 6 to 8 hours apart (≥ 3 years of age)	Headache (7%), other various ocular irritations (< 5%)	1
Rx	Pemirolast	Alamast	Solution, 0.1%; 10 ml	Mast cell stabilizer; inhibits eosinophil chemotaxis	1 to 2 drops in affected eye(s) four times daily (≥ 3 years of age)	Headache, rhinitis, flu-like symptoms (10–25%); other various ocular irritations (< 5%)	1,2
Agents for vernal keratitis, vernal conjunctivitis, and vernal keratoconjunctivitis							
Rx	Cromolyn	Crolom, Opticrom	Solution, 4%; 10 ml	Mast cell stabilizer	1 to 2 drops in each eye four to six times daily (≥ 4 years of age)	Ocular stinging/ burning (frequent); other various ocular irritations (infrequent)	1,2
Rx	Lodoxamide	Alomide	Solution, 0.1%; 10 ml	Mast cell stabilizer	1 to 2 drops in affected eye(s) four times daily (≥ 2 years of age)	Ocular burning/ stinging (15%); other various ocular irritations (< 5%)	1,2

Continued overleaf

Ophthalmic Decongestants

Vasoconstrictors

Rx/OTC	Generic Name	Brand Name	Availability	Pharmacology	Dose/Age Group	Adverse Effects	Comments
OTC	Naphazoline	Allerest, Clear Eyes, Naphcon	Solution, 0.012%; 15 ml	Alpha-1 adrenergic vasoconstriction of conjunctival blood vessels	1 to 2 drops in affected eye(s) up to four times daily	Transient ocular burning/stinging. Increased intraocular pressure (avoid in patients with glaucoma and do not use in narrow-angle glaucoma). Exceeding usual dose/duration may	1
OTC		VasoClear	Solution, 0.02%; 15 ml				
OTC		Naphcon-A	Solution, 0.025%, with pheniramine 0.3%; 15 ml				
OTC OTC	Oxymetazoline	OcuClear, Visine L.R.	Solution, 0.025%; 15 ml, 30 ml		1 to 2 drops in affected eye(s) every 6 hours as needed	produce exaggerated ocular redness/congestion and rebound	1
OTC	Tetrahydrozoline	Visine, generics	Solution, 0.05%; 15 ml, 30 ml		1 to 2 drops in affected eye(s) up to four times daily	hyperemia	1

Comments

1. Contains benzalkonium chloride (or lauralkonium chloride) which adsorbs to contact lenses. Do not use product while lenses are in place; wait 10 minutes after use to insert lenses.

2. Symptom relief may occur within several days but may not be maximal until after several weeks.

3. Phenylephrine 2.5% and 10% solutions (Rx) also available for pupil dilatation and other ophthalmologic procedures or examinations.

Ciprofloxacin/Dexamethasone Otic Combination (CiproDex Otic)

Dose and Administration

Acute otitis externa: Adults and children ≥ 6 months of age: Instill four drops into the affected ear(s) twice daily for 7 days.

Acute otitis media with tympanostomy tubes: Children ≥ 6 months of age: Instill four drops into the affected ear(s) twice daily for 7 days.

Suspension should be shaken before using. Head should be tilted so that the ear is pointing upward. Instill drops and keep the ear tilted up for at least a minute. In addition, for acute otitis media, pump tragus inward five times after instillation to facilitate penetration of drops into the middle ear.

Uses

FDA-approved: Treatment of acute otitis externa and acute otitis media with tympanostomy tubes due to susceptible strains of *Pseudomonas aeruginosa, Staphylococcus aureus, Streptococcus pneumoniae, Haemophilus influenzae,* and *Moraxella catarrhalis*.

Pharmacology

Ciprofloxacin: Fluoroquinolone antibiotic (bactericidal) with a broad *in vitro* spectrum of activity. Inhibits bacterial DNA gyrase and therefore interferes with effective DNA coiling.

Dexamethasone: Synthetic glucocorticoid devoid of mineralocorticoid activity. Possesses anti-inflammatory and immunosuppressive properties. Reduces inflammatory responses accompanying bacterial infection.

Contraindications

Viral infections of the external ear canal, including herpes simplex infections.

Adverse Effects/Precautions

Ear discomfort (3%), ear pain (2.3%), ear pruritus (1.5%), ear precipitate (0.5%), and taste perversion (0.5%).

Pregnancy: FDA category C.

Preparation *Rx*

Otic suspension, per ml: Ciprofloxacin 3 mg/1 mg dexamethasone; 5 ml, 7.5 ml with dropper

Selected Reference

Roland PS, Dohar JE, Lanier BJ, et al. Topical ciprofloxacin/dexamethasone otic suspension is superior to ofloxacin otic solution in the treatment of granulation tissue in children with acute otitis media with otorrhea through tympanostomy tubes. Otolaryngol Head Neck Surg 2004; 130: 736–41.

Ciprofloxacin/Hydrocortisone Otic Combination (Cipro HC Otic)

Dose and Administration

Adults and children aged > 1 year: Instill three drops into affected ear(s) twice daily for 7 days.

Suspension should be shaken before using. Head should be tilted so that the ear is pointing upward. Instill drops and keep the ear tilted up for a few minutes.

Use

FDA-approved: Treatment of acute otitis externa due to susceptible strains of *Pseudomonas aeruginosa*, *Staphylococcus aureus*, and *Proteus mirabilis*.

Pharmacology

Hydrocortisone: Possesses anti-inflammatory, immunosuppressive, and antiproliferative properties.

Ciprofloxacin: Fluoroquinolone antibiotic (bactericidal) with a broad *in vitro* spectrum of activity. Inhibits bacterial DNA gyrase and therefore interferes with effective DNA coiling.

Contraindications

Tympanic membrane perforation, viral infections of the external ear canal.

Adverse Effects/Precautions

Pregnancy: FDA category C.

Headache (1.2%) and pruritus (0.4%) were reported in clinical trials.

Preparation *Rx*

Otic suspension, per ml: Ciprofloxacin 0.2%/hydrocortisone 1%; 10 ml with dropper

Selected Reference

Arnes E, Dibb WL. Otitis externa: clinical comparison of local ciprofloxacin versus local oxytetracycline, polymixin B, hydrocortisone combination treatment. Curr Med Res Opin 1993; 13: 182–6.

Hydrocortisone/Neomycin/Colistin Otic Combination

Dose and Administration

Adults: Instill five drops into affected ear(s) three or four times daily.

Children: Instill four drops into affected ear(s) three or four times daily.

Treatment should not continue for longer than 10 days.

Suspension should be shaken before using. Head should be tilted so that the ear is pointing upward. Instill drops and keep the ear tilted up for a few minutes or insert a cotton plug. If a cotton plug is used, insert the wick into the ear canal and saturate the plug with the suspension. This wick should be kept moist by adding further suspension every 4 hours. The wick should be replaced at least once every 24 hours.

Uses

Treatment of the following infections caused by bacteria susceptible to the preparation's antibiotics: superficial bacterial infections of the external auditory canal, infections of mastoidectomy and fenestration cavities

Pharmacology

Hydrocortisone: Possesses anti-inflammatory, immunosuppressive, and antiproliferative properties.

Neomycin: An aminoglycoside antibiotic (bactericidal). Binds to the 30S subunit of the microbial ribosome, altering mRNA function. Primarily active against gram-negative organisms (except *Pseudomonas aeruginosa*), but does have some activity against gram-positive bacteria (*Staphylococcus aureus*). All streptococci, gram-positive bacilli, and anaerobes are resistant.

Colistin: Bactericidal antibiotic structurally and pharmacologically related to polymyxin B. Cationic surface-active agent (detergent) that interferes with phospholipids of the bacterial plasma membrane. Spectrum of activity limited to gram-negative organisms and primarily includes *Pseudomonas aeruginosa*, *Escherichia coli*, *Klebsiella* species, and *Enterobacter*.

Contraindications

Herpes simplex, vaccinia, varicella.

Adverse Effects/Precautions

Neomycin has been reported to cause contact dermatitis and sensitization reactions. Neomycin has been associated with ototoxicity following oral, topical, aural, and other routes of administration; this adversity is more likely in patients with renal impairment. Limit therapy to 10 days. Caution should be exercised with use in patients with tympanic membrane perforation.

Preparation *Rx*

Otic suspension, per ml: 1% hydrocortisone, 3.3 mg neomycin (as sulfate), 3 mg colistin (as sulfate)

Cortisporin-TC Otic	10 ml, with dropper
Coly-Mycin S Otic	5 ml and 10 ml, with dropper

References

Arnes E, Dibb WL. Otitis externa: clinical comparison of local ciprofloxacin versus local oxy-tetracycline, polymixin B, hydrocortisone combination treatment. Curr Med Res Opin 1993; 13: 182–6.

Rakover Y, Keywan K, Rosen G. Safety of topical ear drops containing ototoxic antibiotics. J Otolaryngol 1997; 26: 194–6.

Smith IM, Keay DG, Buxton PK. Contact hypersensitivity in patients with chronic otitis externa. Clin Otolaryngol 1990; 15: 155–8.

Hydrocortisone/Neomycin/Polymyxin B Otic Combination

Dose and Administration

Adults: Instill four drops into affected ear(s) three or four times daily.

Children: Instill three drops into affected ear(s) three or four times daily.

Treatment should not continue for longer than 10 days.

If using suspension, shake before using. Head should be tilted so that the ear is pointing upward. Instill drops and keep the ear tilted up for a few minutes or insert a cotton plug. If a cotton plug is used, insert the wick into the ear canal and saturate the plug with the suspension. This wick should be kept moist by adding further suspension every 4 hours. The wick should be replaced at least once every 24 hours.

Uses

Treatment of the following infections caused by bacteria susceptible to the preparation's antibiotics: superficial bacterial infections of the external auditory canal (solution or suspension), infections of mastoidectomy and fenestration cavities (suspension only).

Pharmacology

Hydrocortisone: Possesses anti-inflammatory, immunosuppressive, and antiproliferative properties.

Neomycin: An aminoglycoside antibiotic (bactericidal). Binds to the 30S subunit of the microbial ribosome, altering mRNA function. Primarily active against gram-negative organisms (except *Pseudomonas aeruginosa*), but does have some activity against gram-positive bacteria (*Staphylococcus aureus*). All streptococci, gram-positive bacilli, and anaerobes are resistant.

Polymyxin B: Bactericidal antibiotic that is a cationic surface-active agent (detergent). Interferes with phospholipids of the bacterial plasma membrane. Spectrum of activity limited to gram-negative organisms and primarily includes *P. aeruginosa*, *Escherichia coli*, *Klebsiella* species, and *Enterobacter*.

Contraindications

Herpes simplex, vaccinia, varicella.

Adverse Effects/Precautions

Neomycin has been reported to cause contact dermatitis and sensitization reactions. Neomycin has been associated with ototoxicity following oral, topical, aural, and other routes of administration; this adversity is more likely in patients with renal impairment. Limit therapy to 10 days. Caution should be exercised with use in patients with tympanic membrane perforation.

Preparation *Rx*

Per ml: 1% hydrocortisone, 3.5 mg neomycin (as sulfate), 10 000 units polymyxin B (as sulfate)

Solution or suspension	AK-Spore H.C. Otic
	Cortisporin Otic
	Others

Selected References

Arnes E, Dibb WL. Otitis externa: clinical comparison of local ciprofloxacin versus local oxytetracycline, polymyxin B, hydrocortisone combination treatment. Curr Med Res Opin 1993; 13: 182–6.

Rakover Y, Keywan K, Rosen G. Safety of topical ear drops containing ototoxic antibiotics. J Otolaryngol 1997; 26: 194–6.

Smith IM, Keay DG, Buxton PK. Contact hypersensitivity in patients with chronic otitis externa. Clin Otolaryngol 1990; 15: 155–8.

Ofloxacin Otic Solution (Floxin)

Uses, Dose and Administration

Otitis externa due to *Staphylococcus aureus* and *Pseudomonas aeruginosa*:

Adults and children ≥ 12 years of age: Instill 10 drops into affected ear(s) twice daily for 10 days.

Children 1 to 12 years of age: Instill 10 drops into affected ear(s) twice daily for 10 days.

Acute otitis media in pediatric patients 1 to 12 years of age with tympanostomy tubes, due to *S. aureus*, *Streptococcus pneumoniae*, *Haemophilus influenzae*, *Moraxella catarrhalis*, and *P. aeruginosa*:

Instill five drops into affected ear(s) twice daily for 10 days. Drops should be instilled with the affected ear upward. The tragus should be pumped four times to promote solution penetration to the middle ear. Keep head tilted for 5 minutes.

Chronic suppurative otitis media in patients ≥ 12 years of age with perforated tympanic membranes, due to *Proteus mirabilis*, *P. aeruginosa*, and *S. aureus*:

Instill 10 drops into affected ear(s) twice daily for 14 days. Drops should be instilled with the affected ear upward. The tragus should be pumped four times to promote solution penetration to the middle ear. Keep head tilted for 5 minutes.

Pharmacology

Fluoroquinolone antibiotic (bactericidal) with a broad *in vitro* spectrum of activity. Inhibits bacterial DNA gyrase and therefore interferes with effective DNA coiling.

Adverse Effects

Pruritus (4%) and application site reactions (3%) have been reported in patients with intact tympanic membranes. Taste perversion (7%) has occurred in patients with perforated tympanic membranes.

Preparation *Rx*

Otic solution   0.3%   Floxin Otic   5 & 10 ml dropper bottles

References

Goldblatt EL, Dohar J, Nozza RJ, et al. Topical ofloxacin versus systemic amoxicillin/clavulanate in purulent otorrhea in children with tympanostomy tubes. Int J Pediatr Otorhinolaryngol 1998; 46: 91–101.

Jones RN, Milazzo J, Seidlin M. Ofloxacin otic solution for treatment of otitis externa in children and adults. Arch Otolaryngol Head Neck Surg 1997; 123: 1193–200.

Simpson KL, Markham A. Ofloxacin otic solution: a review of its use in the management of ear infections. Drugs 1999; 58: 509–31.

Product	Ingredients	Dose/Administration	Availability	Rx/OTC
Antimicrobial-based preparations				
VoSol Otic Solution	2% acetic acid, 3% propylene glycol diacetate, 0.02% benzethonium chloride, 0.015% sodium acetate	Insert saturated wick. Keep moist 24 h. Remove wick and instill five drops 3 or 4 times daily	15 ml, 30 ml dropper bottles	Rx
VoSol HC Otic Solution	1% hydrocortisone, 2% acetic acid, 3% propylene glycol diacetate, 0.02% benzethonium chloride, 0.015% sodium acetate, 0.05% citric acid	Insert saturated wick. Keep moist for 24 h with 3–5 drops q4–6h. Remove wick and instill five drops 3 or 4 times daily	10 ml dropper bottles	Rx
Domeboro Solution	2% acetic acid in aluminum acetate solution	Insert saturated wick. Keep moist 24 h. Instill 4–6 drops q2–3h	60 ml with dropper	Rx
Analgesics				
Allergen Ear Drops	1.4% benzocaine, 5.4% antipyrine, dehydrated glycerin	Instill drops sufficient to fill auditory canal. Saturate a cotton pledget with the product and insert into ear.	15 ml with dropper	Rx
Auralgan Otic Solution		May repeat as often as q1–2h for relief of pain associated with otitis media. For cerumen removal, instill drops 2–3 times daily for up to 3 days	10 ml with dropper	Rx
Americaine Otic Drops	20% benzocaine, benzethonium chloride 0.1% in a base of glycerin 1% and PEG 300	Instill 4–5 drops into auditory canal. Insert cotton pledget. May repeat as often as q1–2h	15 ml with dropper	Rx
Cerumen emulsifiers				
Cerumenex Eardrops	10% triethanolamine polypeptide oleate-condensate, chlorobutanol 0.5%, propylene glycol	Tilt head to 45° angle and instill drops sufficient to fill auditory canal. Insert cotton plug for 15–30 minutes. Using a rubber syringe, flush ear gently with lukewarm water. Repeat if necessary	6 ml, 12 ml with dropper	Rx
Debrox Drops	6.5% carbamide peroxide, citric acid, glycerin, propylene glycol, sodium stannate	Tilt head to 45° angle, instill 5–10 drops, and allow to remain several minutes. Using a rubber syringe, flush ear gently with lukewarm water. May use twice daily for up to 4 days	15 ml, 30 ml dropper bottles	OTC
Murine Ear Drops	6.5% carbamide peroxide, 6.3% alcohol, glycerin, polysorbate 20		15 ml	OTC

Pigmenting and Depigmenting Agents

β-Carotene

Dose and Administration

Usual dose is 30 to 300 mg orally per day in a single or divided dose with a meal. To achieve optimal photoprotection, serum carotene concentrations should be maintained above 600 g/dl. Two to four weeks of therapy are required before photosensitivity protection is achieved.

Uses

To increase tolerance to sunlight and prevent complications in patients with photosensitivity associated with erythropoietic protoporphyria (EPP). Other uses include the management of polymorphous light eruptions and photosensitivity due to other causes than EPP.

Pharmacology

β-Carotene is a naturally occurring carotenoid pigment that is found primarily in yellow and green vegetables. It is a precursor to vitamin A. Although its exact mechanism for photoprotection in EPP is unknown, it is thought to be related to its ability to scavenge reactive oxygen species.

Hypervitaminosis A resulting from chronic ingestion of β-carotene does not occur. Absorption following oral administration is increased in the presence of fat. β-Carotene is widely distributed in the body and concentrates in the skin and fat.

Adverse Effects/Precautions

Reversible yellowing of the skin (carotenoderma) is the main adverse effect associated with β-carotene. It usually develops within 2 to 6 weeks and is most noticeable on the palms of the hands or soles of the feet. Other adverse effects include diarrhea, ecchymoses, and arthralgia.

Pregnancy: FDA category C.

Special Considerations

Patients should gradually adjust exposure to sunlight. β-Carotene is not a substitute for sunscreen protection. Photosensitivity returns 1 to 2 weeks after therapy is discontinued. β-Carotene 15 mg is considered equivalent to 25 000 international units of vitamin A.

Preparation *OTC*

Capsules	5000 IU
Soft gels	10 000 IU
Soft gels	25 000 IU (15 mg)

Selected References

Mathews-Roth MM, Pathak MA, Fitzpatrick TB, et al. Beta carotene as an oral photoprotective agent in erythropoietic protoporphyria. JAMA 1984; 228: 1004–8.

Rosen CF. Topical and systemic photoprotection. Dermatol Ther 2003; 16: 8–15.

Thomsen K, Schmidt H, Fischer A. Beta-carotene in erythropoietic protoporphyria. 5 years' experience. Dermatologica 1979; 159: 82–6.

Todd DJ. Erythropoietic protoporphyria. Br J Dermatol 1994; 131: 751–66.

Dihydroxyacetone (DHA)

Dose and Administration

Hypopigmentation: Apply to cleansed area to be darkened. Exfoliation of the application area may prevent the appearance of patchy skin and allow for more even application. Apply lightly to rough skin areas (e.g. elbows, knees). Leave on at least 3 hours prior to washing treated area. Multiple applications may be used until the desired color is obtained. Application every 2 to 4 days is required to maintain color.

Turbo-PUVA therapy: Apply DHA Lotion 15% twice weekly for first 3 weeks of PUVA-therapy to the whole body except the face and groin (total of six applications) 12 hours after PUVA treatment. Initial UVA exposure should be based on the following calculation: 0.75 (minimal phototoxic dose x protection factor) with a limit of 32 J/cm^2 for a maximum exposure time of 40 minutes. Liquid 8-methoxypsoralen capsules 0.5 mg/kg should be given orally 1 hour before light treatment with a UVA light cabinet.

Uses

Used for temporary darkening of skin in vitiligo and hypopigmentation disorders. It is the active component in numerous cosmetic preparations for developing an artificial suntan. Another potential use is for enhancement of photochemotherapy with PUVA therapy for stable plaque psoriasis and for photoprotection in variegate porphyria.

Pharmacology

Dihydroxyacetone (DHA) is classified as a pigmenting agent. It induces temporary pigmentation of the skin without the aid of ultraviolet light. It binds to amino acids in the stratum corneum, resulting in a brownish tint following topical application. Repeat application will darken the color but maximal darkening will eventually be achieved with no further darkening with repeat application. Effects last approximately 3 to 10 days with eventual fading as the external epidermal cells are sloughed off. In some patients, a yellow or orange tint may develop.

DHA also offers some protection against UVA light. Its use, however, should never preclude the use of sunscreen. It is an additive in some sunscreens and has been investigated for enhanced photochemotherapy during psoralen-UVA (PUVA) therapy.

Adverse Effects/Precautions

Adverse effects are limited to local reactions, including allergic dermatitis, rashes, and erythema. Effects in pregnancy are unknown.

Special Considerations

Preparations generally do not contain a sunscreen, and thus proper use of sunscreens and sun-protective clothing should be utilized. Following application, clothing should not be worn until adequate drying has occurred. Dihydroxyacetone can stain both clothes and hair. Hands should be washed immediately following application.

Dihydroxyacetone (DHA)

Preparation* *OTC*

Lotion	5%	Vitadye	15 & 60 ml
		Chromelin	30 ml

*Multiple self-tan products contain dihydroxyacetone and are not included in this list.

Selected References

Asawanonda P, Oberlender SY, Taylor C. The use of dihydroxyacetone for photoprotection in variegate porphyria. Int J Dermatol 1999; 38: 916–18.

Levy SB. Dihydroxyacetone-containing sunless or self-tanning lotions. J Am Acad Dermatol 1992; 27: 989–93.

Taylor CR, Kwangsukstith CK, Wimberly J, et al. Turbo-PUVA: dihydroxyacetone-enhanced photochemotherapy for psoriasis: a pilot study. Arch Dermatol 1999; 135: 540–4.

Fluocinolone Acetonide/Hydroquinone/Tretinoin (Tri-Luma)

Dose and Administration

Apply a thin film to cleansed, hyperpigmented areas including about half inch of normal-appearing skin surrounding each lesion once daily at night at least 30 minutes before bedtime. Sun avoidance and use of broad-spectrum sunscreen and sun-protective clothing should be instituted to prevent repigmentation.

Uses

FDA-approved: For short-term and intermittent long-term treatment of moderate to severe melasma of the face.

Pharmacology

Tri-Luma contains fluocinolone acetonide, hydroquinone, and tretinoin. Hydroquinone is a depigmenting agent that produces a reversible depigmentation of the skin via inhibition of the enzymatic oxidation of tyrosine to melanin by tyrosinase. Tretinoin is a retinoid and fluocinolone acetonide is a low-potency (class IV) corticosteroid. The mechanism of action of the active ingredients in Tri-Luma in the treatment of melasma is unknown.

Adverse Effects/Precautions

The most frequently reported adverse events were erythema, desquamation, burning, dryness, and pruritus at the site of application. Systemic absorption of topical corticosteroids can produce reversible hypothalamic–pituitary–adrenal (HPA) axis suppression with the potential for glucocorticosteroid insufficiency after withdrawal of treatment. Tri-Luma contains sodium metabisulfite, a sulfite that may cause allergic reactions including anaphylactic symptoms and life-threatening asthmatic episodes in susceptible people. Rarely causes a gradual blue-black darkening of the skin, in which case the medication should be discontinued.

Pregnancy: FDA category C.

Special Considerations

Improvement is usually seen after 8 weeks. Use as needed until resolution is achieved, then re-treat as necessary if melasma returns. Therapy should include sun protection. Also avoid extreme heat, wind, or cold.

Preparation *Rx*

| Cream | fluocinolone acetonide 0.01%, hydroquinone 4%, tretinoin 0.05% | Tri-Luma | 30 g |

Selected References

Guevara IL, Pandva AG. Melasma treated with hydroquinone, tretinoin, and a fluorinated steroid. Int J Dermatol 2001; 40: 212–15.

Menter A. Rationale for the use of topical corticosteroids in melasma. J Drugs Dermatol 2004; 3: 169–74.

Taylor SC, Torok H, Jones T, et al. Efficacy and safety of a new triple-combination agent for the treatment of facial melasma. Cutis 2003; 72: 67–72.

Hydroquinone

Dose and Administration

Apply to the cleansed affected areas twice daily in the morning and before bedtime. Sun avoidance and use of broad-spectrum sunscreen and sun-protective clothing should be instituted to prevent repigmentation.

Uses

FDA-approved: For gradual bleaching of hyperpigmented skin conditions such as chloasma, melasma, freckles (ephelides), senile lentigines, and other unwanted areas of melanin hyperpigmentation.

Pharmacology

Hydroquinone is a depigmenting agent used for hypermelanosis. It produces a reversible depigmentation of the skin via inhibition of the enzymatic oxidation of tyrosine to melanin by tyrosinase. Inhibition of this reaction results in decreased melanin formation with subsequent reduction in pigmentation. Hydroquinone generally does not completely reverse hyperpigmented skin; however, the results are generally positive for most patients.

Adverse Effects/Precautions

Local irritation is the most common adverse reaction. Specifically, burning, stinging, erythema, and dryness or fissuring of the paranasal and infraorbital areas may occur. On rare occasions, a gradual blue-black darkening of the skin may be noted. Pregnancy: FDA category C.

Special Considerations

Concurrent use of hydroquinone with peroxide-containing products may result in transient dark staining of treated skin due to oxidation of hydroquinone by the peroxide. This transient staining can be removed by discontinuing concurrent usage and normal soap cleansing. Notable treatment effects are generally delayed and may not be seen until 4 months of therapy have elapsed.

Preparation *Rx*   (Products that contain sunscreen are denoted with *)

Cream	1.5%	Esoterica Sensitive Skin *(OTC)*	85 g
Cream	2%	Eldopaque* *(OTC)*	14.2 & 28.4 g
		Eldoquin *(OTC)*	14.2 & 28.4 g
		Esoterica Facial *(OTC)*	90 g
		Esoterica Regular *(OTC)*	85 g
		Solaquin* *(OTC)*	28.4 g
Cream	4%	Alphaquin HP*	28.4 & 56.7 g
		Claripel*	28 & 45 g
		Eldopaque Forte*	30 g
		Eldoquin Forte	28.4 g
		EpiQuin Micro	30 g
		Glyquin*	28 g
		Glyquin-XM*	28 g

		Lustra & Lustra-AF*	28.4 & 56.8 g
		Melpaque HP*	15 & 30 g
		Melquin HP*	15 & 30 g
		Nuquin HP*	15, 30 & 60 g
		Solaquin Forte*	28.4 g
		Various generics	28.4 & 30 g
Gel	2%	Neostrata AHA *(OTC)*	45 g
Gel	4%	Nuquin HP	15 & 30 g
		Solaquin Forte*	30 g
		Various generics	28.35 g
Solution	3%	Melanex	30 ml
		Melquin-3	30 ml
		Various generics	30 ml

Selected References

Amer M, Metwalli M. Topical hydroquinone in the treatment of some hyperpigmentary disorders. Int J Dermatol 1998; 37: 449–50.

Halder RM, Richards GM. Topical agents used in the management of hyperpigmentation. Skin Therapy Lett 2004; 9: 1–3.

Hart LL, Yi Kimberly. Use of hydroquinone as a bleaching cream. Ann Pharmacother 1993; 27: 592–3.

Hydroquinone/Retinol (EpiQuin Micro)

Dose and Administration

Apply to affected areas twice daily, morning and before bedtime. Sun avoidance and use of broad-spectrum sunscreen and sun-protective clothing should be instituted to prevent repigmentation.

Uses

FDA-approved: For gradual treatment of ultraviolet-induced dyschromia and discoloration resulting from the use of oral contraceptives, pregnancy, hormone replacement therapy, or skin trauma.

Pharmacology

EpiQuin Micro contains hydroquinone, which is a depigmenting agent that produces a reversible depigmentation of the skin via inhibition of the enzymatic oxidation of tyrosine to melanin by tyrosinase. Exposure to sunlight or ultraviolet light will cause repigmentation of the bleached areas.

Adverse Effects/Precautions

No systemic reactions have been reported. Occasional cutaneous hypersensitivity may occur, in which case the medication should be discontinued. EpiQuin Micro contains sodium metabisulfite, a sulfite that may cause allergic reactions including anaphylactic symptoms and life-threatening asthmatic episodes in susceptible people. Rarely causes a gradual blue-black darkening of the skin, in which case the medication should be discontinued.

Pregnancy: FDA category C.

Safety and effectiveness in pediatric patients below the age of 12 years have not been established.

Special Considerations

Results are usually seen in 4 weeks with continued improvement over time. EpiQuin Micro is a safe, steroid-free formulation that can be used for both acute and maintenance therapy without the harmful potential side-effects of long-term steroid use. Therapy should include sun protection.

Preparation *Rx*

Cream	hydroquinone 4% and retinol incorporated into patented porous microspheres (Microsponge System)	EpiQuin Micro	30 g

Selected References

Denton C, Lerner AB, Fitzpatrick TB. Inhibition of melanin formation by chemical agents. J Invest Dermatol 1952; 18: 119–35.

Halder RM, Richards GM. Management of dyschromias in ethnic skin. Dermatol Ther 2004; 17: 151–7.

Jimbow K, Obata M, Pathak M, Fitzpatrick TB. Mechanism of depigmentation by hydroquinone. J Invest Dermatol 1974; 62: 436–49.

Mequinol and Tretinoin (Solagé)

Dose and Administration

Apply to the cleansed affected areas using the applicator tip twice daily in the morning and evening, at least 8 hours apart. Sun avoidance and use of broad-spectrum sunscreen and sun-protective clothing should be instituted to prevent repigmentation.

Uses

FDA-approved: Treatment of solar lentigines.

Pharmacology

Mequinol is the monomethyl ether of hydroquinone whereas tretinoin is a retinoid. Mequinol inhibits the enzymatic oxidation of tyrosine to melanin by tyrosinase. Inhibition of this reaction results in decreased melanin formation with subsequent reduction in pigmentation. The mechanism of action of tretinoin as a depigmenting agent is unknown.

Adverse Effects/Precautions

Local irritation is the most common adverse reaction. Frequent adverse effects include erythema, burning, stinging, tingling, desquamation, pruritus, and skin irritation.

Pregnancy: FDA category X based on tretinoin component.

Special Considerations

Notable treatment effects are generally delayed and may not be seen until 6 months of therapy have elapsed. Cosmetics should not be applied until 30 minutes after application. A minimum of 6 hours should elapse before cleansing the treated area.

Preparation *Rx*

Solution   mequinol 2% & tretinoin 0.01%   Solagé   30 ml

Selected References

Fleischer AB, Schwartzel EH, Colby SI, Altman DJ. The combination of 2% 4-hydroxyanisole (Mequinol) and 0.01% tretinoin is effective in improving the appearance of solar lentigines and related hyperpigmented lesions in two double-blind multicenter clinical studies. J Am Acad Dermatol 2000; 42: 459–67.

Griffiths CEM. Drug treatment of photoaged skin. Drugs Aging 1999; 14: 289–301.

Kang S. Photoaging and tretinoin. Dermatol Clin 1998; 16: 357–64.

Monobenzone (Benoquin)

Dose and Administration

Rub into the cleansed affected areas two or three times daily. When the desired degree of depigmentation is obtained, application can be decreased to two times per week.

Uses

FDA-approved: For final depigmentation of normal skin surrounding vitiliginous lesions in patients with disseminated (more than 50% of body surface area) idiopathic vitiligo.

Pharmacology

Monobenzone is the monobenzyl ether of hydroquinone and is classified as a potent depigmenting agent. Although its exact mechanism of action in humans is unknown, increased excretion of melanin from melanocytes has been noted in animal studies. Monobenzone may cause destruction of melanocytes and permanent depigmentation, and therefore it should not be used as a substitute for hydroquinone.

Adverse Effects/Precautions

Mild, transient skin irritation and sensitization, including erythematous and eczematous reactions, have occurred. Areas of normal skin distant to the site of application frequently become permanently depigmented. Careful application is imperative.

Pregnancy: FDA category C.

Special Considerations

Partial depigmentation is usually accomplished after 1 to 4 months of application, whereas permanent depigmentation may take 1 to 2 years. Sun avoidance and use of broad-spectrum sunscreen and sun-protective clothing should be instituted to prevent repigmentation.

Preparation *Rx*

Cream   20%   Benoquin   35.44 g

Selected References

Catona A, Lanzer D. Monobenzone, superfade, vitiligo and confetti-like depigmentation. Med J Aust 1987; 146: 320–1.

Kenney JA Jr. Vitiligo. Dermatol Clin 1988; 6: 425–34.

Njoo MD, Westerhof W, Bos JD, Bossuyt PM. The development of guidelines for the treatment of vitiligo. Arch Dermatol 1999; 135: 1514–21.

Psoriasis Agents

Acitretin (Soriatane)

Dose and Administration

25 or 50 mg orally per day given as a single dose with the main meal. Use of lower doses (25 mg every other day) may be better tolerated and may be beneficial in conjunction with other treatments.

Uses

FDA-approved: Treatment of severe psoriasis, including erythrodermic and generalized pustular psoriasis in adults. Other uses include combination therapy with PUVA or UVB phototherapy in patients with psoriasis, and treatment of ichthyosis, keratoderma, pityriasis rubra pilaris, and cutaneous lupus erythematosus.

Monitoring

Lipid determinations and liver function tests at baseline and then at 1–2-week intervals until the response of the drug is established.

Pharmacology

An oral retinoid. The mechanism in psoriasis is unknown but may involve enhancement of an inflammatory process and promotion of the stratum corneum. Absorption is optimal when given with food. Elimination half life is approximately 48 hours. The drug is eliminated approximately 50% in the feces and 50% in the urine.

Contraindications

Pregnancy: FDA category X. See complete prescribing information for full description of requirements for therapy.

Contraindicated in women who are or may become pregnant during therapy or at any time for at least 3 years following the discontinuation of therapy. Females of reproductive potential should not be given acitretin until pregnancy is excluded and unless the patient meets all of the following conditions: (1) severe psoriasis unresponsive to other therapies; (2) two negative serum pregnancy tests before the first prescription; (3) use of two effective forms of contraception simultaneously; and (4) has signed a Patient Agreement/Informed Consent for Female Patients.

Patients (males or females) should not donate blood for at least 3 years following therapy.

Concomitant therapy with tetracyclines (increased intracranial pressure) or methotrexate (increased risk of hepatitis) is contraindicated. While concomitant use with methotrexate is listed as a contraindication, acitretin and methotrexate have been used together for patients with disease resistant to either drug alone.

Nursing mothers should not receive acitretin.

Adverse Effects/Precautions

Significantly lower doses of phototherapy are required, owing to the drug's effects on the stratum corneum.

Hepatic toxicity may occur, but is generally reversible with discontinuation of the drug. There is no cumulative dose relationship between acitretin dose and hepatic toxicity.

Hypertriglyceridemia and hypercholesterolemia may occur. Reductions in high-density lipoprotein (HDL) have occurred. Pancreatitis may occur in association with elevation of triglycerides, and fatal pancreatitis was reported in one patient.

Depression and other psychiatric symptoms have been reported.

Pseudotumor cerebri may occur, typically when retinoids are used in association with tetracycline. Early signs and symptoms include papilledema, headache, nausea, vomiting, and visual disturbances.

Ophthalmic effects may occur, including dry eyes, irritation to the eyes, and brow and lash loss.

Hyperostosis has been described, but the clinical significance of the changes is not known. Other adverse effects include gingival bleeding, gingivitis, dry mouth, abnormal skin order, changes in hair texture, dry skin, sticky skin, arthritis, myalgias, headache, gastrointestinal disturbances, depression, and sinusitis.

Drug Interactions

When acitretin is present in conjunction with alcohol an esterification may occur to etretinate, which has a much longer half-life than acitretin.

There may be an increased risk of hepatotoxicity in patients treated with both methotrexate and acitretin. Acitretin interferes with the contraceptive effect of micro-dose progestin 'mini pill' preparations. Ethanol potentiates toxicity. Concomitant vitamin A analogues/supplements may result in additive toxic effects. Tetracyclines elevate the risk of increased intracranial pressure.

Preparation *Rx*

Capsules   10 & 25 mg   Soriatane   prescription packs of 30

Selected References

Chou RC, Wyss R, Huselton CA, Wiengand UW. A potentially new metabolic pathway: ethylesterification of acitretin. Xenobiotica 1992; 22: 993–6.

Kullavanijaya P, Kulthanan K. Clinical efficacy and side effects of acitretin on the disorders of keratinization: a one-year study. J Dermatol 1993; 20: 501–6.

Lowe NJ, Prystowsky JH, Bourget T, et al. Acitretin plus UVB therapy for psoriasis. Comparisons with placebo plus UVB and acitretin alone. J Am Acad Dermatol 1991; 24: 591–4.

Mork NJ, Kolbenstvedt A, Austad J. Efficacy and skeletal side effects of two years' acitretin treatment. Acta Derm Venereol (Stockh) 1992; 72: 445–8.

Murray HE, Anhalt AW, Lessard R, et al. A 12-month treatment of severe psoriasis with acitretin: results of a Canadian open multicenter study. J Am Acad Dermatol 1991; 24: 598–602.

Tanew A, Guggenbichler A, Honigsmann H, et al. Photochemotherapy for severe psoriasis without or in combination with acitretin: a randomized, double-blind comparison study. J Am Acad Dermatol 1991; 25: 682–4.

Anthralin (Drithocreme, Psoriatec)

Dose and Administration

Normally applied once daily. Initially, apply for 5 to 10 minutes, increasing to 20 to 30 minutes as tolerated, then wash off.

Uses

FDA-approved for the topical treatment of psoriasis. It is also used to induce irritation as a treatment of alopecia areata.

Pharmacology

The precise mechanism of anthralin's antipsoriatic action is not fully understood, but there is *in vitro* evidence that it inhibits DNA synthesis. Systemic absorption of anthralin after topical application has not been determined in humans.

Contraindications

Contraindicated for patients with acutely inflamed psoriatic lesions or history of hypersensitivity.

Adverse Effects/Precautions

Avoid contact with eyes or mucous membranes. Irritation may occur, particularly to the normal skin surrounding lesions. Anthralin may stain skin, hair, or fabrics. Discoloration of hair and fingernails may occur. Staining of fabrics may be permanent.

Preparation *Rx*

Cream	0.1, 0.5 & 1%	Drithocreme	50 g
	1%	Psoriatec	50 g

Selected References

Gottlieb SL, Heftler NS, Gilleaudeau P, et al. Short-contact anthralin treatment augments therapeutic efficacy of cyclosporine in psoriasis: a clinical and pathologic study. J Am Acad Dermatol 1995; 33: 637–45.

Mahrle G, Bonnekoh B, Wevers A, Hegemann L. Anthralin: how does it act and are there more favourable derivatives? Acta Derm Venereol Suppl (Stockh) 1994; 186: 83–4.

Mustakallio KK. The history of dithranol and related hydroxyanthrones, their efficacy, side effects, and different regimens employed in the treatment of psoriasis. A review. Acta Derm Venereol Suppl (Stockh) 1992; 172: 7–9.

Naldi L, Carrel CF, Parazzini F, et al. Development of anthralin short-contact therapy in psoriasis: survey of published clinical trials. Int J Dermatol 1992; 31: 126–30.

Silverman A, Menter A, Hairston JL. Tars and anthralins. Dermatol Clin 1995; 13: 817–33.

Calcipotriene (Dovonex)

Dose and Administration

Apply twice daily to lesional skin.

Use

FDA-approved for the treatment of plaque psoriasis. Other uses include morphea and vitiligo.

Monitoring

Elevated serum calcium occurs with excessive use of topical calcipotriene. No laboratory monitoring is required with doses of ≤ 100 g/week in adults.

Pharmacology

Calcipotriene is a synthetic analogue of vitamin D_3. Only 6% of the applied dose is absorbed systemically, and much of this is converted to inactive metabolites within 24 hours of application.

Contraindications

Patients with hypercalcemia or evidence of vitamin D toxicity.

Adverse Effects/Precautions

Irritation may occur but may be reduced by concomitant use with a topical corticosteroid.

Reversible elevations of serum calcium may occur with excessive use.

Safety and effectiveness in pediatric patients have not been established. Nevertheless, topical calcipotriene may be one of the safest psoriasis treatments for children with psoriasis.

Pregnancy: FDA category C.

Drug Interactions

Calcipotriene is rapidly inactivated by acid. It should therefore not be mixed with salicylic acid or other acid preparations.

Special Considerations

A combination of topical calcipotriene and topical corticosteroids appears more effective with fewer side-effects than either drug used alone. Topical calcipotriene potentiates improvement in patients treated with UVB and UVA photochemotherapy.

Preparation *Rx*

Ointment	0.005%	Dovonex	30, 60 & 120 g
Cream	0.005%	Dovonex	60 & 120 g
Scalp solution	0.005%	Dovonex	60 ml bottles

Calcipotriene (Dovonex)

Selected References

Bruce S, Epinette WW, Funicella T, et al. Comparative study of calcipotriene (MC 903) ointment and fluocinonide ointment in the treatment of psoriasis. J Am Acad Dermatol 1994; 31: 755–9.

Cullen SI. Long-term effectiveness and safety of topical calcipotriene for psoriasis. Calcipotriene Study Group. South Med J 1996; 89: 1053–6.

Darley CR, Cunliffe WJ, Green CM, et al. Safety and efficacy of calcipotriol ointment (Dovonex) in treating children with psoriasis vulgaris. Br J Dermatol 1996; 135: 390–3.

Green C, Ganpule M, Harris D, et al. Comparative effects of calcipotriol (MC903) solution and placebo (vehicle of MC903) in the treatment of psoriasis of the scalp. Br J Dermatol 1994; 130: 483–7.

Hecker D, Lebwohl M. Topical calcipotriene in combination with UVB phototherapy for psoriasis. Int J Dermatol 1997; 36: 302–3.

Kienbaum S, Lehmann P, Ruzicka T. Topical calcipotriol in the treatment of intertriginous psoriasis. Br J Dermatol 1996; 135: 647–50.

Koo J. Calcipotriol/calcipotriene (Dovonex/Daivonex) in combination with phototherapy: a review. J Am Acad Dermatol 1997; 37: S59–S61.

Lebwohl M, Siskin SB, Epinette W, et al. A multicenter trial of calcipotriene ointment and halobetasol ointment compared with either agent alone for the treatment of psoriasis. J Am Acad Dermatol 1996; 35: 268–9.

Lebwohl M. Topical application of calcipotriene and corticosteroids: combination regimens. J Am Acad Dermatol 1997; 37: S55–S58.

Patel B, Siskin S, Krazmien R, Lebwohl M. Compatibility of calcipotriene with other topical medications. J Am Acad Dermatol 1998; 38: 1010–11.

Speight EL, Farr PM. Calcipotriol improves the response of psoriasis to PUVA. Br J Dermatol 1994; 130: 79–82.

Methoxsalen (Oxsoralen-Ultra Capsules, 8-MOP Capsules, and Oxsoralen Lotion)

Dose and Administration

Oxsoralen-Ultra

Initial dose: Capsules should be taken 1.5 to 2 hours before UVA exposure with some low-fat food or milk according to the following table:

Patient Weight (kg)	Patient Weight (lbs)	Dose (mg)
< 30	< 66	10
30–50	66–100	20
51–65	101–145	30
66–80	146–175	40
81–90	176–200	50
91–115	201–250	60
> 115	> 250	70

Initial Exposure: The initial UVA exposure energy level and corresponding time of exposure is determined by the patient's skin characteristics for sunburning and tanning as follows:

Skin Type	History	Recommended Joules/cm^2
I	Always burn, never tan (patients with erythrodermic psoriasis are to be classed at type I for determination of UVA dosage)	0.5 J/cm^2
II	Always burn, but sometimes tan	1.0 J/cm^2
III	Sometimes burn, but always tan	1.5 J/cm^2
IV	Never burn, always tan	2.0 J/cm^2
	Physician Examination	
V*	Moderately pigmented	2.5 J/cm^2
VI*	Blacks	3.0 J/cm^2

*Patients with natural pigmentation of these types should be classified into a lower skin-type category if the sunburn history so indicates.

Note: If a minimal phototoxic dose (MPD) is assessed, start at 50% of MPD. Also note that 8-MOP capsules have different bioavailability and should not be used interchangeably with Oxsoralen-Ultra.

Oxsoralen lotion may be used topically followed by exposure to a suitable amount of UVA. There should be a conservative dose and should not exceed that which is expected to be 50% of the minimal erythema dose (MED).

Uses

FDA-approved: Methoxsalen is indicated for use in conjunction with long-wave UVA radiation for symptomatic control of severe, recalcitrant, disabling psoriasis not responsive to other therapies. Oxsoralen lotion is indicated as a topical re-pigmenting agent in vitiligo when used in conjunction with controlled doses of UVA light or sunlight. PUVA has been used to treat refractory pruritus and polymorphous light eruption. PUVA may also be used for the treatment of mycosis fungoides and other responsive inflammatory skin conditions. PUVA with systemic psoralen has also been used for re-pigmenting vitiligo. Because the combination of PUVA plus an oral retinoid such as acitretin may improve efficacy and reduce the total dose of UVA required, the combination may have greater safety and efficacy than PUVA alone.

Monitoring

An ophthalmologic examination prior to the start of therapy and yearly thereafter is recommended. Complete blood count, antinuclear antibodies, and liver and renal function tests are recommended prior to the start of therapy and at regular periods thereafter if patients are on extended treatment.

Pharmacology

After photoactivation, methoxsalen conjugates and forms covalent bonds with DNA. Maximal drug levels are reached 0.5 to 4 hours with Oxsoralen-Ultra and 1.5 to 6 hours for 8-MOP when administered with 8 oz of milk. Peak levels are 2–3-fold greater with Oxsoralen-ultra compared with Oxsoralen capsules. The drug half-life is approximately 2 hours, and detectable methoxsalen levels may be present up to 12 hours after the dose. Peak photosensitivity occurs 1.5 to 2 hours after the dose of Oxsoralen-Ultra and approximately 4 hours after Oxsoralen capsules.

Contraindications

Idiosyncratic reactions to psoralen compound, history of photosensitive states, history of melanoma, patients with invasive squamous cell carcinomas, and patients with aphakia (because of risks of retinal damage due to the absence of the lens).

Adverse Effects/Precautions

Serious burns can result from therapy or from other UVA or sunlight exposure.

There is a marked increased risk of squamous cell carcinoma developing in a dose-dependent manner after PUVA exposure. There also is an increased risk of melanoma.

There may be an increased risk of cataracts, and eye shielding is essential during therapy and in the 24 hours following exposure to systemic psoralen. Other adverse reactions include dizziness, headache, malaise, skin tenderness, gastrointestinal disturbances, leg cramps, hypotension, and extension of psoriasis.

Pruritus may occur and may be severe.

If nausea occurs, the drug may be taken with milk or food, or the dose may be divided into two portions taken approximately 30 minutes apart.

Pregnancy: FDA category C.

Drug Interactions

Special care should be exercised in patients who are receiving concomitant therapy with known photosensitizing agents.

Methoxsalen (Oxsoralen-Ultra Capsules, 8-MOP Capsules, and Oxsoralen Lotion)

Special Considerations

Patients with hepatic insufficiency should be treated with caution because hepatic biotransformation is necessary for urinary excretion. Patients with cardiac disease or others who may be unable to tolerate prolonged standing or exposure to heat stress should not be treated in a vertical UVA chamber.

Preparation *Rx*

Capsules	10 mg	Oxsoralen-Ultra	
Capsules	10 mg	8-MOP	
Lotion	1%	Oxsoralen	30 ml

Selected References

Aubin F, Makki S, Humbert P, et al. Treatment of psoriasis with a new micronized 5-methoxypsoralen tablet and UVA radiation. Arch Dermatol Res 1994; 286: 30–4.

Calzavara-Pinton P, Ortel B, Carlino A, et al. A reappraisal of the use of 5-methoxypsoralen in the therapy of psoriasis. Exp Dermatol 1992; 1: 46–51.

Collins P, Rogers S. Bath-water delivery of 8-methoxypsoralen therapy for psoriasis. Clin Exp Dermatol 1991; 16: 165–7.

Morison WL, Baughman RD, Day RM, et al. Consensus workshop on the toxic effects of long-term PUVA therapy. [Review] [44 refs]. Arch Dermatol 1998; 134: 595–8.

Stern RS, Lunder EJ. Risk of squamous cell carcinoma and methoxsalen (psoralen) and UVA radiation (PUVA). A meta-analysis. Arch Dermatol 1998; 134: 1582–5.

Stern RS, Nichols KT, Vakeva LH. Malignant melanoma in patients treated for psoriasis with methoxsalen (psoralen) and ultraviolet A radiation (PUVA). N Engl J Med 1997; 336: 1041–5.

Tazarotene, Topical (Tazorac)

Uses, Dose and Administration

Psoriasis (stable plaque): Begin with 0.05%; increase to 0.1% if needed. Apply once daily, in the evening. Allow skin to dry if recently cleansed; apply emollients at least 1 hour before gel application.

Acne (gel, mild to moderate): Cleanse the face and allow to dry. Apply 0.1% once daily, in the evening, where acne lesions appear.

Other uses include treatment for localized pustular psoriasis and as an irritant for warts refractory to other treatments.

Monitoring

A negative pregnancy test has been recommended for use in women of childbearing potential 2 weeks prior to initiating topical tazarotene therapy.

Pharmacology

Tazarotene is a retinoid prodrug that is converted to an active form that binds to all three members of the retinoid acid receptor family. Its exact mechanism of action in psoriasis and acne is not known. Half-life following topical application is approximately 18 hours. Blood levels of the drug are very low, but the minimal dose required to induce teratogenic effects in humans is unknown.

Contraindications

Pregnancy: FDA category X. Six pregnant women inadvertently exposed to tazarotene in clinical trials delivered healthy babies.

Adverse Effects/Precautions

Topical retinoids can be irritating, and the drug should be applied exclusively to lesional skin. If excessive pruritus, burning, or redness occurs, the medication may be discontinued temporarily. The irritation may be reduced by concomitant use with topical corticosteroids.

Drug Interactions

Other drugs that cause a drying effect to the skin should be avoided. Other photosensitizing agents.

Preparation *Rx*

Gel	0.05 & 0.1%	Tazorac	30 & 100 g
Cream	0.05 & 0.1%	Tazorac	30 & 60 g

Selected References

Bershad S, Singer GK, Parente JE, et al. Successful treatment of acne vulgaris using a new method: results of a randomized vehicle-controlled trial of short-contact therapy with 0.1% tazarotene gel. Arch Dermatol 2002; 138: 481–9.

Kakita L. Tazarotene versus tretinoin or adapalene in the treatment of acne vulgaris. J Am Acad Dermatol 2000; 43: S51–4.

Koo J. Tazarotene in combination with phototherapy. J Am Acad Dermatol 1998; 39: S144–8.

Krueger GG, Drake LA, Elias PM, et al. The safety and efficacy of tazarotene gel, a topical acetylenic retinoid, in the treatment of psoriasis. Acad Dermatol 1998; 134: 57–60.

Lebwohl M, Ast E, Callen JP, et al. Once-daily tazarotene gel versus twice-daily fluocinonide cream in the treatment of plaque psoriasis. J Am Acad Dermatol 1998; 38: 705–11.

Lebwohl MG, Breneman DL, Goffe BS, et al. Tazarotene 0.1% gel plus corticosteroid cream in the treatment of plaque psoriasis. J Am Acad Dermatol 1998; 39: 590–6.

Psychotropic Medications and Sedatives

Amitriptyline (Elavil)

Dose and Administration

Initial oral doses are 75 to 100 mg daily. Doses can be divided or the total dose may be administered at bedtime. Maximum recommended dosing for outpatient therapy is 150 mg per day; however, higher doses may be required. Dose adjustments should be made at bedtime to lessen the effects of sedation on daily activities. Geriatric patients should receive lower initial doses with slow titration to the maximum tolerated effective dose.

Uses

FDA-approved: Treatment of depression. Other uses include various neuropathies and pain syndromes, including postherpetic neuralgia.

Pharmacology

Amitriptyline is a tricyclic antidepressant. Its exact mechanism of action is not known; however, it affects the reuptake of norepinephrine (noradrenaline) and serotonin. It also displays significant anticholinergic activity. Amitriptyline is metabolized in the liver to its active metabolite, nortriptyline. Excretion occurs primarily in the urine.

Adverse Effects/Precautions

Common adverse effects are related to amitriptyline's anticholinergic activity and include dry mouth, constipation, urinary retention, and mydriasis.

Patients with a history of urinary retention, angle-closure glaucoma, or increased intraocular pressure should not receive amitriptyline, because of its anticholinergic properties.

CNS effects are common and include drowsiness, weakness, lethargy, and dizziness.

Adverse cardiovascular effects include postural hypotension, arrhythmias, sinus tachycardia and bradycardia, and conduction disturbances (e.g. atrioventricular (AV) block). Patients with underlying cardiovascular disease may be at higher risk for these adverse effects.

Amitriptyline may lower the seizure threshold and therefore should be avoided in patients at risk for seizure activity.

Pregnancy: FDA category C.

Drug Interactions

Co-administration of amitriptyline and monoamine oxidase inhibitors (MAOIs) should be avoided because hyperpyretic crisis, seizures, and death have occurred. A minimum of 14 days should elapse after discontinuing a MAOI before amitriptyline is taken. Concomitant use of amitriptyline with drugs that inhibit the cytochrome P450 2C9 isoenzyme (e.g. fluconazole) may require lower amitriptyline doses to prevent adverse effects. Combination with drugs known to prolong the QT_c interval should be approached with caution.

Amitriptyline (Elavil)

Special Considerations

Antidepressant effects may not occur until several weeks of therapy have elapsed. Patients receiving high doses for prolonged periods should not abruptly discontinue amitriptyline to prevent symptoms of withdrawal.

Preparation *Rx*

Tablets	10, 25, 50, 75, 100 & 150 mg	Elavil
		Various generics

Selected References

Chouinard G. A double-blind controlled clinical trial of fluoxetine and amitriptyline in the treatment of outpatients with major depressive disorder. J Clin Psychiatry 1985; 46: 32–7.

Egbunike IG, Chaffee BJ. Antidepressants in the management of chronic pain syndromes. Pharmacotherapy 1990; 10: 262–70.

Lancaster T, Wareham D, Yaphe J. Postherpetic neuralgia. Clin Evid 2003; 9: 890–900.

Doxepin (Sinequan)

Dose and Administration

Depression: Usual initial dose is 75 mg by mouth at bedtime. Single doses exceeding 150 mg should be administered in divided doses. The maximum recommended daily dose is 300 mg.

Urticaria and pruritus: Daily doses have ranged from 10 to 75 mg administered in divided doses. An oral regimen of 10 mg three times a day appears to be an optimal dose for most patients; however, greater doses may be required.

Uses

FDA-approved: Treatment of depression and/or anxiety associated with alcoholism, organic disease, and manic-depressive disorders. Other uses include pruritus and urticaria.

Pharmacology

Doxepin is classified as a tricyclic antidepressant, which prevents the reuptake of various neurotransmitters (e.g. norepinephrine, serotonin) and thus potentiates their action in the CNS. Doxepin also has antihistaminic effects and is useful for some histamine-induced dermatologic conditions. It specifically has antagonistic effects at the histamine-1 (H-1) and 2 (H-2) receptors, as well as at muscarinic receptors. *In vitro* data indicate that it has much greater affinity for H-1 receptors than standard antihistamines; however, the clinical significance of this finding is unknown.

Adverse Effects/Precautions

Common adverse effects are related to anticholinergic activity and include dry mouth, blurred vision, constipation, and urinary retention. Patients with a history of urinary retention, angle-closure glaucoma, or increased intraocular pressure should not receive doxepin because of its anticholinergic properties. Drowsiness is also a frequent adverse effect. Adverse cardiovascular effects include postural hypotension, arrhythmias, sinus tachycardia and bradycardia, and conduction disturbances (e.g. AV block). Patients with underlying cardiovascular disease may be at higher risk for these adverse effects. Doxepin may lower the seizure threshold and therefore should be used with caution in patients at risk for seizure activity.

Pregnancy: FDA category C.

Drug Interactions

Doxepin should not be combined with monoamine oxidase inhibitors (MAOIs) because hyperpyretic crisis, seizures, and death have occurred. Two weeks should elapse following discontinuation of a MAOI before initiating doxepin.

Special Considerations

The oral concentrate should be diluted just prior to administration with 120 ml of water, skim or whole milk, orange juice, grapefruit juice, tomato juice, prune juice, or pineapple juice only.

Doxepin (Sinequan)

Preparation *Rx*

Capsules	10, 25, 50, 75, 100 & 150 mg	Sinequan	
		Various generics	
Oral concentrate	10 mg/ml	Sinequan Concentrate	120 ml

Selected References

Goldsobel AB, Rohr AS, Siegel SC, et al. Efficacy of doxepin in the treatment of chronic idiopathic urticaria. J Allergy Clin Immunol 1986; 78: 867–73.

Neittaanmaki H, Myohanen T, Fraki JE. Comparison of cinnarizine, cyproheptadine, doxepin, and hydroxyzine in treatment of idiopathic cold urticaria: usefulness of doxepin. J Am Acad Dermatol 1984; 11: 483–9.

Smith PF, Corelli RL. Doxepin in the management of pruritus associated with allergic cutaneous reactions. Ann Pharmacother 1997; 31: 633–5.

Generic Name	Brand Name	Availability	Indication & Dose	Precautions/Adverse Effects[1]
Citalopram	Celexa	10, 20 & 40 mg tablets 10 mg/5 ml oral solution, 240 ml	*Depression:* Initial dose 20 mg PO QD Maximum daily dose 60 mg PO QD	Common adverse effects include nausea, diarrhea, dry mouth, dizziness, somnolence, and ejaculatory delay. Pregnancy: FDA category C
Duloxetine	Cymbalta	20, 30 & 60 mg delayed release capsules	*Depression:* Initial dose 20 mg PO BID *Diabetic neuropathic pain:* 60 mg PO QD Maximum daily dose 60 mg	Common adverse effects include nausea, dry mouth, constipation, decreased appetite, fatigue, somnolence, and increased sweating. Pregnancy: FDA category C. Do not administer to patients with hepatic insufficiency
Escitalopram	Celexa	5, 10 & 20 mg tablets 1 mg/ml oral solution, 240 ml	*Depression:* Initial dose 10 mg PO QD *Generalized anxiety disorder:* Initial dose 10 mg PO QD Maximum daily dose 20 mg	Common adverse effects include nausea, diarrhea, ejaculation disorders, insomnia, dry mouth, increased sweating, dizziness, and fatigue. Pregnancy: FDA category C
Fluoxetine	Prozac	10, 20 & 40 mg capsules 10 mg tablets 20 mg/5 ml oral solution, 120 ml	*Depression:* Initial dose 20 mg PO qam OR 90 mg PO once per week (Prozac weekly) *Panic disorder:* Initial dose 10 mg PO qam *Obsessive–compulsive disorder:* Initial dose 20 mg PO qam	Common adverse effects include anxiety, nervousness, insomnia, somnolence, tremor, headache, decreased libido, asthenia, anorexia, weight loss, nausea, diarrhea, dry mouth, sweating, rash, and abnormal ejaculation. Pregnancy: FDA category C
	Prozac Weekly	90 mg capsule	*Bulimia nervosa:* Initial dose 60 mg PO qam	
	Sarafem	10 & 20 mg capsules	*Premenstrual dysphoric disorder:* Initial dose 20 mg PO qam Maximum daily dose 80 mg	

Selective Serotonin Reuptake Inhibitors (SSRIs)

Generic Name	Brand Name	Availability	Indication & Dose	Precautions/Adverse Effects[1]
Fluvoxamine	Generic	25, 50 & 100 mg tablets	*Obsessive–compulsive disorder:* Initial dose 50 mg PO QHS. If daily dose exceeds 100 mg, divide the dose & give BID Maximum daily dose 300 mg	Common adverse effects include somnolence, insomnia, nervousness, tremor, nausea, dyspepsia, anorexia, vomiting, dry mouth, abnormal ejaculation, asthenia, sweating, decreased libido, urinary frequency, rhinitis, anorgasmia, and taste perversion Fluvoxamine inhibits the CYP 3A4 isoenzyme system & should be used cautiously with drugs metabolized via this pathway. It can increase alprazolam, midazolam, triazolam, diazepam, theophylline, carbamazepine, cyclopsorine, propranolol and warfarin concentrations requiring a decrease in dose of these drugs. Pregnancy: FDA category C
Paroxetine	Paxil Paxil CR	10, 20, 30 & 40 mg tablets 10 mg/5 ml oral suspension, 250 ml 12.5, 25 & 37.5 mg controlled release tablets	*Depression:* Initial dose 20 mg PO QD. Initial dose 25 mg CR PO QD. *Generalized anxiety disorder:* Initial dose 20 mg PO QD. *Obsessive–compulsive disorder:* Initial dose 20 mg PO QD. Usual maintenance dose 40 mg PO QD. *Panic disorder:* Initial dose 10 mg PO QD. Initial dose 12.5 mg CR PO QD. Usual maintenance dose 40 mg PO QD	Common adverse effects include asthenia, sweating, nausea, decreased appetite, dry mouth, somnolence, insomnia, dizziness, agitation, tremor, impotence, decreased libido, and ejaculatory disturbance. Pregnancy: FDA category C

Continued overleaf

Selective Serotonin Reuptake Inhibitors (SSRIs)

continued

Generic Name	Brand Name	Availability	Indication & Dose	Precautions/Adverse Effects[1]
			Post-traumatic stress disorder: Initial dose 20 mg PO QD *Social anxiety disorder:* Initial dose 20 mg PO QD Initial dose 12.5 mg CR PO QD *Premenstrual dysphoric disorder:* Initial dose 12.5 mg CR PO QD Maximum daily dose regular tablets 60 mg Maximum daily dose CR tablets 75 mg	
Sertraline	Zoloft	25, 50 & 100 mg tablets 20 mg/ml oral concentrate, 60 ml	*Depression:* Initial dose 50 mg PO QD *Obsessive–compulsive disorder:* Initial dose 50 mg PO QD *Panic disorder:* Initial dose 25 mg PO QD Increase to 50 mg PO QD at week 2 *Premenstrual dysphoric disorder:* Initial dose 50 mg PO QD *Post-traumatic stress disorder:* Initial dose 25 mg PO QD Increase to 50 mg PO QD at week 2 *Social anxiety disorder:* Initial dose 25 mg PO QD Increase to 50 mg PO QD at week 2 Maximum daily dose 200 mg PO QD	Common adverse effects include insomnia, somnolence, tremor, anorexia, nausea, diarrhea, dyspepsia, dry mouth, decreased libido, ejaculatory delay, and increased sweating The oral concentrate must be mixed with 120ml of water, ginger ale, lemon–lime soda, lemonade or orange juice only prior to administration. Pregnancy: FDA category C

1. All SSRIs should not be co-administered with a monoamine oxidase inhibitor (MAOI). Allow a washout period of 14 days prior to SSRI therapy.

Select Atypical Antidepressants

Generic Name	Brand Name	Availability	Indication & Dose	Precautions/Adverse Effects[1]
Bupropion	Wellbutrin	75 & 100 mg tablets	*Depression:* Initial dose 100 mg PO BID	Contraindicated in patients with seizure disorders, bulimia or anorexia nervosa. Avoid use in patients with increased risk of seizures (e.g. head trauma, CNS tumor, concomitant medications that lower seizure threshold). Common adverse effects include restlessness, agitation, anxiety, insomnia, sleep disturbances, weight loss, nausea, vomiting, headache, and rash. Pregnancy: FDA category B
	Wellbutrin SR	100, 150 & 200 mg sustained release tablets	On day 4 increase to 100 mg PO TID Initial dose 150 mg SR PO qam On day 4 increase to 150 mg SR PO BID	
	Wellbutrin XL	150 & 300 mg extended release tablets	Initial dose 150 mg XL PO QD On day 4 increase to 300 mg PO QD	
	Zyban	150 mg extended release tablets	*Smoking cessation:* Initial dose 150 mg PO QD for 3 days Maintenance dose 150 mg PO BID Maximum daily dose 450 mg	Initiate treatment for smoking cessation while the patient is still smoking to achieve steady-state concentrations. Smoking should stop during the second week of treatment
Mirtazapine	Remeron Remeron SolTab	15, 30 & 45 mg tablets 15, 30 & 45 mg orally disintegrating tablets	*Depression:* Initial dose 15 mg PO QHS Maximum daily dose 45 mg	Common adverse effects include somnolence, dizziness, increased appetite, weight gain, nausea, increased total cholesterol & triglyceride concentrations. Pregnancy: FDA category C
Nefazodone	Serzone	50, 100, 150, 200 & 250 mg tablets	*Depression:* Initial dose 100 mg PO BID Maximum daily dose 600 mg	Common adverse effects include postural hypotension, somnolence, dry mouth, nausea, dizziness, constipation, asthenia, lightheadedness, blurred vision, confusion, & abnormal vision. Pregnancy: FDA category C

Continued overleaf

255

Select Atypical Antidepressants

continued

Generic Name	Brand Name	Availability	Indication & Dose	Precautions/Adverse Effects[1]
				Nefazodone co-administration with pemozide is contraindicated. Nefazodone inhibits the CYP 3A4 isoenzyme system & should be used cautiously with drugs metabolized via this pathway. Serum concentrations of triazolam, alprazolam & cyclosporine are significantly increased; dose reduction of these drugs is necessary when combining with nefazodone. Avoid concomitant use with simvastatin, lovastatin, or atorvastatin due to increased risk of rhabdomyolysis
Trazadone	Desyrel Desyrel Dividose	50, 100, 150 & 300 mg tablets	*Depression:* Initial dose 50 mg PO TID Maximum daily dose 600 mg	Common adverse effects include blurred vision, constipation, dry mouth, nausea, vomiting, hypotension, confusion, dizziness, drowsiness & nervousness. Priapism may occur & can result in permanent impairment of erectile function. Pregnancy: FDA category C
Venlafaxine	Effexor	25, 37.5, 50, 75 & 100 mg tablets	*Depression:* Initial dose 25 mg PO TID	Common adverse effects include nausea, dry mouth, anorexia, weight loss, abnormal dreams, dizziness, somnolence, insomnia, nervousness, tremor, abnormal vision, abnormal ejaculation, decreased libido, impotence, & anorgasmia. Increased blood pressure occurs in some patients. Pregnancy: FDA category C
	Effexor XR	37.5, 75 & 150 mg extended release capsules	*Depression:* Initial dose 75 mg XR PO QD *Generalized anxiety disorder:* Initial dose 75 mg XR PO QD Maximum daily dose 375 mg	

1. All should not be co-administered with a monoamine oxidase inhibitor (MAOI). Allow a washout period of 14 days prior to initiating therapy.

Alprazolam (Xanax)

Dose and Administration

Anxiety: Initial dose is 0.25 to 0.5 mg by mouth three times a day. In elderly or debilitated patients, initiate therapy at 0.25 mg two or three times a day. The dose may be gradually increased every 3 to 4 days, if needed, to a maximum of 4 mg per day.

Uses

FDA-approved: Anxiety disorder, panic attacks with or without agoraphobia, and short-term relief of symptoms of anxiety. Other uses include alcohol withdrawal and anxiety associated with depression.

Pharmacology

Alprazolam is a short-acting benzodiazepine (BZD) that displays similar activity to other members in the class. The exact mechanism of BZDs and site of action in the CNS are unknown. The pharmacologic activity of these drugs appears, however, to be mediated by the inhibitory neurotransmitter γ-aminobutyric acid (GABA). Specifically, BZD binding to specific receptors within the CNS (e.g. GABA and BZD receptors) is potentiated by the presence of GABA. These interactions result in anti-convulsant, muscle relaxant, sedative, and anxiolytic properties seen with the BZDs. Although alprazolam demonstrates all of these properties, it is primarily utilized for its anxiolytic effects. Alprazolam is extensively metabolized in the liver via cytochrome P450 isoenzyme 3A and is excreted primarily in the urine. It has a plasma half-life of approximately 12 hours.

Adverse Effects/Precautions

Dose-dependent CNS effects are frequent and include drowsiness, fatigue, ataxia, confusion, and dizziness. These may lessen with prolonged therapy or a decrease in dosage.

Alprazolam administration in acute narrow-angle glaucoma is contraindicated.

BZDs may produce physical and psychologic dependence. Therefore, these agents should be used for short-term therapy when possible and should not be abruptly discontinued.

Abrupt discontinuation may result in severe withdrawal including life-threatening symptoms (e.g. seizures). Withdrawal may be more frequent in patients who are receiving doses greater than 4 mg/day and for long periods (more than 12 weeks). However, symptoms have been reported in patients who have received only a few doses of alprazolam.

BZD administration during pregnancy may cause fetal harm and should be avoided.

Pregnancy: FDA category D.

Drug Interactions

Alprazolam administration should be avoided with other CNS-depressant medications and alcohol. Alprazolam should not be combined with potent CYP 3A4 inhibitors (e.g. nefazodone, fluvoxamine, ketoconazole, itraconazole) because its clearance may be reduced with subsequent risk for increased CNS toxicity. Other drugs that may interact with alprazolam include diltiazem, isoniazid, erythromycin,

Alprazolam (Xanax)

clarithromycin, grapefruit juice, sertraline, paroxetine, ergotamine, cyclosporine, amiodarone, nicardipine, and nifedipine. Caution is recommended with co-administration of these drugs with alprazolam.

Special Considerations

If dose reduction or discontinuation of alprazolam is necessary, a decrease of no more than 0.5 mg every 3 days is recommended. More conservative tapering of 0.25 mg every 4 to 7 days may be required in some patients.

Preparation *Rx*

| Tablets | 0.25, 0.5, 1 & 2 mg | Xanax |
| | | Various generics |

Selected References

Hartziekenhuis H. The pharmacology of alprazolam: a review. Clin Ther 1991; 13: 100–17.

Jonas JM, Cohon MS. A comparison of the safety and efficacy of alprazolam versus other agents in the treatment of anxiety, panic, and depression: a review of the literature. J Clin Psychol 1993; 54(Suppl): 24–45.

Tiller JW, Schweitzer I. Benzodiazepines. Depressants or antidepressants. Drugs 1992; 44: 165–9.

Buspirone (Buspar)

Dose and Administration

Anxiety: Give 7.5 mg orally twice daily as an initial dose. If needed, the dose may be increased 5 mg per day every 2 to 3 days. The maximum daily recommended dose is 60 mg.

Uses

FDA-approved: Management of anxiety disorders or the short-term relief of the symptoms of anxiety. Other uses include adjunctive therapy for smoking cessation and anxiety associated with depression.

Pharmacology

Buspirone is a nonbenzodiazepine anxiolytic. Its exact mechanism of action has not been fully elucidated; however, it is thought to exert its anxiolytic effects primarily via the serotonergic and dopaminergic neurotransmitter systems. *In vitro* it has high affinity for serotonin type 1 ($5HT_{1A}$) receptors and acts either as an agonist or mixed agonist–antagonist at these receptors. Additionally, it has moderate affinity for dopamine type 2 (D_2) receptors in the CNS where it displays agonist and antagonist properties. It does not bind to benzodiazepine (BZD) receptors nor does it affect γ-aminobutyric acid (GABA) binding. It has no anticonvulsant or muscle relaxant properties and has a lower propensity to cause impairment of psychomotor skills or sedation as compared with the BZDs. Buspirone undergoes extensive first-pass metabolism following administration. It is extensively metabolized in the liver via the cytochrome P450 3A4 isoenzyme system and is excreted primarily in the urine.

Adverse Effects/Precautions

Common adverse effects include dizziness, nausea, headache, nervousness, lightheadedness, and excitement.

Restlessness may appear after initiating buspirone. The cause is unknown but may be attributed to its effects on the dopaminergic system.

Use with caution in patients with renal or hepatic impairment. Reduced doses should be utilized if prescribing to these patient populations.

Pregnancy: FDA category B.

Drug Interactions

Combining buspirone with a monoamine oxidase inhibitor (MAOI) may result in increased blood pressure and therefore should be avoided. Combinations with CYP 3A4 inhibitors such as itraconazole, nefazodone, or erythromycin can result in significant increases in the serum concentration of buspirone. If concomitant therapy is desired with these medications, a low initial dose of buspirone (2.5 mg twice daily) should be utilized to avoid adverse effects (e.g. lightheadedness, asthenia, dizziness, somnolence).

Special Considerations

Although buspirone is less likely to cause sedation or impairment of psychomotor function, interpatient variability has been noted. Patients should use caution when driving or performing other tasks that require mental alertness and should avoid concomitant alcohol while receiving buspirone. Buspirone's onset of effect may be delayed as compared with the BZDs, and the maximal anxiolytic effect may not occur until 3 to 6 weeks of therapy.

Preparation *Rx*

Tablets	5 & 10 mg	Buspar
		Generic
Tablets	15 & 30 mg	Buspar Dividose
		Generic

Selected References

Apter JT, Allen LA. Buspirone: Future directions. J Clin Psychopharmacol 1999; 19: 86–93.

Fulton B, Brogden RN. Buspirone: an update review of its clinical pharmacology and therapeutic applications. CNS Drugs 1997; 1: 68–88.

Sramek JJ, Frackiewica EJ, Cutler NR. Efficacy and safety of two dosing regimens of buspirone in the treatment of outpatients with persistent anxiety. Clin Ther 1997; 19: 498–506.

Lorazepam (Ativan)

Dose and Administration

Anxiety: Initial oral dose is 2 to 3 mg/day divided in two or three doses. In elderly or debilitated patients, initiate therapy at 1 to 2 mg/day divided in two or three doses. The usual dosage range is 2 to 10 mg daily.

Insomnia: Usual oral dose is 2 to 4 mg at bedtime.

Preoperative use: Give 0.05 mg/kg (not to exceed 4 mg) intramuscularly 2 hours prior to surgery. For intravenous administration, give 0.044 mg/kg (not to exceed 2 mg) 15 minutes prior to surgery.

Status epilepticus: Give 0.05 to 1 mg/kg intravenously, and repeat every 10 to 15 minutes as required.

Uses

FDA-approved:

Oral: Management of anxiety disorders or for the short-term relief of the symptoms of anxiety or anxiety associated with depression.

Injectable: Management of status epilepticus and as a preoperative medication for sedation, anxiolysis, and anterograde amnesia. Other uses for lorazepam include alcohol withdrawal, insomnia, and chemotherapy-induced emesis.

Pharmacology

Lorazepam is a short-acting benzodiazepine (BZD) that displays similar activity to other members in the class. The exact mechanism and site of action of BZDs in the CNS are unknown. The pharmacologic activity of these drugs appears, however, to be mediated by the inhibitory neurotransmitter γ-aminobutyric acid (GABA). Specifically, BZD binding to specific receptors within the CNS (e.g. GABA and BZD receptors) is potentiated by the presence of GABA. These interactions result in anticonvulsant, muscle relaxant, sedative, and anxiolytic properties seen with the BZDs. Lorazepam is metabolized via the liver to an inactive metabolite that is excreted in the urine. It has a plasma half-life of approximately 12 hours.

Adverse Effects/Precautions

CNS effects are common and include sedation, dizziness, weakness, and unsteadiness. These may lessen with continued therapy or a decrease in dosage.

Administer lorazepam injection with caution in patients with respiratory compromise since apnea and hypoxic cardiac arrest may occur.

Lorazepam is contraindicated in acute narrow-angle glaucoma.

BZDs may produce physical and psychologic dependence. Thus, these agents should be used for short-term therapy when possible and should not be abruptly discontinued.

Abrupt discontinuation may result in severe withdrawal including life-threatening symptoms (e.g. seizures). Withdrawal may be more frequent in patients who are receiving higher doses and for long periods. However, symptoms may also occur with short-term therapy.

BZD administration during pregnancy may cause fetal harm and should be avoided. Pregnancy: FDA category D.

Lorazepam (Ativan)

Drug Interactions

Co-administration of lorazepam with other CNS depressant medications and alcohol should be avoided.

Special Considerations

If dose reduction or discontinuation of lorazepam is necessary, a gradual decrease is recommended. If the oral concentrate is used, the dose should be added to at least 30 ml of diluent (e.g. water, juice, soda) or soft food (e.g. apple sauce) prior to administration.

Preparation *Rx*

Tablets	0.5, 1 & 2 mg	Ativan	
		Various generics	
Oral concentrate	2 mg/ml	Lorazepam Intensol	30 ml
Injection	2 mg/ml	Ativan	1 & 10 ml
Injection	4 mg/ml	Ativan	1 & 10 ml

Selected References

Ameer B, Greenblatt DJ. Lorazepam: a review of its clinical pharmacological properties and therapeutic uses. Drugs 1981; 21: 162–200.

Tiller JW, Schweitzer I. Benzodiazepines. Depressants or antidepressants. Drugs 1992; 44: 165–9.

Midazolam (Versed)

Dose and Administration

Injectable: Give 1 to 2.5 mg intravenously over 2 minutes. Patients who are older than 60 years of age, chronically ill and/or debilitated should receive 1 to 1.5 mg as the initial dose. Repeat doses of 1 mg may be given every 2 minutes until desired sedation is achieved up to a maximum total of 5 mg. Higher doses may be required in some patients.

Oral: Give a single dose of 0.25 to 0.5 mg/kg (not to exceed 20 mg) in pediatric patients. Children between 6 months and less than 6 years of age generally require higher doses (1 mg/kg).

Uses

FDA-approved:

Injectable: Used for preoperative/preprocedural sedation, anxiolysis, and amnesia, induction of general anesthesia, continuous infusion for sedation of intubated and mechanically ventilated patients as a component of anesthesia or during treatment in a critical care setting.

Oral: Use in pediatric patients for sedation, anxiolysis, and amnesia prior to diagnostic, therapeutic, or endoscopic procedures or before induction of anesthesia. Another use is for refractory status epilepticus.

Monitoring

Vital signs must be closely monitored during use. Patients should be continuously monitored (e.g. pulse oximetry) for detection of early signs of hypoventilation, airway obstruction, or apnea.

Pharmacology

Midazolam is a short-acting benzodiazepine (BZD) that displays similar activity to other members in the class. The exact mechanism and site of action of the BZDs in the CNS are unknown. The pharmacologic activity of these drugs appears, however, to be mediated by the inhibitory neurotransmitter γ-aminobutyric acid (GABA). Specifically, BZD binding to specific receptors within the CNS (e.g. GABA and BZD receptors) is potentiated by the presence of GABA. These interactions result in anti-convulsant, muscle relaxant, sedative, and anxiolytic properties seen with the BZDs. Midazolam is metabolized via the liver and is excreted in the urine. It has a plasma half-life of approximately 1.5 to 3 hours.

Adverse Effects/Precautions

Frequent adverse reactions include excessive sedation, headache, and drowsiness.

Paradoxical reactions such as agitation and involuntary movements may occur.

Midazolam can cause respiratory depression. Hypoventilation, airway obstruction, and apnea can lead to hypoxia and/or cardiac arrest. The immediate availability of a reversal agent (flumazenil), oxygen, resuscitative drugs, age- and size-appropriate equipment for bag/valve/mask ventilation and intubation, and skilled personnel for the maintenance of a patent airway and support are necessities prior to administration.

Midazolam (Versed)

Patients receiving prolonged continuous intravenous infusion therapy may experience withdrawal symptoms. Discontinuation of the infusion should be gradual.

Midazolam is contraindicated in acute narrow-angle glaucoma.

BZD administration during pregnancy may cause fetal harm and should be avoided. Pregnancy: FDA category D.

Drug Interactions

Co-administration with other CNS depressants should be approached carefully. Caution is advised when midazolam is administered concomitantly with drugs that are known to inhibit the P450 3A4 enzyme. These include, but are not limited to, cimetidine, erythromycin, diltiazem, verapamil, ketoconazole, itraconazole, nelfinavir, and ritonavir. These drug interactions may result in prolonged sedation due to a decrease in plasma clearance of midazolam.

Special Considerations

Midazolam syrup is not intended for chronic administration.

Preparation *Rx*

Injection	1 mg/ml	Generic	2 & 5 ml vial
	5 mg/ml	Generic	1, 2, 5 & 10 ml vial
Oral syrup	2 mg/ml	Generic	118 ml

Selected References

Blumer JL. Clinical pharmacology of midazolam in infants and children. Clin Pharmacokinet 1998;35: 37–47.

Midtling JI. Midazolam: a new drug for intravenous sedation. Anesth Prog 1987; 34: 87–99.

Nordt SP, Clark RF. Midazolam: a review of its therapeutic uses and toxicity. J Emerg Med 1997; 15: 357–65.

Temazepam (Restoril)

Dose and Administration

The usual dose is 15 mg orally at bedtime when needed. In elderly or debilitated patients, an initial dose of 7.5 mg should be utilized. The maximum recommended dose is 30 mg.

Uses

FDA-approved: Short-term treatment of insomnia.

Pharmacology

Temazepam is a long-acting benzodiazepine (BZD) utilized primarily for its hypnotic properties. The exact mechanism and site of action of the BZDs in the CNS are unknown. The pharmacologic activity of these drugs appears, however, to be mediated by the inhibitory neurotransmitter γ-aminobutyric acid (GABA). Specifically, BZD binding to specific receptors within the CNS (e.g. GABA and BZD receptors) is potentiated by the presence of GABA. These interactions result in anti-convulsant, muscle relaxant, sedative, anxiolytic properties seen with the BZDs. Temazepam is metabolized via the liver to an inactive metabolite that is excreted in the urine. It has a plasma half-life of approximately 10 to 20 hours.

Adverse Effects/Precautions

CNS effects are common and include drowsiness, fatigue, headache, dizziness, and nervousness.

BZDs may produce physical and psychologic dependence. Therefore, these agents should be used for short-term therapy when possible and should not be abruptly discontinued.

Abrupt discontinuation may result in severe withdrawal, including life-threatening symptoms (e.g. seizures). Withdrawal may be more frequent in patients who are receiving higher doses and for long periods. However, symptoms may also occur with short-term therapy.

BZD administration during pregnancy may cause fetal harm and should be avoided. Pregnancy: FDA category X.

Drug Interactions

Co-administration of temazepam with other CNS depressant medications and alcohol should be avoided.

Special Considerations

If dose reduction or discontinuation of temazepam is necessary, a gradual decrease is recommended.

Preparation *Rx*

| Capsules | 7.5, 15 & 30 mg | Restoril |
| | | Various generics |

Selected References

Fraschini F, Stankov B. Temazepam: pharmacological profile of a benzodiazepine and new trends in its clinical application. Pharmacol Res 1993; 27: 97–113.

Vogel G. Clinical uses and advantages of low doses of benzodiazepine hypnotics. J Clin Psych 1992; 53(Suppl): 19–22.

Haloperidol (Haldol)

Dose and Administration

Oral: Initial daily doses range from 0.5 to 2 mg divided into two or three doses. Dose adjustments should be performed based on clinical response. Doses up to 100 mg/day may be required in some patients.

IM: Doses of 2 to 5 mg for rapid control in acutely agitated patients with moderately severe to very severe symptoms. Subsequent doses may be administered as often as every hour but 4–8-hour intervals may be satisfactory.

Uses

FDA-approved: Management of manifestations of psychotic disorders, control of tics and vocal utterances of Tourette's disorder, and for severe behavioral problems in children of combative, explosive hyperexcitability (that cannot be accounted for by immediate provocation).

Pharmacology

Haloperidol is a butyrophenone antipsychotic agent that exerts its action via blockade of dopaminergic receptors in the CNS. It also displays weak anticholinergic activity. Because of its strong antidopaminergic activity this agent frequently causes extrapyrimidal reactions, and therefore it is contraindicated for use in patients with Parkinson's disease.

It is well absorbed following oral administration. Parenteral haloperidol is supplied in both regular (haloperidol lactate) and depot (haloperidol decanoate) intramuscular formulations. Following IM administration, the lactate formulation results in control of psychotic symptoms within 30 to 60 minutes. The decanoate formulation, however, is formulated for slow release with peak activity occurring within 6 to 7 days of administration. Haloperidol undergoes metabolism in the liver and is excreted in both the urine and feces.

Adverse Effects/Precautions

Extrapyramidal reactions may occur within the first few days of therapy. These reactions have been categorized generally as Parkinson-like symptoms, akathisia, or dystonias, including opisthotonos and oculogyric crisis. The symptoms may be controlled with dose reduction or benztropine or trihexyphenidyl administration. Tardive dyskinesia may occur in patients on long-term therapy or after drug therapy has been discontinued. Prolactin concentrations may increase with resultant galactorrhea and mastalgia in females. Potential cardiovascular adverse effects include hypotension, tachycardia, and ECG changes.

Pregnancy: FDA category C.

Special Considerations

Although haloperidol lactate injection is not FDA-approved for IV administration, it can be safely administered via the IV route in low doses. The decanoate formulation should never be administered via the IV route. It is designed as a depot formulation for IM administration only. The oral concentrate solution should be diluted with water or juice prior to administration.

Haloperidol (Haldol)

Preparation *Rx*

Tablets	0.5, 1, 2, 5, 10 & 20 mg	Haldol	
		Various generics	
Oral solution	2 mg/ml	Haloperidol Intensol	15 & 120 ml
Injection	5 mg/ml	Haldol	1 & 10 ml
Depot injection	50 & 100 mg/ml	Haldol Decanoate	1 & 5 ml

Selected References

Moller HJ, Kissling W, Lang C, et al. Efficacy and side effects of haloperidol in psychotic patients: oral versus intravenous administration. Am J Psychiatry 1982; 139: 1571–5.

Moller HJ, Kissling W, Riehl T, et al. Double-blind evaluation of the antimanic properties of carbamazepine as a comedication to haloperidol. Prog Neuropsychopharmacol Biol Psychiatry 1989; 13: 127–36.

Van Ameringen M, Mancini C, Oakman JM, Farvolden P. The potential role of haloperidol in the treatment of trichotillomania. J Affect Disord 1999; 56: 219–26.

Pimozide (Orap)

Dose and Administration

Initial daily dose is 1 to 2 mg given orally in divided doses. Dose adjustments can occur every other day based on control of symptoms. Daily doses should not exceed 0.2 mg/kg per day or 10 mg.

Uses

FDA-approved: Use as second-line therapy for patients with Tourette's disorder whose development and/or daily functioning is severely compromised by the presence of motor and phonic tics. It is also used for other psychiatric indications including schizophrenia, psychosis, and delusional disorders, including delusion of parasitosis.

Monitoring

An ECG should be obtained at baseline and periodically thereafter, especially during the period of dose adjustment. Potassium concentrations should be monitored and corrected, since hypokalemia can contribute to the development of ventricular arrhythmias.

Pharmacology

Pimozide is an antipsychotic drug that exerts its action via blockade of dopaminergic receptors in the CNS. It also displays weak anticholinergic activity. Although its exact mode of action has not been established in controlling the motor and phonic tics associated with Tourette's disorder, dopaminergic blockade is likely to be involved.

Pimozide is extensively metabolized in the liver primarily via the CYP 3A enzymatic system and to a lesser extent by CYP 1A2. It is subsequently excreted via the kidney.

Adverse Effects/Precautions

Pimozide prolongs the QT interval and is contraindicated in patients at risk for QT prolongation. These patients include those with congenital long QT syndrome, patients with a history of cardiac arrhythmias, or patients taking other drugs that prolong the QT interval (e.g. tricyclic antidepressants, phenothiazines, antiarrhythmic agents). See **Drug Interactions** below for other contraindications.

Extrapyramidal reactions may occur within the first few days of therapy. These reactions have been generally characterized as Parkinson-like symptoms that have been reversible and mild to moderate in severity. Motor restlessness, dystonia, akathisia, hyperreflexia, opisthotonos, and oculogyric crises have been reported less frequently. Tardive dyskinesia may occur in patients on long-term therapy or after drug therapy has been discontinued. Dry mouth, constipation, and sedation occur frequently and are attributed to pimozide's anticholinergic activity.

Pregnancy: FDA category C.

Drug Interactions

Pimozide is metabolized via the CYP 3A isoenzyme system and it should not be co-administered with inhibitors of this isoenzyme system. It is contraindicated in patients receiving nefazodone, a macrolide antibiotic (i.e. clarithromycin, erythromycin, azithromycin, and dirithromycin);. the azole antifungal agents

Pimozide (Orap)

itraconazole or ketoconazole; and in patients receiving protease inhibitors (e.g. ritonavir, saquinavir, indinavir, nelfinavir, amprenavir).

Preparation *Rx*

Tablets   1 & 2 mg   Orap

Selected References

Koblenzer CS, Bostrom P. Chronic cutaneous dysesthesia syndrome: a psychotic phenomenon or a depressive symptom? J Am Acad Dermatol 1994; 30: 370–4.

Koo J, Lee CS. Delusions of parasitosis. A dermatologist's guide to diagnosis and treatment. Am J Clin Dermatol 2001; 2: 285–90.

Zomer SF, DeWit RF, Van Bronswijk JE, et al. Delusions of parasitosis. A psychiatric disorder to be treated by dermatologists? An analysis of 30 patients. Br J Dermatol 1998; 138: 1030–2.

Miscellaneous Agents

Alendronate (Fosamax)

Uses, Dose and Administration

Treatment of osteoporosis in postmenopausal women: 10 mg orally once daily or 70 mg orally once weekly.

Prevention of osteoporosis in postmenopausal women: 5 mg orally once daily or 35 mg orally once weekly.

Increase bone mass in men with osteoporosis: 10 mg orally once daily or 70 mg orally once weekly.

Treatment of glucocorticoid-induced osteoporosis in men and women receiving glucocorticoids in a daily dosage equivalent to at least 7.5 mg of prednisone and who have low bone mineral density: 5 mg orally once daily (except for postmenopausal women not receiving estrogen who should receive 10 mg).

Paget's disease of bone in men and women: 40 mg by mouth once daily for 6 months.

Patients should receive supplemental calcium and vitamin D if dietary intake is inadequate, particularly patients receiving concomitant glucocorticoids.

Patients must be instructed to take the medication first thing in the morning with a full (6 to 8 ounce) glass of plain (not mineral) water at least 30 minutes before the first food, beverage, or medication of the day. Even dosing with juice or coffee has been shown to markedly reduce absorption. Patients must also be instructed to remain upright and not lie down for at least 30 minutes.

Pharmacology

Bisphosphonate that acts as a specific inhibitor of osteoclast-mediated bone resorption. Analogue of pyrophosphate that binds to hydroxyapatite in bone. Localizes preferentially to resorption sites of active bone turnover. Bone resorption is inhibited at doses that have minimal or no effect on bone mineralization. The half-life of alendronate in bone is up to 10 years. Primarily excreted renally.

Contraindications

Abnormalities of the esophagus which delay esophageal emptying such as stricture or achalasia.

Inability to stand or sit upright for at least 30 minutes.

Patients at increased risk of aspiration should not receive oral solution.

Hypocalcemia.

Adverse Effects/Precautions

The most common adverse effects include headache, musculoskeletal pain, flatulence, acid regurgitation, esophagitis, dysphagia, and abdominal distention.

Alendronate, like other bisphosphonates, may cause local irritation of the upper gastrointestinal mucosa. Esophageal adverse reactions have been reported, and patients must seek medical attention if they develop dysphagia, odynophagia, retrosternal pain, or new or worsening heartburn.

Most excretion occurs via the kidneys, therefore the use of this medication in patients with creatinine clearance of < 35 ml/min is not recommended.

Pregnancy: FDA category C.

Alendronate (Fosamax)

Preparation *Rx*

Tablets	5 , 10, 35, 40 & 70 mg	Fosamax	
Solution	70 mg	Fosamax	single-dose bottles

Selected References

Isenbarger DW, Chapin BL. Osteoporosis: current pharmacologic options for prevention and treatment. Postgrad Med 1997; 101: 129–42.

Phillips E, Knowles S, Weber E, Shear NH. Skin reactions associated with bisphosphonates: a report of 3 cases and an approach to management. J Allergy Clin Immunol 1998; 102: 697–8.

Cevimeline (Evoxac)

Dose and Administration

Adults: 30 mg by mouth three times daily (no information to support doses of > 90 mg/day).

Use

FDA-approved: Treatment of xerostomia (dry mouth) in patients with primary and secondary Sjögren's syndrome.

Pharmacology

Cevimeline binds to muscarinic receptors and acts as a muscarinic receptor agonist. Cevimeline increases the secretion of salivary and sweat glands, and increases smooth muscle tone in the GI tract and urinary tract. Cevimeline is metabolized in the liver by cytochrome P450 isoenzymes CYP2D6 and CYP3A4 and is excreted primarily in the urine.

Contraindications

Patients with uncontrolled asthma and in patients where miosis is undesirable (narrow-angle, angle closure glaucoma and acute iritis).

Adverse Effects/Precautions

Caution in patients with chronic bronchitis; chronic obstructive pulmonary disease (COPD); controlled asthma; cholelithiasis; cholecystis; nephrolithiasis; biliary obstruction; or significant cardiovascular disease, including angina, myocardial infarction, or conduction disturbances.

Patients may experience diaphoresis, excessive salivation, nausea, and rhinitis.

May decrease visual acuity and impair depth perception. Patients should be warned of difficulty driving at night or performing hazardous activities.

Pregnancy: FDA category C.

Drug Interactions

Drugs that inhibit the CYP2D6 or CYP3A4 enzymes may inhibit cevimeline metabolism, thereby increasing the concentration of cevimeline in the blood.

β-Blockers may cause conduction disturbances with concurrent use with cevimeline.

Antimuscarinics may decrease the effects of cevimeline.

Parasympathomimetics may exhibit additive effects with concurrent use with cevimeline.

Preparation Rx

Capsules   30 mg   Evoxac

Selected Reference

Iga Y, Arisawa H, Ogane N, et al. (+/-)-*cis*-2-methylspiro[1,3-oxathiolane-5,3'-quinuclidine] hydrochloride, hemihydrate (SNI-2011, cevimeline hydrochloride) induces saliva and tear secretions in rats and mice: the role of muscarinic acetylcholine receptors. Jpn J Pharmacol 1998; 78: 373–80.

Gabapentin (Neurontin)

Dose and Administration

Postherpetic neuralgia (adults): Day 1, 300 mg once. Day 2, 300 mg twice daily. Day 3, 300 mg three times daily. Titrate to pain relief to a total daily dose of 1800 mg (divided three times daily). Although used in clinical trials, doses greater than 1800 mg/day were not associated with improved efficacy.

Reduce dose for significant renal dysfunction.

Uses

FDA-approved: Postherpetic neuralgia (adults), epilepsy (adults and children).

Pharmacology

Analgesic mechanism of action unknown. Prevents allodynia and hyperalgesia in animal models. Also prevented or decreased pain-related responses in neuropathic pain models and in peripheral inflammation models. Does not alter immediate pain-related behaviors.

Adverse Effects/Precautions

Dizziness (30%), somnolence (20%), peripheral edema (8%), nausea (4%). Safety and efficacy are not established for postherpetic neuralgia in pediatric patients.

Pregnancy: FDA category C.

Drug Interactions

Concentrations increased by hydrocodone (15%) and morphine (44%); hydrocodone concentrations lowered up to 20%. Separate administration time with Maalox.

Preparation *Rx*

(Generic capsules approved October 2004.)
Capsules   100, 300, 400, 600 & 800 mg
Oral solution   250 mg/5 ml

Selected References

Dubinsky RM, Kabbani H, El-Chami Z, et al. Quality Standards Subcommittee of the American Academy of Neurology. Practice parameter: treatment of postherpetic neuralgia: an evidence-based report of the Quality Standards Subcommittee of the American Academy of Neurology. Neurology 2004; 63: 959–65.

Plaghki L, Adriaensen H, Morlion B, et al. Systematic overview of the pharmacological management of postherpetic neuralgia. Dermatology 2004; 208: 206–16.

Rice ASC, Maton S. Gabapentin in postherpetic neuralgia: a randomised, double blind, placebo controlled study. Pain 2001; 94: 215–24.

Rosenberg JM, Harrell C, Ristic H, et al. The effect of gabapentin on neuropathic pain. Clin J Pain 1997; 13: 251–5.

Rowbotham M, Harden N, Stacey B, et al. Gabapentin for the treatment of postherpetic neuralgia: a randomized controlled trial. JAMA 1998; 280: 1837–42.

Singh D, Kennedy DH. The use of gabapentin for the treatment of postherpetic neuralgia. Clin Ther 2003; 25: 852–9.

Glycopyrrolate (Robinul)

Dose and Administration

Adults: 1 to 2 mg orally two to three times daily. Dosages will need to be individualized according to need. Maximum daily dosage is 8 mg.

Uses

FDA-approved: Glycopyrrolate can be used as a gastrointestinal antispasmodic agent as well as an antisialagogue to prevent aspiration pneumonitis during anesthesia. Glycopyrrolate can also be used to treat bronchospasm and hyperhidrosis.

Pharmacology

An antimuscarinic anticholinergic agent that inhibits acetylcholine at autonomic effectors innervated by postganglionic cholinergic nerves. Differs from other anticholinergics, as it contains a polar quartenary ammonium group that prevents it from crossing the blood–brain barrier.

Contraindications

Narrow-angle glaucoma, obstructive uropathy, myasthenia gravis, toxic megacolon, gastrointestinal obstruction, ulcerative colitis.

Adverse Effects/Precautions

Most adverse effects are similar to those with other anticholinergics. These include xerostomia, anhidrosis, blurred vision, ocular hypertension, cycloplegia, mydriasis, palpitations, impairment of taste, headache, nervousness, mental confusion, drowsiness, weakness, dizziness, insomnia, vomiting, nausea, constipation, and suppression of lactation.

Blocks the action of acetylcholine on the heart and may cause tachycardia. It should be used with caution in patients with congestive heart failure, hypertension, coronary heart disease, cardiac arrhythmias, or hyperthyroidism.

Sweat gland suppression is one of the effects of glycopyrrolate; care should be taken in hot or humid environments to prevent hyperthermia.

Pregnancy: FDA category B.

Drug Interactions

Drugs that possess antimuscarinic effects may have additive effects when used concurrently with glycopyrrolate. Examples include tricyclic antidepressants, phenothiazines, antihistamines, cyclobenzaprine, and atropine.

Preparation *Rx*

Tablets	1 mg	Robinul
Tablets	2 mg	Robinul Forte
Injection	0.2 mg/ml	Robinul

Selected References

Olsen AK, Sjögren P. Oral glycopyrrolate alleviates drooling in a patient with tongue cancer. J Pain Sympt Mgmt 1999; 18: 300–2.

Wolff MS, Kleinberg I. The effect of ammonium glycopyrrolate (Robinul)-induced xerostomia on oral mucosal wetness and flow of gingival crevicular fluid in humans. Arch Oral Biol 1999; 44: 97–102.

Pentoxifylline (Trental)

Dose and Administration

Adult: 400 mg orally three times daily with meals.

Uses

FDA-approved: Symptomatic management of intermittent claudication.

Other uses include granuloma annulare, recurrent aphthous stomatitis, Behçet's disease, psoriasis, ischemic lower limb ulcers, and cutaneous vasculitis.

Monitoring

Periodic blood pressure monitoring is recommended, especially for patients receiving antihypertensive therapy.

Pharmacology

Synthetic xanthine derivative shown to produce dose-related hemorheologic effects. Reduces the viscosity of blood and improves flow by increasing the flexibility of red blood cells. Inhibits neutrophil adhesion, activation, and antigen-specific activation of T and B lymphocytes. Has also been shown to inhibit the production of various proinflammatory cytokines, especially tumor necrosis factor (TNF)-α. These properties may be the basis for its therapeutic effect in recurrent aphthous stomatitis and Behçet's disease. Extensively metabolized by the liver and eliminated by the kidneys (caution in patients with renal or hepatic disease).

Contraindications

Recent retinal or cerebral hemorrhage, or hypersensitivity to xanthine derivatives (e.g. caffeine, theophylline).

Adverse Effects/Precautions

Most common adverse effects include dizziness, headache, dyspepsia, nausea, and vomiting. Rare dermatologic adverse effects may include brittle nails, pruritus, rash, urticaria, or angioedema. There have been several reports of angina, hypotension, and arrhythmia.

Use with caution in patients with renal and/or hepatic impairment.

Pregnancy: FDA category C.

Special Considerations

The benefit of using pentoxifylline for recurrent aphthous stomatitis may continue even after discontinuation of the medication. Pentoxifylline may suppress irritant and contact hypersensitivity reactions that may lead to false-negative patch test results.

Preparation *Rx*

Tablets	400 mg	Trental

Selected References

Schwarz A, Krone C, Trautinger F, et al. Pentoxifylline suppresses irritant and contact hypersensitivity reactions. J Invest Dermatol 1993; 101: 549–52.

Wahba-Yahav AV. Pentoxifylline in intractable recurrent aphthous stomatitis. J Am Acad Dermatol 1995; 33: 680–2.

Yasui K, Ohta K, Kobayashi M, et al. Successful treatment of Behçet disease with pentoxifylline. Ann Intern Med 1996; 124: 891–3.

Risedronate (Actonel)

Uses, Dose and Administration

Treatment of osteoporosis in postmenopausal women: 5 mg orally once daily or 35 mg orally once weekly.

Prevention of osteoporosis in postmenopausal women: 5 mg orally once daily or 35 mg orally once weekly.

Treatment of glucocorticoid-induced osteoporosis in men and women receiving glucocorticoids in a daily dosage equivalent to at least 7.5 mg of prednisone and who have low bone mineral density: 5 mg orally once daily.

Paget's disease of bone in men and women: 30 mg by mouth once daily for 2 months.

Patients should receive supplemental calcium and vitamin D if dietary intake is inadequate, particularly patients receiving concomitant glucocorticoids.

Patients must be instructed to take the medication first thing in the morning with a full (6 to 8 ounce) glass of plain (not mineral) water at least 30 minutes before the first food, beverage, or medication of the day. Even dosing with juice or coffee has been shown to markedly reduce absorption. Patients must also be instructed to remain upright and not lie down for at least 30 minutes.

Pharmacology

Bisphosphonate that acts as a specific inhibitor of osteoclast-mediated bone resorption. Analogue of pyrophosphate that binds to hydroxyapatite in bone. Localizes preferentially to resorption sites of active bone turnover. Bone resorption is inhibited at doses that have minimal or no effect on bone mineralization. Primarily excreted renally.

Contraindications

Inability to stand or sit upright for at least 30 minutes.

Hypocalcemia.

Adverse Effects/Precautions

The most common adverse effects include musculoskeletal pain, headache, nausea, diarrhea, and abdominal pain.

Risedronate, like other bisphosphonates, may cause local irritation of the upper gastrointestinal mucosa. Esophageal adverse reactions have been reported, and patients must seek medical attention if they develop dysphagia, odynophagia, retrosternal pain, or new or worsening heartburn.

Most excretion occurs via the kidneys, therefore the use of this medication in patients with creatinine clearance of < 30 ml/min is not recommended.

Pregnancy: FDA category C.

Preparation *Rx*

| Tablets | 5, 30 & 35 mg | Actonel |

Selected References

Crandall C. Risedronate: a clinical review. Arch Intern Med 2001; 161: 353–60.

Delmas PD. Treatment of postmenopausal osteoporosis. Lancet 2002; 359: 2018–26.

Saag KG. Prevention of glucocorticoid-induced osteoporosis. South Med J 2004; 97: 555–8.

Agent	Select Availability/Brands		Uses	Adverse Effects	Comments
Benzalkonium chloride	0.13% (with lidocaine 2.5%) liquid	Bactine First Aid Liquid	A cationic detergent useful for topical disinfection and as a solution preservative. Also in many combination products containing topical anesthetics or anti-infectives. Activity against a wide variety of bacteria, fungi, and protozoa; however, bacterial endospores, viruses, certain gram-negative bacteria generally considered resistant. Disinfection of surgical equipment (1:500); preoperative skin preparation, treatment of minor wounds and lacerations (1:750); vaginal douches (1:2000 to 1:5000); deep infected wounds (1:3000 to 1:20000); preservative for ophthalmic solutions (1:5000 to 1:7500); denuded skin, mucous membranes, eye irrigation (1:5000 to 1:10000); bladder and urethral irrigation (1:5000 to 1:20000); bladder retention lavage (1:20000 to 1:40000)	Contact dermatitis has been reported	Do not use ophthalmic preparations containing this agent while contact lenses are in the eye Prepare diluted solutions with Sterile Water for Injection or distilled water (not tap water). Use more dilute solutions on inflamed skin
	13% spray 17% solution (concentrate)	Zephiran chloride Various			
	1:750 solution, tincture, spray	Zephiran chloride			
Chlorhexidine gluconate	2% liquid (w/4% isopropyl alcohol)	Bactoshield, Dyna-Hex 2 Skin Cleanser	An antiseptic/antimicrobial skin cleanser for use as a surgical scrub, hand-washing by medical personnel, for preoperative skin preparation, and for skin wound and general skin cleansing. Active against gram-positive and gram-negative bacteria, facultative anaerobes and aerobes, and yeast	Irritation, sensitization, generalized allergic reactions have been reported, especially in the genital areas; incidence is low	
	4% liquid (w/4% isopropyl alcohol)	Bactoshield, Betasept, Dyna-Hex, Hibiclens			

Continued overleaf

Topical Antiseptics

Agent	Select Availability/Brands	Uses	Adverse Effects	Comments
Hexachlorophene	3% liquid 0.23% foam	pHisoHex Septisol	Surgical scrub and skin cleanser	Photosensitivity has been reported	Activity against gram-positive organisms. Low activity against gram-negative organisms. Less effective than povidone iodine
Iodine	2% iodine and 2.4% sodium iodide in purified water	Iodine topical solution	Skin disinfection. Iodine is active against all bacteria, fungi, protozoa, viruses, and yeasts. Elemental iodine solutions (except povidone iodine) are only active on	Urticaria, hyper-sensitivity reactions may occur	Iodine solution and tincture should not be confused with Strong Iodine Solution (Lugol's
	2% iodine and 2.4% sodium iodide in 47% alcohol, purified water	Iodine tincture	the tissue surface 2% aqueous solution: decontamination of minor wounds. 2% tincture in an alcoholic vehicle: disinfection of intact skin		Solution, 5% iodine and 10% potassium iodide in water), used in the treatment of thyroid disorders
	5% iodine & 10% potassium iodide in water	Strong Iodine (Lugol's Solution)	2% solution of iodine in glycerin: disinfection of mucous membranes		Topically applied iodine should not be covered with occlusive dressings.
	7% iodine & 5% potassium iodide in 83% alcohol	Strong Iodine tincture	2% tincture: skin cleansing prior to venipuncture		A 7% tincture is also available, but it may be associated with increased adversities (e.g. severe burns), and use should be limited

Agent	Select Availability/Brands	Uses	Adverse Effects	Comments
Povidone Iodine	10% ointment 10% solution, and swabsticks, gauzepads 10% gel (vaginal) 10% suppositories (vaginal, 7s) 7.5% surgical scrub 5% cream 1% solution	ACU-Dyne, Betadine, Iodex-p, Povidine; various generics Betadine, Betagen, Povidine; various generics Betadine Betadine Betadine Betadine ACU-Dyne	Primary use is disinfection of skin, particularly preoperatively. Commonly used for vaginitis. Active against all bacteria, fungi, protozoa, viruses, and yeasts	Local irritation, itching, and burning are the most common effects. Contact dermatitis has occurred. Vaginal administration results in systemic iodine absorption	Reported as superior to chlorhexidine gluconate and benzalkonium chloride against nosocomial micro-organisms (e.g. methicillin-resistant *Staphylococcus aureus*)
Thimerosal	2% swabs (10s) 1:1000 solution 1:1000 tincture (contains 50% alcohol) 1:1000 spray (with 72% alcohol)		Bacterial and fungistatic mercurial antiseptic used pre-surgically and for first aid uses (e.g. lacerations). Also as a preservative in pharmaceutical products (e.g. contact lens solutions)	Hypersensitivity may occur, manifested by erythematous, papular, and vesicular eruptions	
Oxychlorosene sodium	2 g powder for solution	Clorpactin WCS-90	A chlorine-releasing antiseptic with the general properties of chlorine. Activity against bacteria, fungi, viruses, mold, yeast and spores. Used for superficial and localized infections (e.g. urologic, ophthalmic). Also pre- and postoperatively to prevent infection	Chlorine-releasing antiseptics are generally regarded as irritating	Typically used as 0.4% solution for wound cleansing and as a 0.1% to 0.2% solution for urologic and ophthalmic indications

Continued overleaf

continued

Agent	Select Availability/Brands	Uses	Adverse Effects	Comments
Silver nitrate	10% ointment 10% solution 25% solution 50% solution 75% with 25% potassium nitrate, with applicators	An antiseptic, germicidal, astringent, and caustic (escharotic) agent	Skin discoloration has occurred with repeated ingestion or absorption of small quantities of silver through mucous membranes; routine use is not typically associated with this reaction. Will stain clothing (prior to drying). Methemoglobinemia has occurred in septic patients	A 1% ophthalmic preparation is available for prevention of gonorrheal ophthalmia neonatorium
Sodium hypochlorite	0.25%, 0.5% solution Dakin's	A disinfectant and antiseptic with the actions of chlorine. Primarily used to prevent wound infections (e.g. post-surgical)	Tissue damage, reduced wound epithelialization	Many authors, as well as results of *in vitro* tests, suggest use of dilute solutions (must be compounded). A concentration of 0.025% has been shown to balance antimicrobial efficacy with minimal cellular toxicity

Rx/OTC	Generic	Availability	Administration	Adverse Effects
Rx	Mafenide acetate	Sulfamylon cream: 2 oz, 4 oz, 16 oz	Apply with sterile gloved hand 1–2 times daily, to a thickness of 1/16″. Dressings are not required	Fatal hemolytic anemia has been reported (probably due to G-6-PD deficiency). Inhibits carbonic anhydrase which may result in metabolic acidosis; caution in patients with extensive burns, renal or pulmonary impairment. Pain on application. Dermatologic/allergic reactions may occur
		Sulfamylon topical solution (5% when mixed): packets, 50 g*	Cover grafted area with one layer of fine mesh gauze. Wet an eight-ply dressing with the solution, secure to the area, and wrap. Keep wet	
Rx	Nitrofurazone	Ointment (and with soluble dressing), 0.2%: 30 g, 454 g. Topical solution, 0.2%: 480 ml	Apply directly with spatula or after applying to gauze. May use gauze impregnated with soluble dressing. Solution may be sprayed directly on lesion. Reapply once daily or every few days	Allergic contact dermatitis. Caution in G-6-PD deficiency. Ointment contains polyethylene glycol (PEG) which may be absorbed through denuded skin; renally impaired patients may not eliminate PEG normally, leading to metabolic acidosis
Rx	Silver sulfadiazine	Cream, 1% (Silvadene, SSD, Thermazene, and generics): 20 g, 50 g, 85 g, 400 g, 1000 g	Apply with sterile gloved hand 1–2 times daily, to a thickness of 1/16″. Dressings are not required	Caution in G-6-PD deficiency. May be absorbed and accumulate in renally impaired patients. Leukopenia. Irritation, itching, burning, although not the pain on application with mafenide.

*Each packet should be mixed aseptically with 1 liter sterile H_2O or NS for irrigation and filtered; use within 48 hours.

Amount of Topical Medication to Prescribe Based on Body Surface Area Affected

	Hands, Face, Scalp, or Genitals	One Upper Extremity or One Side of Trunk	One Lower Extremity	Entire Body
	3% BSA	*10% BSA*	*20% BSA*	*100% BSA*
One application	1 g	3 g	5 g	30–60 g
Twice daily for 1 week	15 g	45 g	60 g	1 pound
Twice daily for 1 month	30 g	180 g	240 g	5 pounds

Index

Index

A/T/S 12
Abreva 186
Accutane 6, 7
Acitretin 238, 239
Acne 246
Acne conglobata 6
Acne rosacea 14, 16
Acne vulgaris 2, 8, 10, 12, 14, 15, 16, 40, 42, 44, 50, 205
Acticin 166
Actinic keratosis 62, 78, 97, 98, 189
Actinic prurigo 110
Actonel 278
Acular 218
Acyclovir, topical 183
Acyclovir, oral and injection 180, 181, 182
Adalimumab 58
Adapalene 2
Advil 146, 147
Agitation 266
AIDS-associated proctitis 110
Akne-Mycin 12
Alamast 219
Alavert 142
Alcohol withdrawal 261
Aldactone 205, 206
Aldara 189, 190
Alefacept 59, 60
Alendronate 272, 273
Aleve 148, 149
Alitretinoin gel 61
Allegra 139
Allerest 220
Allergic conjunctivitis 218
Alomide 219
Alopecia areata 204, 240
Alphaquin HP 232
Alprazolam 257, 258
Amevive 59, 60
Aminolevulinic acid 62
Amitriptyline 248, 249
Ampicillin 20, 21
Anaerobic infections 50
Anal warts 197
Analgesic 146, 148
Anaprox 148, 149

Anaprox DS 149
Androgenetic alopecia 203, 204, 205
Anesthetic 171, 172, 173
Ankylosing spondylitis 105
Annular elastolytic giant cell granuloma 71
Anthralin 240
Antihistamine 134, 140
Anxiety 257, 259, 261
Anxiety disorder 257, 259
Arava 91
Artificial suntan 229
Atabrine 102
Atarax 140
Ativan 261, 262
Atopic dermatitis 71, 101, 109, 134, 170
Avar 16
Avita 17, 18
Azathioprine 63, 64
Azelaic acid 3
Azelastine 218
Azelex 3
Azithromycin 29, 30
Azulfidine 105, 106

Bacitracin/polymyxin B 216
Bacterial conjunctivitis 208, 210, 211, 212
Bacterial endocarditis prophylaxis 20
Bacterial prostatitis 36, 38
Bacterial vaginosis 50
Bactrim 48, 49
Bactroban 53
Basal cell carcinoma 184, 189
Behçet's syndrome 68, 71, 86, 110, 277
Benadryl 138, 169
Benoquin 236
Benzac AC 4
Benzac W 4
BenzaClin 4
Benzamycin 4
Benzashave 4
Benzoyl peroxide 4, 5
β-Carotene 228
Bexarotene, systemic 65, 66
Bexarotene, topical 67
Biaxin 31, 32

Index

Biaxin XL 32
Bicillin L-A 27
Blastomycosis 118, 120
Blenoxane 184, 185
Bleomycin 184, 185
Bleph-10 212, 215
Blephamide 217
Brevoxyl 4, 5
Bronchitis 22, 29, 29, 48
Bulimia nervosa 252
Bullous pemphigoid 46, 71, 110
Bupropion 255
Burns 54, 55
Buspar 259, 260
Buspirone 259, 260

Calcipotriene 241, 242
Candidiasis 114, 120
Candiduria 120
Capsaicin 168
Ceftin 22, 23
Cefuroxime axetil 22, 23
Celexa 252
CellCept 100
Cephalexin 24
Cervicitis, chlamydial 29
Cetirizine 134
Cevimeline 274
Chancroid 29, 36
Chemotherapy-induced emesis 261
Chickenpox 180
Chlamydia trachomatis infection 40
Chloasma 232
Chlorpheniramine 135
Chromelin 229
Chromomycosis 120
Chronic idiopathic urticaria 134, 137, 139, 142
Chronic mucocutaneous candidiasis 120
Chronic pigmented purpura 71
Chronic urticaria 71
Cicatricial pemphigoid 110
Ciclopirox 8% lacquer 123
Ciloxan 208, 214
Cipro HC Otic 222

Cipro 36, 37
CiproDex Otic 221
Ciprofloxacin 36, 37
Ciprofloxacin/dexamethasone otic combination 221
Ciprofloxacin/hydrocortisone otic combination 222
Ciprofloxacin ophthalmic solution and ointment 208, 214
Citalopram 252
Clarinex 137
Claripel 232
Clarithromycin 31, 32
Claritin 142
Clear Eyes 220
Cleocin 50, 51
Cleocin T 10, 11
Clinac BPO 5
Clinda-Derm 11
Clindagel 10
ClindaMax 10
Clindamycin phosphate 50, 51
Clindamycin phosphate, topical 10, 11
Clindets 10
Clofazimine 52
Clotrimazole 124, 125
Coccidioidomycosis 120
Colchicine 68, 69
Cold sores 186
Colonization, nasal 53
Coly-Mycin S Otic 223
Community-acquired pneumonia 29, 31
Condylomata acuminata 88, 189, 192, 194
Condylox 192, 193
Corneal ulcer 208
Cortisporin 210, 211, 217
Cortisporin Otic 224
Cortisporin-TC Otic 223
Crohn's disease 105
Crolom 219
Cromolyn 219
Cromolyn oral concentrate 136
Cryptococcal meningitis 114
Cutaneous candidiasis 124
Cutaneous T-cell lymphoma 65, 67, 73, 86

Index

Cyclophosphamide 70
Cyclosporine 71, 72
Cymbalta 252
Cystitis 24, 36, 38
Cytoxan 70

Dapsone 46, 47
Darier's disease 6
Decadron 216
Deltasone 150, 151
Delusional disorders 268
Denavir 191
Denileukin diftitox 73, 74
Depression 250, 252, 253, 254, 255,256
Dermatitis 170
Dermatitis herpetiformis 46, 68, 103, 105
Dermatomycosis 124
Dermatomyositis 71
Dermatophyte infections 120
Desloratadine 137
Desquam-E 4
Desquam-X 5 4, 5
Desyrel 256
Dexamethasone 216
DHA 229, 230
Diarrhea, traveler's 48
Differin 2
Diflucan 114, 115
Dihydroxyacetone 229, 230
Diphenhydramine 138
Diphenhydramine, topical 169
Discoid lupus erythematosus 46, 52, 80, 105, 110
Dissecting folliculitis 6
Docosanol 186
Dovonex 241, 242
Doxepin 250, 251
Doxepin, topical 170
Doxy 100 41
Doxycycline 40, 41
Drithocreme 240
Droxia 82, 83
Duac 4
Duloxetine 252
Dynacin 43
Dyschromia 234

E.E.S. 34
Eczema 170
Efalizumab 75
Effexor 256
Effexor XR 256
Eflornithine cream 202
Efudex 78, 79
Elavil 248, 249
Eldopaque 232
Eldopaque Forte 232
Eldoquin 231
Eldoquin Forte 231
Elestat 218
Elidel 101
Elimite 166
Emadine 218
Emedastine 218
Emgel 12
EMLA 172, 173, 174
Enbrel 76, 77
Endocarditis prophylaxis 50
Enteritis 48
Enteritis, sexually transmitted 40
Enterococcal infections 26
Ephelides 232
Epidermolysis bullosa acquisita 71
Epididymitis 40
Epinastine 218
EpiQuin Micro 232, 234
ERYC 34
Erycette 12
EryDerm 12
Erygel 12
EryPed 34
Ery-Tab 34
Erythema multiforme 110
Erythema nodosum leprosum 52, 110
Erythrocin 34, 35
Erythromycin 33, 34, 35
Erythromycin ophthalmic ointment 209, 214
Erythromycin, topical 12
Erythropoietic protoporphyria 228
Esophageal candidiasis 118
Esoterica 232

Index

Etanercept 76, 77
Evoxac 274

Famciclovir 187, 188
Familial Mediterranean fever 68
Famvir 187, 188
Febrile neutropenia 36
Fexofenadine 139
Finacea 3
Finasteride 203
Flat warts 17
Floxin 38, 39, 225
Fluconazole 114, 115
Fluocinolone
    acetonide/hydroquinone/tretinoin 231
Fluoroplex 79
Fluorouracil 86, 87
5-*Fluorouracil* 78, 79
Fluoxetine 252
Fluvoxamine 253
Fosamax 272, 273
Freckles 232
Fulvicin P/G 116, 117
Fulvicin UF 117

Gabapentin 275
Garamycin 214
Gastrocrom 136
Generalized anxiety disorder 252, 253,
    256
Gengraf 72
Genital herpes 180, 183, 187, 198
Genital warts 88, 189, 190, 192, 193, 194,
    197
Genoptic 214
Gentacidin 214
Gentamicin 214
Glycopyrrolate 276
Glyquin 232
Glyquin-XM 232
Gonorrhea 22
Gonorrhea, uncomplicated cervical
    and urethral 36, 38
Graft-versus-host disease 71, 110
Granuloma annulare 71, 277
Granuloma inguinale 48

Grifulvin V 116, 117
Griseofulvin 116, 117
Gris-PEG 116, 117
Gyne-Lotrimin 125

Hailey–Hailey disease 71
Hair removal 202
Haldol 266, 267
Haloperidol 266, 267
Helicobacter pylori eradication 31
Herpes keratitis 213
Herpes labialis 183, 191
Herpes simplex 180, 181, 183, 187, 191,
    198
Herpes zoster 180, 187, 198
Hidradenitis suppurativa 6, 71
Hirsutism 203, 205
Histoplasmosis 118, 120
HSV 180, 181, 183, 187, 191, 198
Human papilloma virus 194
Humira 58
Hydrea 82, 83
Hydrocortisone/neomycin/colistin otic
    combination 223
Hydrocortisone/neomycin/polymyxin B
    otic combination 224
Hydroquinone 232, 233
Hydroquinone/retinol 234
Hydroxychloroquine sulphate 80, 81
Hydroxyurea 82, 83
Hydroxyzine 140, 141
Hydroxyzine pamoate 141
Hyperhidrosis 276
Hypermelanosis 232
Hypersensitivity 138
Hypopigmentation 229

Ibuprofen 146, 147
Ichthyosis 6, 238
Idiopathic thrombocytopenic purpura 68
IL-2 fusion protein 73
Ilotycin 209
Imiquimod 189, 190
Impetigo 22, 53
Imuran 63, 64
Infectious diarrhea 36

Index

Infliximab 84, 85
Insomnia 261, 265
Interferon α-2a 86, 87
Interferon α-2b 88, 89, 90
Intra-abdominal infections 36
Intron A 88, 89, 90
Iquix 215
Ischemic leg ulcers 277
Isotretinoin 6, 7
Itraconazole 118, 119
Ivermectin 162

Jessner–Kanof disease 110
Joint infections 36

Kaposi's sarcoma 61, 65, 86, 88, 184
Keflex 24
Keftab 24
Kenalog 160
Keratitis 213
Keratoconjunctivitis 213
Keratoderma 238
Keratosis, actinic 62, 78, 97, 98, 189
Ketoconazole 120, 121
Ketorolac 218
Ketotifen 218
Klaron 15
Kwell 163, 164

Lamisil 122
Lamprene 52
Latent syphilis 40
Leflunomide 91
Legionnaires' disease 33
Leprosy 46, 52
Leucovorin calcium 92
Levocabastine 219
Levofloxacin 215
Levulan Kerastick 62 Lichen planus 6, 71
Lichen simplex chronicus 170
Lidocaine patch 171
Lidocaine/prilocaine cream 172, 173, 174
Lidoderm 171
Lindane 163, 164
Livostin 219
Lodoxamide 219

Loratadine 142
Lorazepam 261, 262
Lotrimin 125
Lupus erythematosus 102, 238
Lustra & Lustra AF 233
Lyme disease 22
Lymphogranuloma venereum 40
Lymphoma 67
Lymphoma, T-cell 65, 73

Malathion 165
Mastocytosis 136
Mechlorethamine, topical 93, 94
Melanex 233
Melanoma 88
Melasma 3, 17, 231, 232, 234
Melpaque HP 233
Melquin HP 233
Melquin-3 233
Mequinol and tretinoin 235
Methicillin-resistant *Staphylococcus aureus* eradication 53
Methotrexate 95, 96
Methotrexate toxicity 92
Methoxsalen 243, 244, 245
8-Methoxypsoralen (MOP) capsules 243, 244, 245
Methyl aminolevulinate 97, 98, 99
MetroCream 14
MetroGel 14
MetroLotion 14
Metronidazole, topical 14
Metvix 97, 98, 99
Midazolam 263, 264
Minocin 42, 43
Minocycline 42, 43
Minoxidil topical solution 204
Mirtazapine 255
Mixed infections of the urethra and cervix 38
Monobenzone 236
Morphea 241
Motrin 146, 147
Moxifloxacin 214
Mupirocin 53
Mustargen 93, 94

Index

Mycelex 125
Mycobacterium avium complex infection 29, 31, 52
Mycophenolate mofetil 100
Mycophenolic acid 100
Mycosis fungoides 93, 95, 244
Myfortic 100

Naphazoline 220
Naphcon 220
Naphcon-A 220
Naprelan 148, 149
Naprosyn 148, 149
Naprosyn EC 149
Naproxen/naproxen sodium 148, 149
Necrotizing vasculitis 68
Nefazodone 255
NeoDecadron 217
Neomycin/dexamethasone 217
Neomycin/polymyxin B/bacitracin 216
Neomycin/polymyxin B/bacitracin/hydrocortisone ophthalmic ointment 210, 217
Neomycin/polymyxin B/hydrocortisone ophthalmic suspension 211, 217
Neoral 71, 72
Neosporin 54
Neosporin, AK-Spore 216
Neostrata AHA 233
Neuralgia 168
Neurontin 275
Nicosyn 16
Nitrogen mustard 93, 94
Nix 166
Nizoral 120, 121
Nodular basal cell carcinoma 62, 98
Nongonoccal nonchlamydial urethritis 40
Nongonoccal urethritis and cervicitis 38
Norgestimate–ethinyl estradiol 8, 9
Noritate 14
Nosocomial pneumonia 36
Nuquin HP 233

Obsessive–compulsive disorder 252, 253, 254
OcuClear 220

Ocuflox 215
Ofloxacin 38, 39
Ofloxacin otic solution 215, 225
Olopatadine 219
Onchocerciasis 162
Ontak 73, 74
Onychomycosis 114, 118, 122, 123
Ophthalmia neonatorum 209
Ophthalmic ointment 210
Opticrom 219
Optivar 218
Oral thrush 120
Orap 268, 269
Orasone 150, 151
Oropharyngeal candidiasis 118, 124
Ortho Tri-Cyclen 8, 9
Osteoarthritis 146, 148
Osteomyelitis 24
Osteoporosis 272, 278
Otitis externa 221, 222
Otitis media 22, 24, 26, 29, 31, 221, 225
Ovide 165
Oxsoralen 243, 244, 245
Oxsoralen-Ultra capsules 243, 244, 245
Oxymetazoline 220
Oxytetracycline/polymyxin B 216

Paget's disease of the bone 272, 278
Pain 171
Palmoplantar pustulosis 68, 110
Panic attacks 257
Panic disorder 253, 254
Panretin 61
Paracoccidioidomycosis 120
Parasitosis 268
Paroxetine 253
Patanol 219
Paxil 253
PCE Dispertab 34
Pediculosis capitis 163, 166
Pediculosis humanis capitis 165
Pediculosis pubis 163
Pelvic inflammatory disease 29, 38
Pemirolast 219
Pemphigus vulgaris 46, 71, 103
Pen VK 26, 27, 28

Index

Penciclovir 191
Penicillin 26, 27, 28
Penlac 123
Pentoxifylline 277
Pen-Vee K 28
Perianal warts 189
Permethrin 166
Pertussis 33
Pharyngitis 22, 24, 31
Photoaging 17
Photodermatosis 71
Photoprotection 229
Pimecrolimus 101
Pimozide 268, 269
Pityriasis lichenoides chronica 71
Pityriasis rubra pilaris 6, 238
Pityriasis versicolor 124
Plaque psoriasis 76
Plaquenil 80, 81
Plexion 16
Pneumocystis carinii pneumonia 48
Pneumonia 26
Podocon-25 194
Podofilox 192, 193
Podophyllin 194
Podophyllum resin 194
Polyarticular course juvenile rheumatoid
 arthritis 76
Polymorphous light eruption 228, 244
Polymyxin B sulfate/bacitracin zinc 55
Polymyxin B sulfate/bacitracin
 zinc/neomycin sulfate 54
Polymyxin B/neomycin/gramicidin 216
Poly-Pred 217
Polysporin 55, 216
Polytrim 216
Porphyria cutanea tarda 80
Postherpetic neuralgia 110, 168, 171, 172,
 248, 275
Post-traumatic stress disorder 254
Pred-Forte 216
Pred-G 217
Pred-Mild 216
Prednisolone 216
Prednisolone/gentamicin 217
Prednisolone/neomycin/polymyxin B 217

Prednisone Intensol 151
Prednisone 150, 151
Premenstrual dysphoric disorder 254
Preoperative sedation 261
Preprocedural sedation 263
Primary or secondary syphilis 40
Principen 20, 21
Proctitis, sexually transmitted 40
Proctocolitis, sexually transmitted 40
Prograf 107, 108
Propecia 203
Prophylaxis of organ rejection 71
Proscar 203
Prostatitis 24
Protopic 109
Prozac 252
Prurigo nodularis 110
Pruritus 139, 166, 170, 244, 250
Pseudofolliculitis barbae 202
Psittacosis 52
Psoralen 244
Psoriasis 6, 52, 58, 59, 68, 71, 73, 75, 76, 82,
 91, 95, 100, 107, 109, 112, 238, 240, 241,
 243, 244, 246
Psoriatec 240
Psoriatic arthritis 58, 76, 105
Psychotic disorders 266
Pyelonephritis 36, 38
Pyoderma gangrenosum 52, 68, 71, 103,
 105, 110

Quinacrine 102
Quixin 215

Raptiva 75
Recalcitrant nodular acne 6
Recurrent aphthous stomatitis 277
Refractory rosacea 6
Remeron 255
Remicade 84, 85
Renova 17, 18
Respiratory tract infections 20, 33
Restoril 265
Retin-A 17, 18
Retin-A Micro 17, 18

Index

Rheumatoid arthritis 63, 76, 80, 91, 105, 110, 146, 148, 150
Rheumatrex 95, 96
Rhinitis 135, 138
Ringworm 116
Risedronate 278
Robinul 276
Roferon-A 86, 87
Rogaine 204
Rosacea 3
Rosula 16

Sandimmune 71, 72
Sarafem 252
Sarcoidosis 70, 95, 110
Sarcoma, Kaposi's 61, 65, 86, 88, 184
Scabies 162, 163, 166
Schizophrenia 268
Scleroderma 68, 71
Seborrheic dermatitis 16
Senile lentigines 232
Septra 48, 49
Sertraline 254
Severe rheumatoid arthritis 71
Severe, recurrent aphthous stomatitis 110
Sinequan 250, 251
Sinusitis 22, 31, 48
Sjögren's syndrome 274
Skin and skin structure infections 20, 22, 24, 26, 29, 31, 33, 36, 38
Skin hyperpigmentation 231, 232
Skin infections 53
Skin wounds, surgical 54, 55
Skin wounds, traumatic 53, 54, 55
Smoking cessation 255, 259
Social anxiety disorder 254
Sodium sulfacetamide, topical 15
Solagé 235
Solaquin 233
Solaquin Forte 233
Solar keratosis 78
Solar lentigines 235
Soriatane 238, 239
Spironolactone 205, 206
Sporanox 118, 119
Squamous cell carcinoma 184

Staticin 12
Status epilepticus 261, 263
Stongyloidiasis 162
Streptococcal infections 26
Stromectol 162
Subcorneal pustular dermatosis 103
Sulfacetamide 215
Sulfacetamide/prednisolone 217
Sulfacetamide sodium
    ophthalmic solution and ointment 212
Sulfacet-R 16
Sulfapyridine 103, 104
Sulfasalazine 105, 106
Sulfoxyl Regular 5
Sulfoxyl Strong 5
Sulfur and sodium sulfacetamide, topical 16
Sumycin 44, 45
Suntan, artificial 229
Superficial basal cell carcinoma 62, 78, 98
Superficial ocular infections 209
Syphilis 26, 44
Systemic fungal infections 120
Systemic lupus erythematosus 46, 63, 70, 71, 80, 95

Tabloid 112
Tacrolimus, systemic 107, 108
Tacrolimus, topical 109
Targretin 65, 66, 67
Tazarotene, topical 246
Tazorac 246
TCAA 197
T-cell lymphoma 65, 73
Temazepam 265
Terak 216
Terbinafine 122
Tetracycline, oral 44, 45
Tetrahydrozoline 220
Thalidomide 110, 111
Thalomid 110, 111
Theramycin Z 12
Thioguanine 112
Tinea 116
Tinea barbae 116
Tinea capitis 116

Index

Tinea corporis 116, 124
Tinea cruris 116, 124
Tinea pedis 116, 124
Tinea unguium 116
Tinea versicolor 120
TobraDex 217
Tobramycin 216
Tobramycin/dexamethasone 217
Tobrex 216
Tonsillitis 22, 24, 26, 29, 31
Topical salicylic acid preparations 195, 196
Tourette's disorder 266, 268
Trachoma 212
Trazadone 256
Trental 277
Tretinoin, topical 17, 18
Triamcinolone acetonide injection 160
Triaz 4, 5
Trichloroacetic acid topical solution 197
Trifluridine 213
Tri-Luma 231
Trimethoprim/polymyxin B 216
Trimethoprim–sulfamethoxazole 48, 49
Trivagizole 125
T-Stat 12
Typhoid fever 36

Ulcerative colitis 105
Uremic pruritus 110
Urethritis, chlamydial 29
Urinary tract infections 20, 36, 38, 48
Urticaria 134, 250
Uveitis 210, 211

Valacyclovir 198, 199
Valtrex 198, 199
Vaniqa 202

Varicella-zoster viruses 181, 183
Variegate porphyria 229
Vasculitis 63, 70, 95, 277
VasoClear 220
Veetids 28
Venlafaxine 256
Vernal conjunctivitis 219
Vernal keratitis 219
Vernal keratoconjunctivitis 219
Versed 263, 264
Vibramycin 40, 41
Vibra-Tabs 41
Vigamox 214
Viroptic 213
Visine 220
Visine L.R. 220
Vistaril 141
Vitadye 229
Vitiligo 71, 229, 236, 241, 244
Vulvovaginal candidiasis 124

Warts 184, 195, 196, 246
Wellbutrin 255
Wellbutrin SR 255
Wellbutrin XL 255

Xanax 257, 258
Xerostomia 274

Zaditor 218
Zetacet 16
Zithromax 29, 30
Zoloft 254
Zonalon 170
Zostrix 168
Zovirax 180, 181, 182, 183
Zyrtec 134